The Complete Diagnosis Coding Book

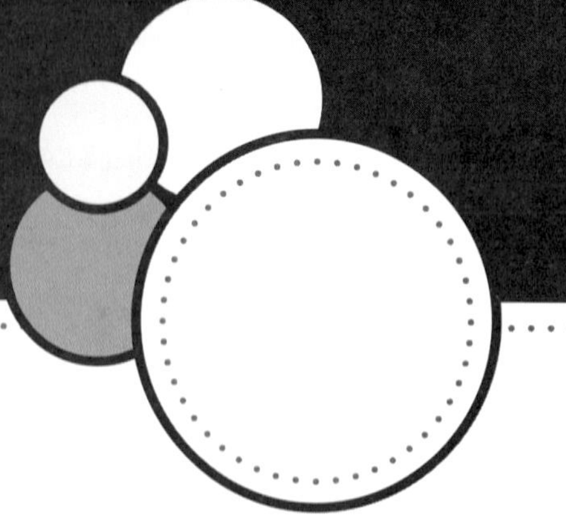

SECOND EDITION

Shelley C. Safian

MAOM/HSM, CCS-P, CPC-H, CPC-I, CHA
AHIMA-Approved ICD-10-CM/PCS Trainer

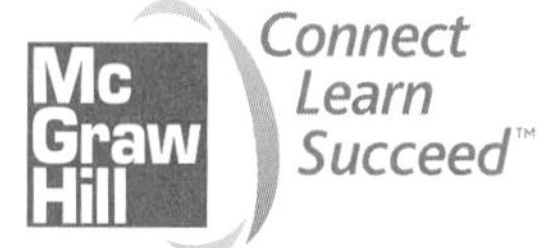

The McGraw-Hill Companies

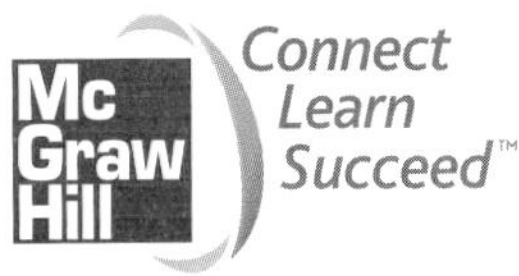

THE COMPLETE DIAGNOSIS CODING BOOK

Published by McGraw-Hill, a business unit of The McGraw-Hill Companies, Inc., 1221 Avenue of the Americas, New York, NY, 10020.

This book is printed on acid-free paper.

2 3 4 5 6 7 8 9 0 DOW/DOW 1 0 9 8 7 6 5 4 3 2

ISBN 978-0-07-337451-2
MHID 0-07-337451-2

Vice president/Editor in chief: *Elizabeth Haefele*
Vice president/Director of marketing: *Alice Harra*
Publisher: *Kenneth S. Kasee Jr.*
Senior sponsoring editor: *Natalie J. Ruffatto*
Development editor: *Raisa Priebe Kreek*
Executive marketing manager: *Roxan Kinsey*
Lead digital product manager: *Damian Moshak*
Director, Editing/Design/Production: *Jess Ann Kosic*
Project manager: *Jean R. Starr*
Buyer: *Susan Culbertson*
Senior designer: *Marianna Kinigakis*
Lead photo research coordinator: *Carrie K. Burger*
Digital production coordinator: *Brent dela Cruz*
Cover design: *Alexa R. Viscius*
Typeface: *10.5/13 Melior*
Compositor: *Aptara, Inc.*
Printer: *RR Donnelley*
Credits: The credits section for this book begins on page 407 and is considered an extension of the copyright page.

Library of Congress Cataloging-in-Publication Data

Safian, Shelley C., author.
The complete diagnosis coding book / Shelley C. Safian, MAOM/HSM, CCS-P, CPC-H, CHA, AHIMA-Approved ICD-10-CM/PCS Trainer. —Second edition.
p. ; cm.
Includes index.
ISBN-13: 978-0-07-337451-2 (alk. paper)
ISBN-10: 0-07-337451-2 (alk. paper)
1. Nosology—Code numbers. 2. Clinical medicine—Code numbers. I. Title.
[DNLM: 1. Forms and Records Control. 2. Medical Records. W 80]
RB115.S34 2012
651.5'04261—dc22

2010048333

CPT codes are based on CPT 2011. ICD-9-CM codes are based on ICD-9-CM 2011.
All names, situations, and anecdotes are fictitious. They do not represent any person, event, or medical record.

www.mhhe.com

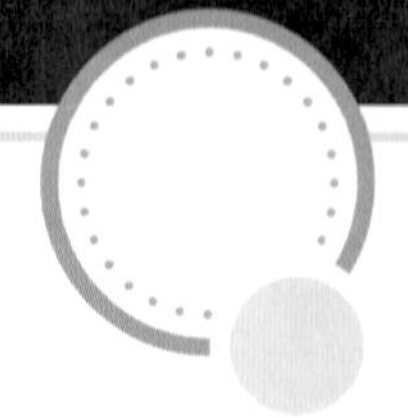

About the Author

Shelley C. Safian has been teaching medical coding and health information management for more than a decade, at both on ground and online campuses. In addition to her regular teaching responsibilities at Herzing University, Berkeley College Online, and Dover Business College, she often presents seminars sponsored by AHIMA, AAPC, and Kaplan University, writes regularly about coding for the *Just Coding* newsletter, and has written articles published in AAPC *Coding Edge, SurgiStrategies,* and *HFM* (Health care Financial Management) magazine. Safian is the course author for several AHIMA distance education courses on various coding topics including ICD-10-CM, ICD-10-PCS, and HCPCS Level II coding.

Safian is a Certified Coding Specialist-Physician-based (CCS-P) from the American Health Information Management Association and a Certified Professional Coder-Hospital (CPC-H) and a Certified Professional Coding Instructor (CPC-I) from the American Academy of Professional Coders. She is also a Certified HIPAA Administrator (CHA), and has earned the designation of AHIMA-Approved ICD-10-CM/PCS Trainer.

Safian completed her Graduate Certificate in Health Care Management in June 2005 at Keller Graduate School of Management. The University of Phoenix awarded her Master of Arts/Organizational Management degree in 2002. She is currently working on the dissertation for her Ph.D. in Health Care Administration with a focus in Health Information Management.

Brief Contents

Contents

CHAPTER 5 Coding Neoplasms 120

CHAPTER 6 Coding Poisonings and Adverse Reactions 144

CHAPTER 7 Coding Burns 169

CHAPTER 8 Coding Musculoskeletal Conditions 192

CHAPTER 9 Coding Obstetrics and Gynecology 216

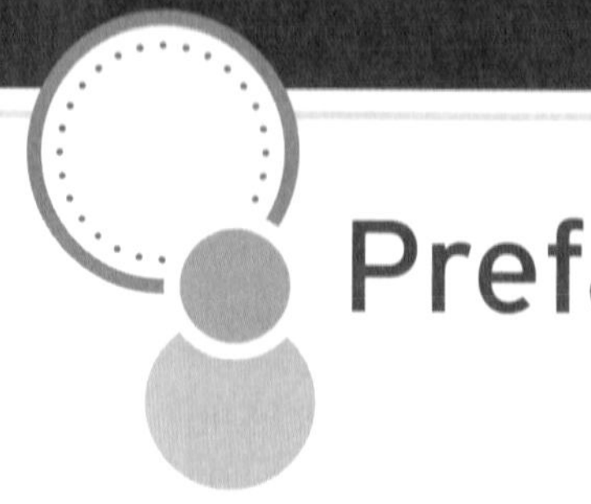

Preface

Welcome to *The Complete Diagnosis Coding Book*! This book is part of a three-book series that instructs students on how to become proficient in medical coding—a health care field that continues to be in high demand. The Bureau of Labor Statistics notes the demand for health information management professions (which includes coders) will continue to increase incredibly through 2018 and beyond.

This series of books was written to speak directly to the medical coding student using step-by-step instructions and conversational language to maximize understanding. Built into the structure of these texts are many opportunities for students to practice coding and apply what they have learned. Students will also have the chance to practice abstracting with real-world health professionals' documentation and accurately translating these facts into the best, most accurate codes.

TO THE STUDENT

Your medical coding classes introduce you to the skills you will need to work in the health information management field. A fundamental role of an insurance coding and medical billing specialist's job is to work with the insurance companies that will reimburse the health care facility for the services and treatments provided to patients. You may be employed by a hospital, clinic, doctor's office, health maintenance organization, mental health care facility, insurance company, government agency, or long-term care facility. Your career will be challenging, interesting, and one of the top ten fastest-growing Allied Health professions.

Before you begin your adventure, here are some tips to help you succeed:

- First, take a deep breath. Coding is complex and is not like anything else you have tackled before. Remember that you are learning a new skill! Give yourself some time to become proficient.
- Second, *never* code directly from the alphabetic index. *Always* look the code up in the tabular list before deciding on a code. If you remember this rule, you will always head in the right direction.
- Third, when you encounter a word or abbreviation that you don't understand, stop and look it up in your medical dictionary. Your instructor can recommend a medical dictionary for you, or you can purchase McGraw-Hill's *Medical Dictionary for Allied Health* (ISBN: 0-07-351096-3).
- Fourth, after you finish coding the case studies, scenarios, or whatever you are coding, put it all aside. Then, later or the next day, go back and do "back coding." In the tabular list, look up each code

you came up with and match the code description carefully with the case study or scenario words. This is a very effective way to double-check your answers. Your fresh eyes will enable you to see words and notations you may have missed before.

- Finally, reevaluate your work by checking each and every question to make certain you understand how you found your answer. When you find you have gotten an exercise, test question, or other activity wrong, try to figure out what happened. Make sure you ask your instructor for help when you need it!

Good luck on your medical coding journey!

TO THE INSTRUCTOR

Shelley Safian's Medical Coding series includes three books:

The Complete Diagnosis Coding Book (ISBN: 0-07-337451-2)
The Complete Procedure Coding Book (ISBN: 0-07-337450-4)
You Code It! Abstracting Case Studies Practicum (ISBN: 0-07-337452-0)

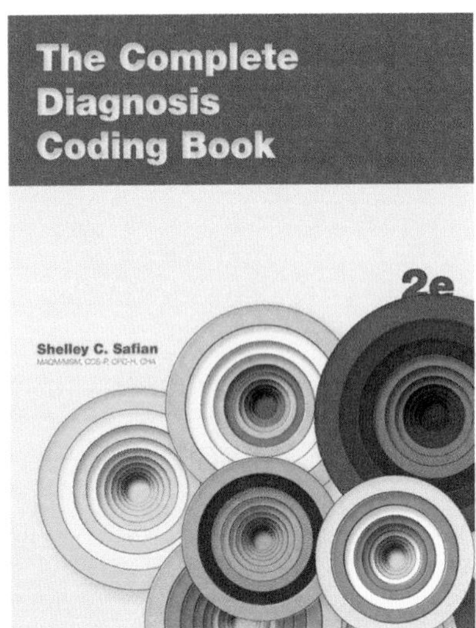

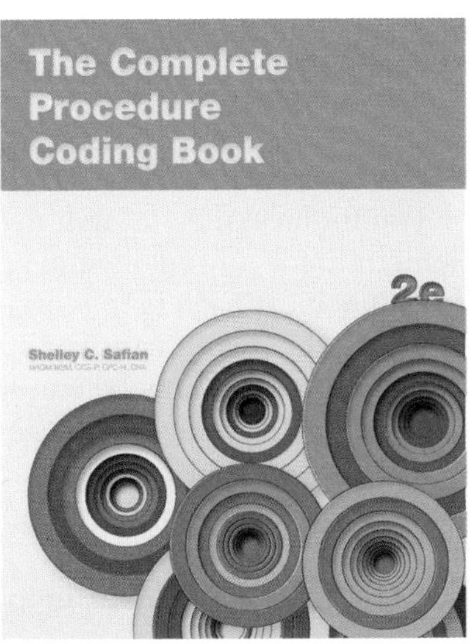

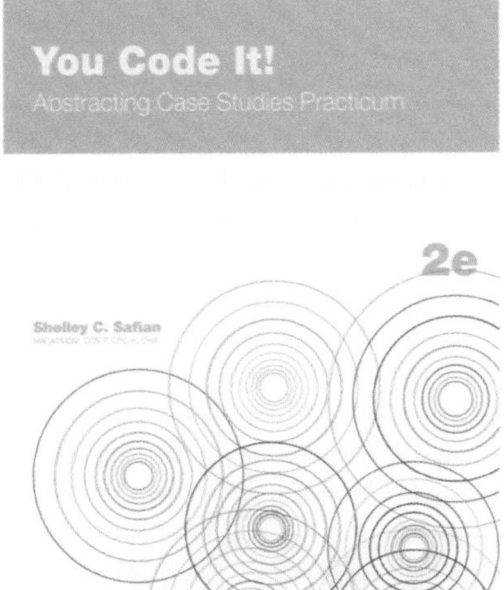

These books are designed to give your students the medical coding experience they need in order to pass their first medical coding certification exams, such as the CCS/CCS-P or CPC/CPC-H. The books offer students a variety of practice opportunities by reinforcing the learning outcomes set forth in every chapter. The chapter materials are organized in short bursts of text followed by practice—keeping students active and coding!

Instructor Resources

McGraw-Hill offers extensive resources on the Online Learning Center for our textbooks. After obtaining the instructor username and password from your McGraw-Hill sales representative, access our instructor resources here: **www.mhhe.com/safian2e.**

Online Learning Center Features

- Instructor's Manual—this manual includes the answers to the end-of-chapter exercises as well as a chapter outline with overviews, discussion activities, and additional resources.
- Instructor's PowerPoint® slides—organized by the chapter learning outcomes, these slides help reinforce the text content and make your course prep a breeze!
- Test Bank—our test bank is available in both EZ-Test Online and Word document formats. Organized by chapter, learning outcome, level of difficulty, and Bloom's taxonomy, this test bank is sure to help with assessment.

LearnSmart: Medical Insurance Billing and Coding

Mc Graw Hill LearnSmart

McGraw-Hill's LearnSmart diagnoses students' skill levels to determine what they know and what they don't and delivers customized learning content based on their strengths and weaknesses. Visit **www.mhhe.com/learnsmart** to try it yourself!

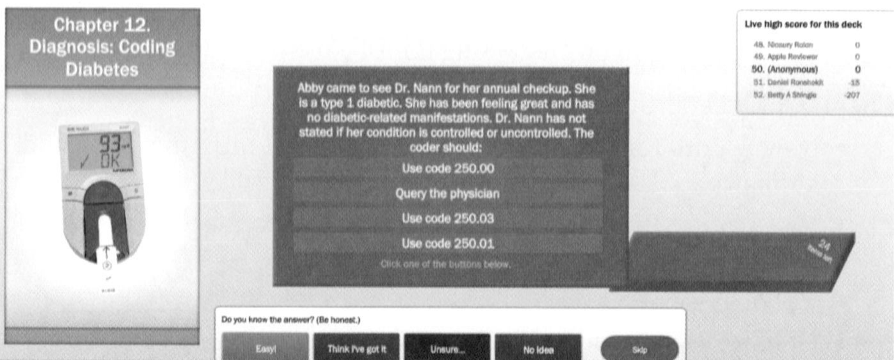

WHAT'S NEW IN OUR SECOND EDITION

The Complete Diagnosis Coding Book, second edition, has been revised to include a greater number of realistic scenarios and case studies for students to gain hands-on learning with the popular **Let's Code It!** scenarios and **You Code It!** case studies. **Keys to Coding**—a new feature for this edition—make it easier for students to connect learning concepts and specific official guidelines to critical thinking. Another new feature, **Bridge to ICD-10,** prepares students for transition to ICD-10. Throughout the book, more anatomy and physiology descriptions, as well as more information on inclusive signs and symptoms, enhance students' comprehension of the diagnosis coding process.

The entire text has been updated using 2011 ICD-9-CM codes. The new instructor's manual features a 2011-compliant answer key to all end-of-chapter tests: **Chapter Reviews** (multiple-choice questions), **You Code It! Practice** (short scenarios), and end-of-chapter **You Code It! Simulation** (full physician's notes/operative reports).

Chapter-by-Chapter Updates

Chapter 1: Introduction to Diagnostic Coding

- Key Terms include additional ICD-10-CM key term
- New feature Keys to Coding includes critical thinking paths and guidance
- New feature Bridge to ICD-10-CM includes connections between coding from ICD-9-CM and ICD-10-CM
- Updated Coding from Physician's Notes
- Updated and expanded Rules for Ethical and Legal Coding
- Updated AHIMA Standards of Ethical Coding
- Updated AAPC Code of ethical standards

Chapter 2: Introduction to ICD-9-CM

- New feature Keys to Coding includes critical thinking paths and guidance
- New feature Bridge to ICD-10-CM includes connections between coding from ICD-9-CM and ICD-10-CM
- Updated section on Format of the ICD-9-CM
- Updated section on Dissecting the Diagnostic Statement

Chapter 3: General Guidelines and Notations

- New feature Keys to Coding includes critical thinking paths and guidance
- New feature Bridge to ICD-10-CM includes connections between coding from ICD-9-CM and ICD-10-CM
- Updated section on Notations
- Updated section on Multiple and Additional Codes

Chapter 4: Coding Circulatory and Cardiovascular Conditions

- New feature Keys to Coding includes critical thinking paths and guidance
- New feature Bridge to ICD-10-CM includes connections between coding from ICD-9-CM and ICD-10-CM
- New sections on Heart Failure, Myocardial Infarction, Disease of Veins, Late Effects of Cerebrovascular Disease
- Additional Let's Code It! and You Code It! exercises
- Two new cases in You Code It! Simulation

Chapter 5: Coding Neoplasms

- New feature Keys to Coding includes critical thinking paths and guidance
- New feature Bridge to ICD-10-CM includes connections between coding from ICD-9-CM and ICD-10-CM
- New section on Remission

Chapter 6: Coding Poisonings and Adverse Reactions

- New feature Keys to Coding includes critical thinking paths and guidance

- New feature Bridge to ICD-10-CM includes connections between coding from ICD-9-CM and ICD-10-CM
- New sections on Patient Non-Compliance and Sequencing Codes

Chapter 7: Coding Burns

- New feature Keys to Coding includes critical thinking paths and guidance
- New feature Bridge to ICD-10-CM includes connections between coding from ICD-9-CM and ICD-10-CM
- New section on Solar and Radiation Burns
- New subsections on Multiple Burns and sequencing multiple codes
- Additional Let's Code It! activity

Chapter 8: Coding Musculoskeletal Conditions

- New feature Keys to Coding includes critical thinking paths and guidance
- New feature Bridge to ICD-10-CM includes connections between coding from ICD-9-CM and ICD-10-CM
- New sections on Complications of Fractures
- New subsection on Multiple Fractures Combination Category
- Updated section on Aftercare for Fractures
- Additional Let's Code It! and You Code It! exercises

Chapter 9: Coding Obstetrics and Gynecology

- New feature Keys to Coding includes critical thinking paths and guidance
- New feature Bridge to ICD-10-CM includes connections between coding from ICD-9-CM and ICD-10-CM
- New subsections on Normal Pregnancy, High-Risk Pregnancy, and Incidental Pregnancy
- New case in You Code It! Simulation

Chapter 10: Coding Congenital and Pediatric Conditions

- New feature Keys to Coding includes critical thinking paths and guidance
- New feature Bridge to ICD-10-CM includes connections between coding from ICD-9-CM and ICD-10-CM
- Additional Let's Code It! exercise
- New case in You Code It! Simulation

Chapter 11: Coding Infectious Diseases

- New feature Keys to Coding includes critical thinking paths and guidance
- New feature Bridge to ICD-10-CM includes connections between coding from ICD-9-CM and ICD-10-CM
- New section on Methicillin-Resistant *Staphylococcus aureus*
- New subsections on Viral Hepatitis

Chapter 12: Coding Conditions of the Endocrine and Metabolic Systems

- Additional Key Terms
- New feature Keys to Coding includes critical thinking paths and guidance
- New feature Bridge to ICD-10-CM includes connections between coding from ICD-9-CM and ICD-10-CM
- New sections on The Endocrine System, Secondary Diabetes Mellitus, Weight Factors, Other Metabolic Disorders, and Thyroid Disorders
- New subsections on Obesity, Body Mass Index, and Underweight
- Additional You Code It! exercises

Chapter 13: Coding Respiratory Conditions

- New feature Keys to Coding includes critical thinking paths and guidance
- New feature Bridge to ICD-10-CM includes connections between coding from ICD-9-CM and ICD-10-CM
- New sections on Pleural Disorders, Pulmonary Embolism, and Respiratory Failure
- New subsections on Respiratory Syncytial Virus Infections and Pulmonary Fibrosis
- Additional You Code It! exercises

Chapter 14: Hospital (Inpatient) Diagnosis Coding

- **New chapter!**
- New feature Keys to Coding includes critical thinking paths and guidance
- New feature Bridge to ICD-10-CM includes connections between coding from ICD-9-CM and ICD-10-CM
- New sections on Concurrent & Discharge Coding, Official Coding Guidelines, Present on Admission (POA) Indicators, Diagnostic-Related Groups (DRG), and Uniform Hospital Discharge Data Set (UHDDS)
- New subsections on Uncertain Diagnosis, Patients Receiving Diagnostic Services Only, General Reporting Guidelines, POA Indicators, Principal Diagnosis, and Complications and Co-Morbidities (MCC)

Chapter 15: You Code It! Practice and Simulation

- New cases

CODEITRIGHTONLINE™: YOUR ONLINE CODING TOOL

So that your students can gain experience with the use of an online coding tool, they will have access for a 14-day period to CodeitRightOnline, produced by Contexo Media, a division of Access Intelligence. CodeitRightOnline offers a comprehensive search function for CPT, HCPCS Level II, and ICD-9-CM codes, along with ICD-10-CM/PCS code sets. It

ICD-10-PCS (International Classification of Diseases–10th revision–Procedure Coding System). [On October 1, 2013, ICD-10-PCS will replace ICD-9-CM volume 3.]

For services provided in an outpatient setting, such as a physician's office, a clinic, or an ambulatory care center, you will probably use CPT.

Remember: Whether you are coding diagnoses or procedures using the ICD-9-CM, ICD-10-CM, ICD-9-CM Volume 3, ICD-10-PCS, or CPT, each set of numbers and letters is so specific that a code number just one digit off could mean something totally different. That difference could cause the claim to be rejected, resulting with your patient being labeled with a disease he or she does not have, and/or your facility not being paid for the work it provided. This is why it is very critical to be careful and accurate when coding and always *double-check* your codes.

These procedure code sets are mentioned here so you will be familiar with their names and what they represent. This book, however, focuses solely on the diagnosis coding portion of a professional coding specialist's job.

SEVEN STEPS TO ACCURATE CODING

Here is a seven-step process that you can follow to code a health care encounter in the approved manner. As you gain experience, it will take you less time to go through these steps. However, remember that time is not the number one consideration when coding—no matter what anyone says, *accuracy* is the most important factor.

THE SEVEN STEPS

1. Read completely through the superbill (see Fig. 1-1) and the physician's notes for the encounter, from beginning to end. Make a copy of the pages relating to the visit so that you can write on the copies without marking the originals. If you prefer, you can use scratch paper on the side.
2. Reread the physician's notes and highlight key words regarding diagnoses and procedures directly relating to the encounter. Pulling out the key words is also called *abstracting* physician's notes. You will need to evaluate the key words and distinguish between diagnostic statements and procedural statements.
3. Make a list of any questions you have regarding unclear or missing information necessary to code the encounter. Query, or confer with, the health care provider who treated the patient. Never assume or try to guess. Code only what you know from actual documentation. If it is not written down, it did not happen, and you cannot code it!

«« KEYS TO CODING

Is it a diagnosis or a procedure?

A. **Do the key words tell you WHY or WHAT?**

a. A **diagnostic statement** will explain WHY the physician cared for the patient, saw the patient, and/or provided a service or treatment or performed a procedure.

b. A **procedural statement** will explain WHAT the physician did for, or to, the patient.

B. **Look at the parts of the medical term.** There are parts of medical terms that are specific to a diagnosis or a procedure.

Examples:

A diagnostic term might have a suffix like

-dynia, meaning pain (a condition or something wrong)

-lepsy, meaning seizure (a condition or something wrong)

A diagnostic term might have a prefix like

macro-, meaning large (a condition or something wrong)

ankyl-, meaning fused or stiffened (a condition or something wrong)

whereas a procedural term might have a suffix like

-tomy, meaning incision (an action)

-scopy, meaning to view (an action)

«« CODING TIP

One absolute rule for coders: "If it's not documented, it didn't happen! So you can't code it!"

BRIDGE TO ICD-10-CM/PCS:

Both ICD-10-CM and ICD-10-PCS code descriptions will require more details and additional specifics to determine the most accurate code. Therefore, querying the physician may become more frequent until new habits in documentation become second nature. This may be something that the professional coding specialist must prompt. Remember, you know what information is required for the code determination, the provider may not.

CODING TIP »»

Use a medical dictionary to learn the true meaning of a medical term. If you don't know what the term means, you will have a problem interpreting it into an accurate code.

EXAMPLE

Dr. Mandell diagnosed Ilona with malignant neoplasm of the brain (brain cancer). The code category for this is 191 Malignant neoplasm of the brain. However, you need a fourth digit. As you read down the list of code descriptions for the four-digit codes in this category, you will notice that each one identifies WHERE in the brain the tumor (the neoplasm) is located. Rather than report code 191.9 Malignant neoplasm of the brain, unspecified, you need to query the physician to add this specific information to the patient's documentation.

Why go through all this effort when you have heard that the insurance company has paid the claim with a diagnosis code of 191.9 (or other unspecified code)? Two reasons:

1. Next week, Dr. Mandell may want to perform a procedure on Ilona that would NOT be supported for medical necessity with an unspecified code.
2. Unspecified codes are virtually non-existent in ICD-10-CM. You want to begin learning coding processes now in preparation for the transition. This way,ICD-10-CM will be easier for you and your facility.

CODING TIP »»

A great way to help assure you have all the necessary diagnosis codes to tell the whole story - take a look at all of the procedures, services, and treatments (WHAT was done for the patient) and confirm that you have at least one diagnosis code to support providing that procedure. This works well even when you are not responsible for coding procedures.

CODING TIP »»

Code backward: Instead of beginning with the alphabetic index, look up the numbers you have chosen in the tabular list and make certain the description in the code book matches the physician's notes. This is one method of confirming that your codes are correct.

4. Code each diagnosis and/or appropriate signs or symptoms describing *why* the health care provider treated this patient during this encounter, as documented in his or her notes. Use the best, most accurate code available based on that documentation.
   a. Assign codes to the greatest specificity (highest level of detail) of confirmed diagnoses, signs, symptoms, and other conditions that are connected to, or related to, services and procedures provided at this visit
   b. Code only those documented conditions that require or influence treatment at this encounter
   c. Include as many codes as necessary to report the reasons *why* completely (to tell the whole story).
5. Code each procedure, as stated in the notes, describing *what* the provider did for the patient. Use the best, most accurate codes available based on the documentation. There are similar steps to determining the procedure code to report. These are reviewed at length in the companion book *The Complete Procedure Coding Book.*
6. Link each and every procedure code to at least one diagnosis code to verify medical necessity.
7. Double-check your codes. Go back into the books you have used, and reread the code descriptions of the codes you have assigned and match them with the notes—one more time.

Following these steps will help you code precisely, resulting in a greater number of your claims getting paid quickly. That is much better than having the claims rejected or denied and dealing with the same case again.

Family Doctors Associates
123 Main Street • Anytown, FL 32711
(407) 555-1200

Date: September 16, 2011 Attending Physician: J. Healer, MD

Patient Name: Sasha White

CPT DESCRIPTION	CPT DESCRIPTION	CPT DESCRIPTION
OFFICE/HOSPITAL	PATHOLOGY/LAB/RADIOLOGY	PROCEDURES/TESTS
☐ 99201 OFFICE-NEW; FOCUSED	☒ 71020 X-RAY CHEST TWO VIEWS	☐ 12011 SIMPLE SUTURE, FACE
☒ 99202 OFFICE-NEW; EXPANDED	☒ 72040 X-RAY SPINE-C, TWO VIEWS	☐ 29125 SPLINT-SHORT ARM
☐ 99203 OFFICE-NEW; DETAILED	☒ 73030 X-RAY SHOULDER COMP	☐ 29355 WALKER CAST-LONG LEG
☐ 99204 OFFICE-NEW; COMPREHEN	☐ 76085 MAMMOGRAM-COMP DET	☐ 29540 STRAPPING-ANKLE
☐ 99205 OFFICE-NEW; COMPREHEN	☐ 76092 MAMMOGRAM SCREENING	☐ 45378 COLONOSCOPY-DIAGNOSTIC
☐ 99211 OFFICE-ESTB; MINIMAL	☐ 80050 BLOOD TEST-GEN HEALTH	☐ 45385 COLONOSCOPY-POLYP REM.
☐ 99212 OFFICE-ESTB; FOCUSED	☐ 80061 BLOOD TEST-LIPID PANEL	☐ 50390 ASPIRATION, RENAL CYST
☐ 99213 OFFICE-ESTB; EXPANDED	☐ 82947 BLOOD TEST-GLUCOSE	☐ 90703 TETANUS INJECTION
☐ 99214 OFFICE-ESTB; DETAILED	☐ 83718 BLOOD TEST-HDL	☐ 92081 VISUAL FIELD EXAM
☐ 99215 OFFICE-ESTB; COMPREHEN	☐ 85025 BLOOD TEST-CBC	☐ 93000 ECG, 12 LEADS, W/RPT
☐ 99281 EMER DEPT; FOCUSED	☐ 86403 STREP TEST, QUICK	☐ 93015 TREADMILL STRESS TEST
☐ 90844 COUNSELING – 50 MIN.	☐ 87430 ENZY IMMUNOASSAY-STREP	☐ 99173 VISUAL ACUITY SCREEN

ICD DESCRIPTION	ICD DESCRIPTION	ICD DESCRIPTION
☐ 034.0 STREP THROAT	☐ 522 LOW RED BLOOD COUNT	☐ V01.5 RABIES EXPOSURE
☐ 042 HUMAN IMMUNO VIRUS	☐ 538.8 STOMACH PAIN	☐ V16.0 FAMILY HISTORY-COLON
☐ 250.51 DIABETES W/VISION	☐ 643 HYPEREMESIS	☐ V16.3 FAMILY HISTORY- BREAST
☐ 250.80 DIABETES, TYPE II	☐ 707.14 ULCER OF HEEL/MID FOOT	☐ V20.2 WELL CHILD
☐ 307.51 BULIMIA NON-ORGANIC	☐ 788.30 ENURESIS	☐ V22.0 PREGNANCY-FIRST NORM
☐ 354.0 CARPEL TUNNEL SYNDROME	☐ 815.00 FRACTURE, HAND	☐ V22.1 PREGNANCY-NORMAL
☐ 362.01 RETINOPATHY (DIABETIC)	☐ 823.20 FRACTURE, TIBIA	☐ E816.2 MOTORCYCLE ACCT
☐ 401.9 HYPERTENSION, UNSPEC	☐ 831.00 DISLOCATION, SHOULDER	☐ E826.1 FALL FROM BICYCLE
☐ 482.30 PNEUMONIA	☐ 845.00 SPRAINED ANKLE	☐ E849.0 PLACE OF OCCUR-HOME
☐ 490 BRONCHITIS, UNSPECIFIED	☐ 880.03 OPEN WOUND UPPER ARM	☐ E881.0 FALL FROM LADDER
☐ 493.92 ASTHMA, UNSPECIFIED	☒ 912.0 ABRASION, SHOULDER	☐ E906.0 DOG BITE

FOLLOW-UP

PRN ______________

WEEKS ______________

NXT APPT. ______________

TIME ______________

Figure 1-1 An Example of a Superbill.

CODING FROM PHYSICIAN'S NOTES

As mentioned earlier in this chapter, you, as the professional coding specialist, will need all of the details and specifics about what occurred between the health care professional and the patient during an encounter,

KEYS TO CODING »»

The Official ICD-9-CM Guidelines state, *"The entire record should be reviewed to determine the specific reason for the encounter and the conditions treated."*

and why. The best way to gather this information is to review the physician's notes, lab reports, superbill/encounter form, and *all* documentation for that encounter. When you read *exactly* what the physician thought, heard, and observed in his or her own words, you will have more specific information to help you determine the most accurate code. The more complete the communication between the providing professional and the professional coding specialist, the more accurate the codes will be—ensuring optimal reimbursement.

Whether you are using ICD-9-CM or ICD-10-CM, your diagnosis codes will be more accurate and will report medical necessity for the procedures, services, and treatments provided when you access all the documentation. After all, how can you report the *whole story* if you don't know the *whole story?*

EXAMPLE

Janelle's facility has her use information from the office's preprinted encounter form rather than waiting for the doctor to dictate his notes from the encounter. However, that superbill only offers one choice for a diagnosis of hypertension and one code for heart disease, to save room on the one-page encounter form:

401.9 Essential hypertension, unspecified

429.9 Heart disease, unspecified

After reading the notes, Janelle discovered that the actual diagnosis written by the physician was hypertensive heart disease, changing the correct code to:

402.90 Hypertensive heart disease, without heart failure

The difference between these two codes could dramatically affect whether or not the facility gets paid for the procedures provided.

OFFICIAL ICD-9-CM GUIDELINES FOR CODING AND REPORTING

In the front of your ICD-9-CM book, you will find the Official Guidelines for Coding and Reporting as issued by the Centers for Medicare and Medicaid Services (CMS) and the National Center for Health Statistics (NCHS), two departments within the U.S. government's Department of Health and Human Services (HHS). You will learn all about them as you study this book. The guidelines will literally guide you toward the best, most accurate code and make coding decisions easier.

The guidelines are divided into four sections:

I. Conventions, General Coding Guidelines, and Chapter-Specific Guidelines

II. Selection of Principal Diagnosis

III. Reporting Additional Diagnoses

IV. Diagnostic Coding and Reporting Guidelines for Outpatient Services

The guidelines are the same for, and are applicable to, both inpatient (those patients admitted into the hospital) and outpatient (outpatient departments, same-day surgical centers, physicians offices, etc.) coding with a few exceptions. The exceptions are important.

> *Section II. Selection of Principal Diagnosis. Subsection H. Uncertain Diagnosis.* The guidelines state that with regard to a diagnosis documented as "probable," "suspected," "likely," "questionable," "possible," or "still to be ruled out," you should "code the condition as if it existed or was established."

Now, consider the following.

> *Section IV. Diagnostic Coding and Reporting Guidelines for Outpatient Services. Subsection I.* The guidelines state, "Do not code diagnoses documented as 'probable,' 'suspected,' 'questionable,' 'rule out,' or 'working diagnosis.' Rather, code the condition(s) to the highest degree of certainty for that encounter/visit."

The differences between these two rules is that when you are coding for a hospital inpatient, you are permitted to code those conditions stated as possible or likely, but not when you are coding for a physician or outpatient service. These guidelines are always right there, in your ICD-9-CM book, for you to reference at any time.

In the Official Guidelines, section I, "Convention, General Coding Guidelines and Chapter-Specific Guidelines," Subsection C, lists detailed rules affecting your decisions when coding certain diseases, conditions, illnesses, and injuries. The headings, or sections, of the guidelines are very specific:

- C1. Infectious and Parasitic Diseases
- C2. Neoplasms
- C3. Endocrine, Nutritional, and Metabolic Diseases and Immunity Disorders
- C4. Diseases of Blood and Blood-Forming Organs
- C5. Mental Disorders
- C6. Diseases of the Nervous System and Sense Organs
- C7. Diseases of the Circulatory System
- C8. Diseases of the Respiratory System
- C9. Diseases of Digestive System
- C10. Diseases of Genitourinary System
- C11. Complications of Pregnancy, Childbirth, and the Puerperium
- C12. Diseases of Skin and Subcutaneous Tissue
- C13. Diseases of Musculoskeletal and Connective Tissue
- C14. Congenital Anomalies
- C15. Newborn (Perinatal) Guidelines
- C16. Signs, Symptoms, and Ill-Defined Conditions
- C17. Injury and Poisoning
- C18. Classification of Factors Influencing Health Status and Contact with Health Services
- C19. Supplemental Classification of External Causes of Injury and Poisoning

We review all these guidelines in the chapters to come.

RULES FOR ETHICAL AND LEGAL CODING

As a coder, you have a very important responsibility—to yourself, your patients, and your facility. The work you do results in the creation of health claim forms and other reports that are legal documents. What you do can contribute to your facility staying healthy (businesswise) or being fined and possibly shut down by the Office of the Inspector General and your state's attorney general. You might make an error that could cause a patient to be unfairly denied health insurance coverage. It is important that you clearly understand the ethical and legal aspects of your new position.

1. It is very important that the codes indicated on the health claim form represent the services actually performed and the reasons why they are provided as supported by the documentation in the patient's health record. Don't use a code on a claim form without assuring the **supporting documentation** is there in the file.

Supporting documentation

The paperwork in the patient's file that corroborates the codes presented on the claim form for a particular encounter.

EXAMPLE

Stephanie Zambro's file indicates that Dr. Villa ordered a blood test to determine whether or not she is pregnant. There is no report showing the results of the test. You see Dr. Villa, and he tells you that Stephanie is pregnant and you should go ahead and code that diagnosis so the claim can be sent in. He promises to place the lab report and update the notes in her file later. Until the physician documents that the patient is pregnant, you are not permitted to code the pregnancy.

Coding for coverage

Choosing a code on the basis of what the insurance company will cover (pay for) rather than accurately reflecting the truth.

2. Some health care providers may improperly encourage **coding for coverage.** This term refers to the process of determining diagnostic and procedural codes not by the accuracy of the code but with regard to which the insurance company will pay for or "cover." That is dishonest and is considered fraud. If you find yourself in an office or facility that insists you "code for coverage" rather than code to accurately reflect the documentation and the services actually performed, you should immediately discuss your situation with your instructor or someone you trust. Some providers will rationalize the process by saying they are doing it so the patients can get the treatment they really need paid for by the insurance company. Altruism aside, it is still illegal and once discovered, financial penalties and possible jail time, can be assessed.

EXAMPLE

Kyle Ford wants a nose job (rhinoplasty); however, he cannot afford it. The insurance carrier will not pay for cosmetic surgery, so the coder changes the code to indicate that Kyle has a deviated septum requiring surgical correction so that the insurance carrier will pay for the procedure. That is coding for coverage and is fraud.

3. If you find yourself in an office or facility that insists that you include codes for procedures that you know, or believe, were never performed,

talk to someone you trust about what you suspect. This might be fraudulent behavior, known as **upcoding**—the process of using a code that claims a higher level of service, or a more severe illness, than is true. Upcoding is considered falsifying records. Even if all you do is fill out the claim form, you are participating in something unethical and illegal.

Upcoding

Using a code on a claim form that indicates a higher level of service, or a more severe aspect of disease or injury than that which was actual and true.

EXAMPLE

Tracey Mendez, a 71-year-old female, in the hospital for a broken hip, had her glucose level checked by the nurse, and it was at an abnormal level. Dr. Basso ordered additional tests to rule out diabetes mellitus. Coding that Tracey has diabetes is upcoding her condition and will fraudulently increase reimbursement from Medicare by changing the diagnosis-related group (DRG). In addition, placing a chronic disease on her health chart, when she doesn't have it, will cause her problems later on.

4. It is not permissible to code and bill for individual (also known as component) elements when a comprehensive or combination (bundle) code is available. This is referred to as **unbundling** and is illegal.

Unbundling

Coding the individual parts of a specific diagnosis or procedure rather than one combination or bundle that includes all of those components.

EXAMPLE

Dr. Cooke's notes indicate that Sabrina was experiencing nausea and vomiting. Instead of coding 787.01 Nausea with vomiting, the coder unbundles, coding 787.02 Nausea alone and 787.03 Vomiting alone.

5. You must code all conditions or complications that are relevant to the current encounter. Failure to do so can be considered unethical.
6. Separating the codes relating to one specific encounter and placing them on several different claim forms over the course of several different days is neither legal nor ethical. It not only indicates a lack of organization of the office but also can cause suspicion of duplicating service claims, known as **double billing.** Even if you are reporting procedures that were actually done for diagnoses that actually exist, remember that the claim form is a legal document. All data on that claim form, including dates of service, must be accurate. Do not submit the claim form until you are certain it is complete, with all diagnoses and procedures listed. If it happens that, after you submit a claim, an additional service provided comes to light (such as a lab report with an extra charge that didn't come across your desk until after you filed the claim), then you must file an amended claim. While not illegal because you are identifying that the claim contains an adjustment, most third-party payers really dislike amended claims. You can expect an amended claim to be scrutinized.

Double billing

Sending a claim for the second time to the same insurance company, for the same procedure or service, provided to the same patient on the same date of service.

All the activities mentioned here are considered fraud and are against the law. The Health Insurance Portability and Accountability Act (HIPAA) created the Health Care Fraud and Abuse Control Program (HCFACP). This program, under the direction of the Attorney General and the secretary of the HHS, acts in accordance with the Office of the Inspector

General (OIG) and coordinates with federal, state, and local law enforcement agencies to discover those who attempt to defraud or abuse the health care system, including Medicare and Medicaid patients and programs.

By catching those who submitted fraudulent claims, approximately $723 million was returned to the Medicare Trust Fund in 2003 and another $151.6 million was reimbursed to the Centers for Medicare and Medicaid Services (CMS). The federal government deposited approximately $2.51 billion to the Medicare Trust Fund in fiscal year 2009, plus more than $441 million of federal Medicaid funds were brought into the United States Treasury. Since it was created in 1997, the HCFACP has collected more than $15.6 billion to the Medicare Trust Fund—money improperly received by health care professionals filing fraudulent claims. The statistics show that for every $1.00 (one dollar) spent to pay for these investigations and prosecutions, the government actually brings in about $4.00 (four dollars) in money returned.

Also, in 2003, 362 criminal indictments were filed in health care fraud cases, and 437 defendants were convicted for health care fraud-related crimes. Another 231 civil cases were filed, and 1,277 more civil matters were pending during this same year. These investigations also prohibited 3,275 individuals and organizations from working with any federally sponsored programs (such as Medicare and Medicaid). Most of these were as a result of convictions for Medicare or Medicaid-related crimes, including patient abuse and patient neglect, or as a result of providers' licenses having been revoked.

In 2009, 1,014 new investigations were started by the Fraud Section of the criminal division in conjunction with the U.S. Attorneys' offices. These investigations involve 1,786 defendants, while the federal prosecutors filed criminal charges involving 803 defendants in 481 cases and had another 1,621 health care fraud investigations involving 2,706 potential defendants. At the same time, the Department of Justice had 1,155 civil health care fraud cases pending and 886 new civil investigations opened.

When you compare the 2003 numbers with the 2009 numbers you can see that an increasing number of people are being caught trying to get money for health care services to which they are not entitled. This is an important reminder that if individuals try to get you to participate in illegal or unethical behaviors, the question is not "will you be caught?" but "*when* will you be caught?'

It is not worth breaking the law and being charged with any of these penalties just to hang onto a job.

CODING TIP »»

Always read the complete description in the provider's notes in addition to referencing the encounter form or superbill, and then carefully find the best available code that supports medical necessity according to the documentation.

RESOURCES

Using the ICD-9-CM to identify the correct diagnosis code is like a treasure hunt. Sometimes it is very easy to find the best, most appropriate code as documented in the physician's notes. Other times, it may seem as though the code isn't there. However, you must remember that if the health care provider can diagnose it—the code is in the book!

To help you in your search use the following references: you may find these resources helpful:

- A medical dictionary: to find an alternate term that might be easier to find in the ICD-9-CM book

- The *Merck Manual:* to determine which signs and symptoms are included in a diagnosis and which should be coded separately
- The *Physician's Desk Reference* (PDR): to find alternate or generic names for drugs or other chemicals
- Publications including the *Coding Clinic* and the *Correct Coding Initiative,* as well as *CodeWrite,* a free electronic newsletter from the American Health Information Management Association (AHIMA)
- The official guidelines focusing on the sections that directly relate to your workplace's health care specialty
- Professional websites, including www.cms.hhs.gov, www.ahima.org, www.aapc.com, and www.dhhs.gov
- And, of course, the health care provider who saw the patient can help answer any questions and provide additional details

AMERICAN HEALTH INFORMATION MANAGEMENT ASSOCIATION CODE OF ETHICS

The American Health Information Management Association (AHIMA) is the preeminent professional organization for health information workers, including insurance coding specialists.

The AHIMA House of Delegates considers its Code of Ethics (Box 1-1) and Standards of Ethical Coding (Box 1-2) as being critical to the highest level of honorable behavior for its members.

AAPC CODE OF ETHICAL STANDARDS

AAPC is another influential organization in the health information management industry. Its members, and its certifications, are well respected throughout the United States and the world. Its Code of Ethical Standards, shown in Box 1-3, also highlights the importance of an insurance coding and billing specialist exhibiting the most ethical and moral conduct.

CHAPTER SUMMARY

It is your responsibility, as a professional in the health information management industry, to ensure that you always behave in an ethical and legal manner. Doing so will protect you, your health care facility, and your patients.

Once you assign a diagnosis or procedure code to a patient's claim form, it becomes a legal document and a permanent part of the patient's health care record. Coding is a very important part of the health care industry's process of caring.

BOX 1-1 AHIMA Code of Ethics

PREAMBLE

This Code of Ethics sets forth ethical principles for the health information management profession. Members of this profession are responsible for maintaining and promoting ethical practices. This Code of Ethics, adopted by the American Health Information Management Association, shall be binding on health information management professionals who are members of the Association and all individuals who hold an AHIMA credential.

ETHICAL PRINCIPLES

The following ethical principles are based on the core values of the American Health Information Management Association and apply to all health information management professionals.

Health information management professionals:

1. Advocate, uphold and defend the individual's right to privacy and the doctrine of confidentiality in the use and disclosure of information.
2. Put service and the health and welfare of persons before self-interest and conduct themselves in the practice of the profession so as to bring honor to themselves, their peers, and to the health information management profession.
3. Preserve, protect, and secure personal health information in any form or medium and hold in the highest regard the contents of the records and other information of a confidential nature, taking into account the applicable statutes and regulations.
4. Refuse to participate in or conceal unethical practices or procedures.
5. Advance health information management knowledge and practice through continuing education, research, publications, and presentations.
6. Recruit and mentor students, peers and colleagues to develop and strengthen professional workforce.
7. Represent the profession accurately to the public.
8. Perform honorably health information management association responsibilities, either appointed or elected, and preserve the confidentiality of any privileged information made known in any official capacity.
9. State truthfully and accurately their credentials, professional education, and experiences.
10. Facilitate interdisciplinary collaboration in situations supporting health information practice.
11. Respect the inherent dignity and worth of every person.

BOX 1-2 AHIMA Standards of Ethical Coding

The Standards of Ethical Coding are based on the American Health Information Management Association's (AHIMA's) Code of Ethics. Both sets of principles reflect expectations of professional conduct for coding professionals involved in diagnostic and/or procedural coding or other health record data abstraction.

A Code of Ethics sets forth professional values and ethical principles and offers ethical guidelines to which professionals aspire and by which their actions can be judged. Health information management (HIM) professionals are expected to demonstrate professional values by their actions to patients, employers, members of the healthcare team, the public, and the many stakeholders they serve. A Code of Ethics is important in helping to guide the decision-making process and can be referenced by individuals, agencies, organizations, and bodies (such as licensing and regulatory boards, insurance providers, courts of law, government agencies, and other professional groups).

The AHIMA Code of Ethics (available on the AHIMA web site) is relevant to all AHIMA members and credentialed HIM professionals and students, regardless of their professional functions, the settings in which they work, or the populations they serve. Coding is one of the core HIM functions, and due to the complex regulatory requirements affecting the health information coding process, coding professionals are frequently faced with ethical challenges. The AHIMA Standards of Ethical Coding are intended to assist coding professionals and managers in decision-making processes and actions, outline expectations for making ethical decisions in the workplace, and demonstrate coding professionals' commitment to integrity during the coding process, regardless of the purpose for which the codes are being reported. They are relevant to all coding professionals and those who manage the coding function, regardless of the healthcare setting in which they work or whether they are AHIMA members or nonmembers.

These Standards of Ethical Coding have been revised in order to reflect the current healthcare environment and modern coding practices. The previous revision was published in 1999.

STANDARDS OF ETHICAL CODING

Coding professionals should:

1. Apply accurate, complete, and consistent coding practices for the production of high-quality healthcare data.
2. Report all healthcare data elements (e.g. diagnosis and procedure codes, present on admission indicator, discharge status) required for external reporting purposes (e.g., reimbursement and other administrative uses, population health, quality and patient safety measurement, and research) completely and accurately, in accordance with regulatory and documentation standards and requirements and applicable official coding conventions, rules, and guidelines.
3. Assign and report only the codes and data that are clearly and consistently supported by health record documentation in accordance with applicable code set and abstraction conventions, rules, and guidelines.
4. Query provider (physician or other qualified healthcare practitioner) for clarification and additional documentation prior to code assignment when there is conflicting, incomplete, or ambiguous information in the health record regarding a significant reportable condition or procedure or other reportable data element dependent on health record documentation (e.g., present on admission indicator).
5. Refuse to change reported codes or the narratives of codes so that meanings are misrepresented.
6. Refuse to participate in or support coding or documentation practices intended to inappropriately increase payment, qualify for insurance policy coverage, or skew data by means that do not comply with federal and state statutes, regulations and official rules and guidelines.
7. Facilitate interdisciplinary collaboration in situations supporting proper coding practices.
8. Advance coding knowledge and practice through continuing education.
9. Refuse to participate in or conceal unethical coding or abstraction practices or procedures.
10. Protect the confidentiality of the health record at all times and refuse to access protected health information not required for coding-related activities (examples of coding-related activities include completion of code assignment, other health record data abstraction, coding audits, and educational purposes).
11. Demonstrate behavior that reflects integrity, shows a commitment to ethical and legal coding practices, and fosters trust in professional activities.

Revised and approved by the House of Delegates 09/08

*The Cooperating Parties are the American Health Information Management Association, American Hospital Association, Health Care Financing Administration, and National Center for Health Statistics.

BOX 1-3 AAPC Code of Ethics

Members of the AAPC shall be dedicated to providing the highest standard of professional coding and billing services to employers, clients and patients. Professional and personal behavior of AAPC members must be exemplary.

AAPC members shall maintain the highest standard of personal and professional conduct. Members shall respect the rights of patients, clients, employers and all other colleagues.

Members shall use only legal and ethical means in all professional dealings and shall refuse to cooperate with, or condone by silence, the actions of those who engage in fraudulent, deceptive or illegal acts.

Members shall respect and adhere to the laws and regulations of the land and uphold the mission statement of the AAPC.

Members shall pursue excellence through continuing education in all areas applicable to their profession.

Members shall strive to maintain and enhance the dignity, status, competence and standards of coding for professional services.

Members shall not exploit professional relationships with patients, employees, clients or employers for personal gain.

Above all else we will commit to recognizing the intrinsic worth of each member.

This code of ethical standards for members of the AAPC strives to promote and maintain the highest standard of professional service and conduct among its members. Adherence to these standards assures public confidence in the integrity and service of professional coders who are members of the AAPC.

Failure to adhere to these standards, as determined by AAPC, will result in the loss of credentials and membership with the AAPC.

Chapter 1 Review
Introduction to Diagnostic Coding

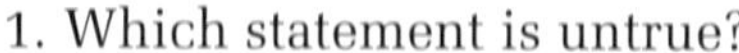

1. Which statement is untrue?
   a. ICD-10-CM will replace ICD-9-CM as the code set to report diagnoses.
   b. ICD-10-CM will be implemented in the United States on January 1, 2013
   c. The coding process is the same for both ICD-9-CM and ICD-10-CM
   d. ICD-10-CM codes will require more specific information.

2. The most important factor in coding is
   a. Speed of coding process.
   b. Accuracy of codes.
   c. Quantity of codes.
   d. Level of codes.

3. When you find unclear or missing information in the physician's notes, you should
   a. Ask a coworker.
   b. Figure it out yourself. You should know what the doctor is thinking.
   c. Query the physician.
   d. Place the file at the bottom of the pile.

4. Diagnostic codes identify
   a. What the provider did for the patient.
   b. Who the policyholder is.
   c. At which facility the patient was seen by the provider.
   d. Why the provider cared for the patient.

5. Procedure codes identify
   a. What the provider did for the patient.
   b. Who the policyholder is.
   c. At which facility the patient was seen by the provider.
   d. Why the provider cared for the patient.

6. It is important to read the physician's encounter notes so you will know
   a. The deadline for filing the claim.
   b. Insurance information.
   c. Predetermined general codes.
   d. Details to code accurately.

7. ICD-9-CM Official Guidelines
   a. Are generalized and do not provide details about any one section of the book.
   b. Identify specific rules for coding.
   c. Only apply to hospital coders.
   d. Only apply to coders working in physician's offices.

8. ICD-9-CM Official Guidelines
   a. Must be memorized by professional coders.
   b. Can be found in the front of every CPT-4 book.
   c. Can be found in the front of the ICD-9-CM book.
   d. Can be found in the front of the ICD-9-CM section.

9. When ICD-9-CM codes support medical necessity, it means that
   a. A licensed health care professional was involved.
   b. There was a valid health care reason to provide services.
   c. The patient was seen in a hospital.
   d. A preexisting condition was treated.

10. The implementation of ICD-10-CM means
    a. More details will be required from the documentation.
    b. You will not be able to do your job.
    c. Diagnosis codes will not be needed anymore.
    d. You will have to learn new anatomy.

11. Changing a code to one you know the insurance company will pay for is called
    a. Coding for coverage.
    b. Coding for packaging.
    c. Unbundling.
    d. Double billing.

12. Unbundling is an illegal practice that has coders
    a. Bill for services never provided.
    b. Bill for services with no documentation.
    c. Bill using several individual codes instead of one combination code.
    d. Bill using a code for a higher level of service than what was actually provided.

13. Upcoding is an illegal practice that has coders
    a. Bill for services never provided.
    b. Bill for services with no documentation.
    c. Bill using several individual codes instead of one combination code.
    d. Bill using a code for a higher level of service than what was actually provided.

14. When reading the physician's notes to abstract key words with regard to diagnostic coding, you must look for
    a. Confirmed diagnoses relating to why the physician is caring for the patient at this visit.
    b. Signs relating to why the physician is caring for the patient at this visit.
    c. Symptoms relating to why the physician is caring for the patient at this visit.
    d. All of these.

15. Coding improperly on a claim form can cause that claim to be
    a. Rejected.
    b. Denied
    c. Published in a journal
    d. (*a*) and (*b*) only.

YOU CODE IT! Simulation

Chapter 1. Introduction to Diagnostic Coding

Below and on the following pages are some health care scenarios. Determine the best course of action that you, as the health information management professional for the facility, should take. Identify any legal and/or ethical issues that may need to be considered and explain how you would deal with the situation.

CIPHER, VICTORS, & ASSOCIATES
A Complete Health Care Facility
234 MAIN STREET • ANYTOWN, FL 32711 • 407-555-1234

PATIENT: HAVERLAND, JULIANNA
MRN: HAVEJU001
Date: 5 April 2011

Attending Physician: Valerie R. Victors, MD

This 3-year-old female is the daughter of your best friend, Sarah. Sarah comes to see you after she finishes Julianna's checkup with the doctor. Julianna has not yet begun to speak, and Dr. Victors is concerned that she may have a developmental disorder.

The correct ICD-9-CM diagnosis code for Julianna's condition is

315.31 Expressive language disorder, developmental aphasia

However, Sarah is very concerned about a mental disorder being placed on her daughter's chart. She is afraid of the stigma that may follow her daughter throughout her life and the things she might be denied in the future. However, with a diagnosis of

389.11 Sensory hearing loss, bilateral

Julianna can still get the therapy she needs to help her without the mental disorder status. Sarah begs you to change the code in Julianna's file.

All you need to do is change the one code.

What should you do?

____

____

____

CIPHER, VICTORS, & ASSOCIATES
A Complete Health Care Facility
234 MAIN STREET • ANYTOWN, FL 32711 • 407-555-1234

PATIENT: DARDEN, CONNER
MRN: DARDCO001
Date: 15 October 2011

Attending Physician: James I Cipher, MD

Dr. Cipher performs a rhinoplasty on this 16-year-old male because of low self-esteem. However, cosmetic surgery is not reimbursable by the insurance carrier. So the physician writes a diagnosis of

Deviated Septum

to support medical necessity and get the insurance carrier to pay for the procedure. There is nothing at all in the rest of the documentation, including the encounter notes and lab reports, to support the diagnosis.

What should you do?

____

____

____

This matches the physician's notes perfectly.

Occasionally, you have to look a little further. Suppose you read that "Dr. Farina removed a splinter from Jaleel Waters's finger."

When you look in the alphabetic index under splinter, you discover a *see* reference:

Splinter—*see* Injury, superficial, by site.

Therefore, you turn to

Injury
Superficial
Finger(s) (nail) (any) 915

Read back up the indented words, and it becomes: "Superficial injury to any finger or fingernail 915."

You might think you are done, but you are not. Turn to the tabular list (volume 1) and you will find that you do not yet have the complete, valid code. In the tabular list, turn to code 915:

√4th 915 Superficial injury of finger(s)

Notice the little symbol to the left of the number 915. This is the ICD-9-CM telling you that you need a fourth digit. Continue reading down the indented list below the subheading, you see

915.6 Superficial foreign body (splinter) without major open wound, without mention of infection

Code 915.6 is not only the complete code, you will notice it actually does tell the *whole story*. There is more specific detail in code 915.6 when you compare it to code 915, and while you may not understand why this additional information matters, the book says it does, so it does.

«« CODING TIP

Never, never, never code *only* from the alphabetic index (volume 2, Index to Diseases). *Always check* the code in the tabular list (volume 1) and read the entire code description and all notations before deciding it is the most accurate code.

Finding the most accurate code can be like looking for a contact lens on the carpet—you have to really look carefully and think about what the problem really is.

Example

Darlene Samanski broke a drinking glass in her hand. She was pretty certain she got all the glass out and cleaned the wound well, but two days later, her hand was still hurting. She went to Dr. Mahoney, who removed several tiny shards of glass from the wound.

You have to think about this carefully and realize that the glass is actually a foreign body. In addition, you must figure out that the glass is not actually in Darlene's hand; it is in her soft tissue. Now, you will be able to find this in the alphabetic index:

Foreign Body, In, Soft Tissue (residual) 729.6

Other times, you may have to use alternate terms from those in the notes to find the correct listing. A medical dictionary will help you. Also, practicing so you can familiarize yourself with the terms used and the thinking process that is a part of coding.

Example

Stephan Lewis fell off of his bicycle and scraped his knee very badly, so he came to see Dr. Martinez.

Scrape is not in the alphabetic index. Another term for scrape is *abrasion*. Turn to *abrasion* in the alphabetic index, and it will direct you to *Injury, Superficial, by site*. Eventually you arrive at Injury, Superficial, Knee 916.

Remember that accuracy is the *most* important issue here. It is not a race. You need to be careful and meticulous.

LET'S CODE IT! SCENARIO

Jerry Califon, a 47-year-old male, came to see his regular physician, Dr. Warren. Jerry has a family history of pancreatic cancer, so he is very diligent about his checkups.

Let's Code It!

As you read through the notes, you can see that Dr. Warren identified the reason for Jerry's visit. He has a "family history of pancreatic cancer."

There are four key words: *family, history, pancreas,* and *cancer.* Let's look them up in the alphabetic index one at a time.

Cancer: When you look up the word *cancer* in the alphabetic index, you find that the ICD-9-CM book refers you to *see also Neoplasm, by site, malignant.* (You may remember from your medical terminology class that *malignant neoplasm* is the proper term for what is commonly called cancer.) But be careful! Jerry does *not have* a malignant neoplasm, just a family history. If you follow this lead and go to the neoplasm listings, you will see that there is nothing that indicates a family history. You now know that this key word will not lead to the correct ICD-9-CM code for this particular encounter.

(Note: Don't worry about that M8000/3 code shown here. That is a special code, and you will learn all about it in Chap. 5, "Coding Neoplasms.")

Go to the next key word.

Pancreas: Find the word *pancreas* in the alphabetic index, and you read the direction to *see condition.* This does not mean to go to the listing for the word *condition;* it means that you should go back to the physician's notes and look for the condition of Jerry's pancreas. What is wrong with his pancreas? Well, there really isn't anything indicating that there is anything wrong with his pancreas. So this is not going to get you any closer to the correct code because the alphabetic index does not include code listings by **anatomical site.**

Anatomical site

A specific location or part of the human body.

Don't get frustrated. Look at this like a treasure hunt. The correct answer is here in this book. You just have to find it. Let's go to the next key word: family.

Family: Next to the word *family,* the book directs us to *see also condition.* Underneath, there are codes indicated for

Family disruption V61.09

Family planning advice V25.09

Family problem V61.9

Family problem specified circumstance NEC V61.8

None of these possibilities comes close to the reason why Jerry came to see Dr. Warren. So let's move on to the last key word.

History: Looks like you struck gold! There are over a page and a half of codes listed under *History (personal) of.* The first question you need to answer is what kind of history does this individual have: a *family* history. Look down the column at the long list of words indented under the word *history* until you reach *family.*

You will notice under the word *family* there is an indented column, in alphabetical order, of codes for different conditions. Let's go ahead and look down the list to see if the word *pancreas* appears. It does not. A person can't have a family history of having a pancreas. Everyone has one! What does the individual actually have? A *family history* of a *malignant neoplasm* of the pancreas. Aha! Let's continue down the list:

History
  Family
    Malignant neoplasm (of) NEC V16.9

This is read as "family history of a malignant neoplasm not elsewhere classified (NEC)." But that's not our situation. Let's keep going down the list indented under *malignant neoplasm:*

Pancreas V16.0

This is read as "family history of a malignant neoplasm, pancreas." Finally! We found it!!

As you can see, each word or phrase indented below another word or phrase includes the one above.

Look above to *family* indented once under the heading *history.* You read this as "family history." Then *malignant neoplasm* is indented once under *family* that is indented once under *history.* So we read this as "family history of malignant neoplasm." This can get a little confusing, so use a ruler or your finger to keep track of what is indented at which level. If you let your eyes jump ahead, you might accidentally look at the next column under history that says "malignant neoplasm (of) V10.90." If you look at the indentations of the columns, you will see that this means a *history of malignant neoplasm* (indicating that the patient had been previously diagnosed) but not a *family* history of a malignant neoplasm (indicating that someone in the family, not this individual, was diagnosed). A *big* difference!

Now turn to the tabular list (volume 1), and look for code V16.0 to make certain this is the best, most specific code available. You read:

√4th V16 Family history of malignant neoplasm
    V16.0 Gastrointestinal tract
    Family history of condition classifiable to 140–159

You read the tabular list (volume 1) in the same way you read the indented lists in the alphabetic index. Each indented phrase includes the description above it at the margin. Therefore, the complete description is read as "V16.0 Family history of malignant neoplasm, gastrointestinal tract."

«« KEYS TO CODING

Family is a description of a type of history.

Malignant is a description of a type of neoplasm.

Open is a description of a type of wound.

«« CODING TIP

Once you find the appropriate main key word from the notes in the alphabetic index, the next item you want to identify is the adjective, or descriptor, used by the provider.

CODING TIP »»

When looking through these long lists with lots of indentations, you must be conscientious and go down the columns carefully. Use a ruler or your finger to keep things in line.

But Jerry has a family history of pancreatic cancer. Is that in the gastrointestinal tract? Take a look at the notation indented below the code description

Family history of condition classifiable to 140–159

This means that the original diagnosis would have come from the code range of 140 through 159. As you read through the descriptions of all the codes in that range, take a look at code 157, Malignant neoplasm of pancreas. That is what someone in Jerry's family had; therefore, V16.0 is correct. (See Fig. 2-1.)

KEYS TO CODING »»

The alphabetic index will suggest a possible diagnosis code. Then, you must find the code suggested by the alphabetic index in the Tabular list (volume 1) of ICD-9-CM. This step is not a suggestion . . . this is mandatory. The Tabular list of ICD-9-CM provides more detail for the code description, as well as additional notations such as *includes* and *excludes* notes and directives for the requirement of additional digits and codes. *NEVER, NEVER, NEVER code from the alphabetic index.*

Confirmed

Found to be true or definite.

Outpatient services

Health care services provided to individuals without an overnight stay in the facility.

The Tabular List

Volume 1 of the ICD-9-CM book lists all the codes and their descriptions. However, it lists all its information in numeric order, starting at 001 and running all the way through to 999.99. These are followed by the V codes listed in numerical order from V01 through V99, and these are followed by the E codes in numerical order, E000 through E999. This section is called the *tabular list.* Let's investigate the different types of codes shown in the list and discuss when you would use each kind.

ICD-9-CM Codes

As discussed previously in this chapter, the majority of the ICD-9-CM book contains codes that are three-, four-, or five-digit numbers that identify specific, **confirmed** diagnoses of illness (disease) or injury.

When coding **outpatient services,** you must be certain that the patient's file, including the physician's notes, verify that the patient actually has the condition, disease, illness, or injury. The guideline (Section IV. I. Uncertain diagnosis) states that you are to use the code or codes that identify the condition to its highest level of certainty. This means that

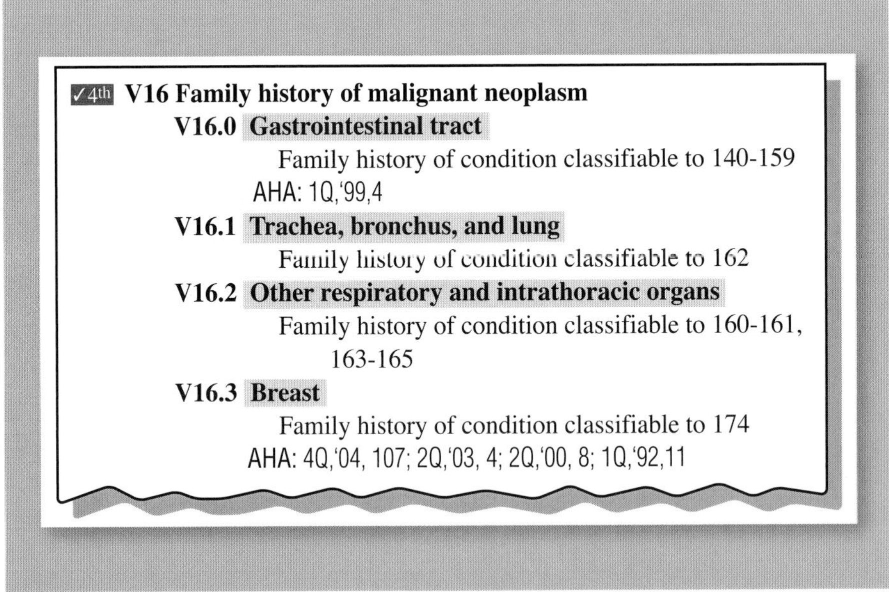
✓4th **V16 Family history of malignant neoplasm**
V16.0 Gastrointestinal tract
Family history of condition classifiable to 140-159
AHA: 1Q,'99,4
V16.1 Trachea, bronchus, and lung
Family history of condition classifiable to 162
V16.2 Other respiratory and intrathoracic organs
Family history of condition classifiable to 160-161, 163-165
V16.3 Breast
Family history of condition classifiable to 174
AHA: 4Q,'04, 107; 2Q,'03, 4; 2Q,'00, 8; 1Q,'92,11

Figure 2-1 V Code for Family History of Malignant Neoplasm.

you code only what you know for a fact. You are *not permitted* to assign an ICD-9-CM diagnosis code for a condition that is described by the provider as *probably, suspected, possible, questionable,* or *to be ruled out.* If the health care professional has not been able to confirm a diagnosis, then you must code the signs, symptoms, abnormal test results, or other element stated as the reason for the visit.

Example

Larry Glass, a 39-year-old male, came to see Dr. Walden, in his office, because of a sharp pain in his abdomen. After doing a thorough examination, Dr. Walden suspects that Larry may have enteritis due to the Norwalk virus, so he orders a blood test. If the blood test comes back *positive* to confirm enteritis due to the Norwalk virus (after the physician documents it in the file), you would use the following code:

008.63 Enteritis due to Norwalk virus

If the blood test comes back *negative*, meaning Larry does *not* have enteritis due to the Norwalk virus (after the physician documents it in the file), then you would use code

558.9 Enteritis, NOS (not otherwise specified)

The rules for coding uncertain diagnoses for patients of an **inpatient facility** are different from those for outpatients. As directed by the guideline (Section II, H. Uncertain diagnosis), when at the time of discharge the diagnosis is described as probable, possible, suspected, likely, or still to be ruled out, you must code that condition as if it did exist. This directive applies only when you are coding services provided in a short-term, acute, long-term care, or psychiatric hospital or facility. It is one of the few circumstances where you will find the guidelines differ between coding for outpatient and inpatient services.

Inpatient facility

An establishment that provides acute care services to individuals who stay overnight on the premises.

YOU CODE IT! CASE STUDY

Jenna Butler, a 59-year-old female, was admitted to the hospital for observation after she complained of having severe chest pain radiating to her left shoulder and down her arm. Dr. Halberton discharged her the next day with a diagnosis of probable variant angina pectoris.

You Code It!

As the hospital's coder, go through the steps of coding, and determine the diagnosis code that should be reported for this encounter between Dr. Halberton and Jenna Butler.

Step 1: Read the case completely.

Step 2: Abstract the notes: Which key words can you identify relating to why Dr. Halberton cared for Jenna?

____

Step 3: Query the provider, if necessary.

Step 4: Code the diagnosis or diagnoses.

Step 5: Code the procedure(s): One-night hospital stay for observation.

Step 6: Link the procedure codes to at least one diagnosis code to confirm medical necessity.

Step 7: Back code to double-check your choices.

Answer

Did you find the correct code?

413.1 Prinzmetal angina

Good job!

V Codes

There are times when an individual comes to see a health care provider without having a particular illness or injury. In such cases, you might assign a V code, which describes an encounter between a provider and an individual who does not have a current health condition.

CODING TIP »»

The *V* in V code stands for Validate. This code is used for a patient who doesn't have a current disease or injury but comes to see the physician to validate his or her current healthy status—to prevent something from going wrong or to ensure continued health.

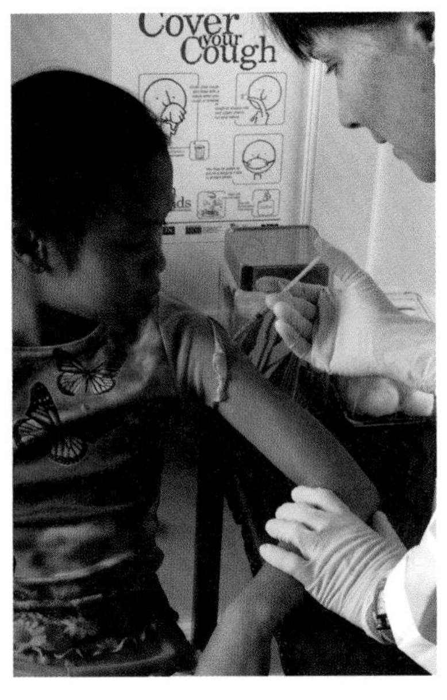

1. A healthy person might go to see a physician for the following reasons:
   a. Preventive care such as a flu shot or vaccination: codes V03.0 through V06.9
   b. Routine and administrative exams, such as an annual physical or a well-baby checkup: codes V20, V21, and V70.0 - V72.9 (except V72.5 and V72.6)
   c. Monitoring care and screenings for someone:
      i. With a personal history of a condition: codes V10.00 through V15.9
      ii. With a family history: codes V16.0 through V19.8
      iii. In a population subgroup, such as mammograms for women over 40 or prostate examinations for men over 50: codes V76.1*x* and V76.44
   d. Counseling for the patient and/or family members relating to the circumstances involved with an illness or injury or to help with family problems or social concerns such as contraceptive or procreative management: codes throughout the V code section
   e. Organ donation (to be a donor): codes V59.01–V59.9

Example

Kinley Washington finds out his brother has end-stage renal disease (ESRD). He comes in today to be tested to see if he can donate his kidney: code V59.4

2. A person might require continuous care for the following:
   a. Chronic illness or injury

b. Healing illness or injury requiring aftercare, such as follow-up after surgery: codes V51 through V58.9

c. Status identification, which is a follow-up for someone who is a carrier of a disease, has residual effects of a past condition, or has a prosthetic or mechanical device: status codes throughout the V code section

d. Follow-up examinations for a condition that has already been treated or no longer exists: codes V24.0–V24.2 or V67.00–V67.9

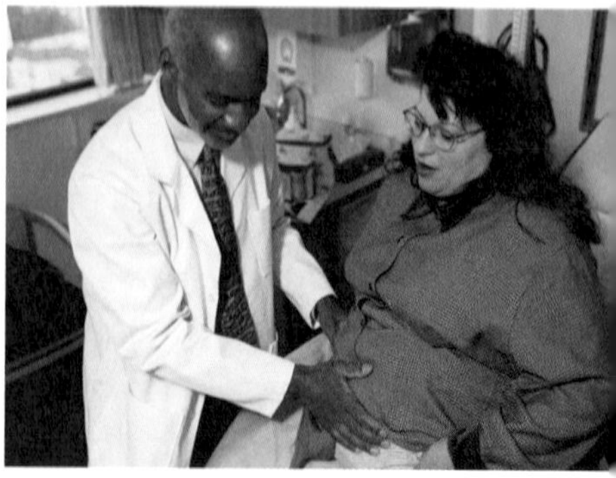

Example

Dr. Rosin sees Don Bowlin in the office six weeks after performing a carpal tunnel release before closing this case . . . code V67.09

3. A person without any signs or symptoms of a disease but who comes to the health care professional because he or she
   a. Was exposed to an infected individual: codes V01.0–V01.9
   b. Might be a carrier or suspected carrier of a disease: codes V02.0– V02.9
   c. Needs to be observed for a suspected condition that is ruled out: codes V29.0–V29.9 or V71.0–V71.9

Example

Robert Boatman, a 19-year-old male, discovers that his roommate has been diagnosed with tuberculosis. He visits his physician to find out what he should do: code V01.1

4. Obstetrics and neonatal evaluations and circumstances including regularly planned, periodic checkups, the outcome of delivery, birth status, and health supervision and observations of an infant or child may be reported with a V code. These related codes range from V22.0 through V39.

Example

Tiffany Sherwood, a 29-year-old female, is seven weeks pregnant with her first child. She has an appointment with Dr. Nelson today for her regularly scheduled prenatal checkup: code V22.0

5. When coding a visit for routine lab work or radiology services, when there are no current signs, symptoms, or related diagnosis, report the visit using either code V72.5 or V72.6x.

Example

Rhonda Shultz comes in for a routine chest x-ray. She does not see Dr. Fahey or have any other services provided: code V72.5

6. When routine testing is performed during an encounter at which an unrelated sign, symptom, or diagnosis is evaluated. Code both the V code for the routine test and the reason for the evaluation.

«« KEYS TO CODING

When you identify why the physician cared for the patient, ask yourself, "Is the patient currently sick or injured?" If this is not a current, active issue, then there is a good chance the medical necessity for this encounter will be reported with a V code. Another question you can ask yourself is, "Did the patient have signs or symptoms or did the patient come to the encounter because the calendar said to?" The calendar tells patients to come in for an annual exam, seasonal flu vaccine, or a 12-week prenatal exam. These are all reported with V codes.

«« BRIDGE TO ICD-10-CM

Reasons other than current disease or injury to have contact with the health care industry are reported with codes from Chap. 21 codes Z00-Z99 Factors Influencing health status and contact with health services.

Example

Kallie Pasternak, a 25-year-old female, is here for her annual well-woman exam. She asks Dr. Walli to do a genetic disease test because she and her husband are discussing beginning a family: codes V72.31 (routine gynecological examination) and V26.31 (testing of female for genetic disease carrier status).

LET'S CODE IT! SCENARIO

Lewis Elliott brings his daughter Marissa to Dr. Cruse, her pediatrician, for a rubella vaccination. Marissa is 4 years old and will be going to preschool next month. The school requires just this one shot. Marissa chooses a sunflower sticker as her prize for being a good patient.

Let's Code It!

CODING TIP »»

Remember that a diagnostic code identifies the reason *why* the physician treated this patient during this encounter. In Marissa's case this is because she *needed* to have the vaccination. That is the reason that the code reads "Need for." The diagnostic code is not the code for the actual provision of the injection. That will come from the procedure coding book. This is just the *why*, not the *what*.

Marissa did not come to Dr. Cruse because she was ill or injured. She came so that he could *prevent* her from becoming ill. Dr. Cruse indicates that the reason why he saw Marissa today was to give her a *vaccination* to prevent her from getting *rubella*. Let's go to the alphabetic index.

Looking up the key word *rubella*, you see the code

Rubella (German measles) 056.9

Using this code indicates that Marissa had been confirmed to have a diagnosis of rubella. But she does not. The physician's notes document that she has come for a vaccination to prevent her from getting rubella. So let's look up *vaccination*. You see a long list indented below the key word, most of which are shown below another indented word *prophylactic* (another word for preventive). Underneath, you find

Rubella (alone) V04.3

Go to the tabular list to confirm this code. Find

√4th V04 Need for prophylactic vaccination and inoculation against certain viral diseases

Below this three-digit code category is an excludes notation. This is telling you that reporting vaccinations against combinations of diseases is reported from a different code category (V06.0–V06.9). This means, if the patient was receiving an MMR vaccination (measles, mumps, rubella), then a code from the V06 code category would be more accurate. That is not the case here, so let's stay in V04. To the left of the V04 code, you see a symbol that tells you this code needs a fourth digit. This is mandatory, so read down the column and find the fourth digit that most accurately identifies what type of vaccination Marissa received.

V04.3 Need for prophylactic vaccination, rubella alone

Some V codes cover a variety of miscellaneous issues: problems relating to lifestyle (V69) or encounters for administrative purposes (V68). Take a few minutes to look through the V code section of your ICD-9-CM book. Get a feeling for the category headlines and sections. The descriptions for all V codes are included in the alphabetic index, and the ICD-9-CM book will guide you as to when to use them.

LET'S CODE IT! SCENARIO

After having surgery to remove a cancerous tumor, Caroline completed her planned sequence of chemotherapy treatments. She comes to see Dr. Masters for a follow-up.

Let's Code It!

Caroline has completed her treatments, so she is technically no longer ill. However, it would be remiss of Dr. Masters not to examine her to ensure that she is doing as well as expected and that the treatments worked. You cannot report the visit with a code for cancer, because Caroline no longer has cancer. This visit is a follow-up as a part of her completed treatment, so she actually does not yet qualify for a personal history code. Let's try the best key word we have: *follow-up*. In the alphabetic index, you see

Follow-up (examination) (routine) (following) V67.9

Cancer chemotherapy V67.2

In the tabular (numeric) listing, reading from the top of the subsection, you see

√4th V67 Follow-up examination

INCLUDES surveillance only following completed treatment

Excludes surveillance of contraception (V25.40–V25.49)

Keep reading down the column to

V67.2 Following chemotherapy

Cancer chemotherapy follow-up

That is a perfect match to the notes. Good job!

YOU CODE IT! CASE STUDY

Augustina Saciolo, a 36-year-old female who is approximately 12 weeks pregnant with her first baby, comes to see Dr. Apple for a routine pregnancy checkup. The sonogram shows no abnormalities with a fetus that appears to be appropriate size and growth for the approximated gestation.

You Code It!

Go through the steps of coding, and determine the diagnosis code that should be reported for this encounter between Dr. Apple and Augustina.

Step 1: Read the case completely.

Step 2: Abstract the notes: Which key words can you identify relating to why Dr. Apple cared for Augustina?

____

Step 3: Query the provider, if necessary.

Step 4: Code the diagnosis or diagnoses.

Step 5: Code the procedure(s): Regular pregnancy checkup; sonogram.

Step 6: Link the procedure codes to at least one diagnosis code to confirm medical necessity.

Step 7: Back code to double-check your choices.

Answer

Did you find the correct code?

V23.81 Supervision of high-risk pregnancy, elderly primigravida

Good job!

BRIDGE TO ICD-10-CM

External causes of injury and poisoning are reported with codes from Chapter 20 V01-Y99 External causes of morbidity.

Adverse effect

The harm a patient experiences by a medication that has been prescribed by a health care professional and taken as instructed; an unexpected reaction to a drug taken for therapeutic purposes.

External cause

An event, outside the body, that causes injury, poisoning, or an adverse reaction.

E codes

Codes that report *how* and/or *where* an injury or poisoning happened.

CODING TIP

The E code explains the *external* cause of the individual's injury, poisoning, or adverse reaction.

E Codes

When an individual has an injury, has been poisoned, or has had an **adverse effect,** something had to cause it. You can't catch a broken leg or wake up with a case of poisoning. Something outside of the body caused the problem. There has to be an **external cause. E codes** are used, along with ICD-9-CM and/or V codes, to explain exactly what has happened. (See Fig. 2-2.)

Example

How was Mickey poisoned by that drain cleaner? E864.2 Accidental poisoning by corrosives and caustics, caustic alkalis

Where was Mickey when he got poisoned? E849.0 Home

How did Rosanne aspirate all that water? E910.0 Accidental drowning and submersion while water-skiing

Where did Rosanne almost drown? E849.4 Place for recreation and sport

How did Arthur get that rash? E930.4 Adverse effects in therapeutic use, tetracycline group

Where was Arthur when he got that rash? When using therapeutic use codes, you do not need a place of occurrence code.

How did Ruth break her ankle? E880.0 Fall on an escalator

Where was Ruth when she was on that escalator? E849.6 Public building, store (mall)

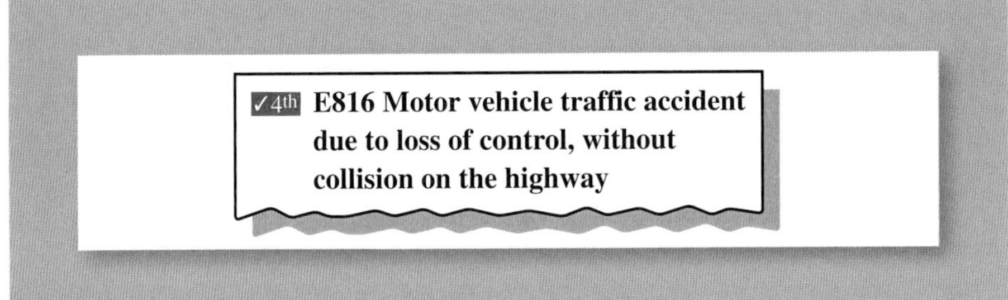

✓4th E816 Motor vehicle traffic accident due to loss of control, without collision on the highway

Figure 2-2 Example of an E Code, Including Both How and Where.

LET'S CODE IT! SCENARIO

Ellen Depew was brought to Dr. Davis's office with a bad headache. She had been riding her bicycle in the park and had fallen off her bicycle and hit her head fiercely against the ground. After x-rays have been taken, Dr. Davis determines that Ellen has a brain concussion.

Let's Code It!

Why do the claim forms and the reports need to identify *how* or *where* Ellen got hurt? The answer is that the situation responsible for Ellen's concussion affects which insurance carrier's policy pays the medical expenses. If Ellen hit her head:

At work, then *workers' compensation* insurance would pay the medical bills, not her health care plan.

While shopping at a store, the store's *liability insurance* might pay for the medical bills.

In an automobile accident, then her *automobile insurance* would probably be billed.

In her own home, then her own *health care policy* would be billed first.

Therefore, as a coding specialist, you must use codes to explain what happened so that it will be clear which insurance carrier is responsible for, and should receive, the medical bills. In addition, your state or federal agencies may need to know the circumstances for statistical analysis or other research purposes.

You will use E codes, *after* the diagnosis code(s), to provide this important information. Now, let's look back at Ellen Depew's scenario and pick out the key words that will lead us to the correct codes. With our diagnosis codes and E codes, the entire story must be reported to explain *why* Ellen came to see Dr. Davis for this visit. As you learned, because Ellen has an injury, you must also report *how* and *where* she became injured.

Dr. Davis's notes tell us that Ellen had a headache that turned out to be a concussion: "Dr. Davis determines that Ellen has a *brain concussion.*" In the alphabetic index, find

Concussion (current) 850.9

Without loss of consciousness 850.0

Now turn to the tabular list, and find

√4th 850 Concussion

Beneath this code you can see an *includes* note and some *excludes* notes. None of these relate to Ellen's diagnosis, so continue reading down the column looking at all of the fourth-digit choices.

850.0 Brain concussion, with no loss of consciousness

The notes do not mention anything about her losing consciousness after she hurt her head, so it is the most accurate code. Now, you know that a concussion is an injury, so you will need to explain *how* and *where* she hurt her head. Go back to the notes, and find the documentation to explain how she injured herself: "*She had fallen off her bicycle and hit her head fiercely against the ground.*" For the correct code to report the *how* and *where* information about an injury, you will need to look this up in the E code alphabetic index in Volume 2, Section 3, and then confirm it in the E code tabular list. Let's begin with the *how*. . . . In the Alphabetic Index to External Causes of Injury and Poisoning (E Codes), find

Fall, falling (accidental) E888.9

Read down the indented list under this key term, and find the item from which she fell:

Fall, falling (accidental) E888.9

bicycle E826

Turn to the tabular list for the E codes, found in your ICD-9-CM book after the regular codes and then after the V codes. Find

√4th E826 Pedal cycle accident

The *includes* note shows "fall from pedal cycle" so you know you are in the right place. Now, you need to look for that required fourth digit. There are no fourth digit choices shown below code E826, so you will need to look above. In the box above code E826 you will see:

> The following fourth-digit subdivisions are for use with categories E826–E829 to identify the injured person:
>
> .0 Pedestrian
>
> .1 Pedal cyclist
>
> .2 Rider of animal
>
> .3 Occupant of animal-drawn vehicle
>
> .4 Occupant of streetcar
>
> .8 Other specified person
>
> .9 Unspecified person

The notes tell you that she was riding a bicycle, so the correct fourth digit is one, giving you the correct code:

E826.1 Pedal cycle accident, pedal cyclist injured

You need one more code to explain *where* Ellen was when she was injured. It is called a *place of occurrence* code. Let's look at the notes, and find out where she got hurt: "riding her bicycle in the park." When you go to the E code alphabetic index, look up P for place of occurrence. This listing directs you to *Accident (to), occurring (at) (in).*

Go back to A for accident, and look down the columns until you reach the first indented word: *occurring (at) (in).*

Go down the indented column underneath the phrase until you get to *park (public) E849.4.* Confirm it in the tabular list to find that the code accurately reports *where* Ellen was when she got hurt.

E849.4 Place of occurrence, place for recreation and sport

Now, with those three codes, you can accurately and completely report the reasons *why* Ellen came to see Dr. Davis for this visit and identify the medical reason for Dr. Davis ordering the x-ray.

850.0 Brain concussion, with no loss of consciousness

E826.1Pedal cycle accident, pedal cyclist injured

E849.4 Place of occurrence, place for recreation and sport

CODING TIP »»

An E code can *never* be a principal, or first-listed, code. In other words, it cannot be first code on a claim form and it can never be the only diagnosis code on a claim form.

You may have to ask the intake nurse, the attending physician, or the patient him or herself to obtain all the information you need to code an injury properly. However, in some circumstances, additional information may not be available. If the patient is unconscious, for example, you may know the *how* with regard to the event (e.g., fell off a ladder, in an automobile accident, overdose of aspirin?) but not have a confirmation on the intent (e.g., was the injury or poisoning an accident, assault, or attempted suicide?). In such cases, you can use a code from the following:

E980.0–E989 Injury undetermined whether accidentally or purposely inflicted

Although less likely, the reverse may occur. You may know the intent but not the event. In such cases, you may choose the most appropriate code:

E928.9 Unspecified accident

E958.9 Suicide and self-inflicted injury by unspecified means

E968.9 Assault by unspecified means

Undetermined and unspecified codes should only be used as a last resort, when you have no way of getting additional information. Most insurers are wary of such codes and will typically pull claims using them for further investigation. It will delay payment.

Occasionally, the ICD-9-CM book will actually remind you to include an E code.

Example

995.5*x* Child maltreatment syndrome

Use additional E code to identify:

nature of abuse (E960-E968)

perpetrator (E967.0-E967.9)

Most of the time, however, you have to use your judgment as to whether an E code is necessary. These code descriptions are *not* included in the main alphabetic index. So once you have determined that an E code is necessary, you will begin the search for the most accurate E code in Section 3 of Volume 2: the *Index to External Causes,* the alphabetic index of E code descriptions.

In some cases, one E code will include both the how and the where:

√4th E815 Other motor vehicle traffic accident involving collision on the highway

The one E code explains *how* the individual got injured (a motor vehicle accident) and *where* it happened (on the highway).

Example

Selene Judd sustained a simple fracture of her ulna when she fell off her skateboard while practicing flips at City Park. The codes required are

813.82 Fracture of ulna (alone), unspecified part, closed

E885.2 Fall from skateboard

E849.4 Place of occurrence, place for recreation and sport

««« BRIDGE TO ICD-10-CM

The codes may begin with an X or a V, but these codes will still provide the same information as ICD-9-CM's E codes . . . explaining *how* and *where* the injury or poisoning happened.

««« CODING TIP

In some circumstances, you might need to include multiple E codes to tell the whole story—the how and the where. Some codes include both in their description. Read carefully.

««« CODING TIP

An E code can be added to any ICD-9-CM code (from 001 through V91) that designates an injury, poisoning, or adverse effect. The code should be included on the claim form, or the statistical report, only for the *first* encounter when the condition is treated by the health care professional, not the follow-up encounters.

KEYS TO CODING »»

Review the **ICD-9-CM Coding Guidelines, Section 1. B. General Coding Guidelines, subsection 12. Late Effects** for more input on identifying what to code and what not to code. Use this to support your reading here, and as a reminder booster later on.

Late effect

Cause-and-effect relationship between an original condition, illness, or injury and an additional problem caused by the existence of that original condition. Time is not a requirement for a diagnosis as a late effect because the additional concern may be present at any time.

CODING TIP »»

PaCE the coding of the late effect of an injury or poisoning as follows:

P Problem being treated (scarring, mental retardation, paralysis, etc.)

C Cause (what caused the problem), late effect code (905–909)

E E code (late effect code to explain *how* the "cause" occurred)

CODING TIP »»

When the problem was *not* caused by injury or poisoning, you will not need an E code. Such late effects will have two diagnostic codes:

P Problem being treated (scarring, mental retardation, paralysis, etc.)

C Cause (what caused the problem), late effect code (905-909)

Remember: The main purpose of the E code is to help guide you in your determination as to which insurance policy should be responsible for paying the bill. Therefore, be certain you know the whole story so that your codes can tell the whole story. While E codes are not required in all states or by all insurance carriers, including the codes on your health claim form will speed the process along and get your claim paid faster. And that's what this is all about!

LATE EFFECTS

A patient may come to see a health care professional for the treatment of a **late effect** of an illness, injury, or a poisoning. It can be difficult to know whether to report this as a manifestation or a late effect. The guidelines direct you to code the condition as a late effect *only* in the following situations:

- Scarring, as the result of a burn, laceration, wound, or other injury
- Nonunion or malunion of a fracture
- As specifically stated by the physician or health care professional as a late effect

Coding the treatment of a late effect will require at least two codes, in the following order:

1. The late effect, which is the condition that resulted and that is being treated
2. The late effect code that refers to the original condition

As with any rule, there is always an exception. When coding a late effect whose code is followed by an additional digit (fourth or fifth digit to the code) to identify a manifestation or when a separate manifestation code is required, the code for the original illness or injury is not reported with a code for the late effect.

Late effect E codes E929.0–E929.9, E959, E969, E977, E989, and E999.0–E999.1 should be used for the treatment of the late effect of an injury or poisoning for the first and any subsequent encounters. Unlike original E codes, late effect E codes are *not* reported when the original condition was an adverse effect. In addition, you will *not* assign a late effect E code for any condition resulting from a medical misadventure or a surgical complication.

Cerebrovascular disease can often cause other problems in the patient. When the physician identifies any condition as a late effect of cerebrovascular disease, a cardiovascular accident (CVA) or other diagnosis originally described with codes from the 430–437 range, report code 438.*xx* to connect the current problem with the specific late effect.

There are times when a patient experiences a complication with her pregnancy or the birth of the child and/or a complication of the puerperium, and that complication creates a condition that requires treatment or services later on. Even when that treatment occurs after the initial postpartum period, if the condition is identified as a late effect of a pregnancy complication, you will use code 677.

LET'S CODE IT! SCENARIO

Bruce Bucholz, a 27-year-old male, comes to see Dr. Walker for treatment of adherent scars on the back of his hand. Bruce is a firefighter and suffered third-degree burns on his right hand last year when he reached in to save a child from a burning house. Dr. Walker evaluates Bruce's scars and proceeds to plan out a series of plastic surgeries.

«« CODING TIP

Code V12.59 History of cerebrovascular disease is only reported when the patient has no neurological deficits as a result.

Let's Code It!

Remember from previously in this chapter, scarring is automatically reported as a late effect. Therefore, because this is an injury, you can use the PaCE memory tip to help you recall that, in addition to the code for Bruce's scars (the problem), you have to include a late effects code to relate how Bruce got the scars in the first place (the cause), and because it was an injury, you need a late effects E code.

Let's begin with the problem being treated, the "*adherent scars on the back of his hand*". In the alphabetic index, find

Scar, scarring—see also Cicatrix 709.2
  Adherent 709.2

In the tabular list, find

√4th 709 Other disorders of skin and subcutaneous tissue
709.2 Scar conditions and fibrosis of skin . . . adherent scar (skin)

Next, you need to find the late effects code to report this scarring is the late effect of a burn on his hand, so in the alphabetic index, find

Late—see also condition
  Effect(s) (of) (see also condition)
    burn (injury classifiable to 948–949) 906.9
      extremities NEC (injury classifiable to 943 or 945) 906.7
        hand or wrist (injury classifiable to 944) 906.6

This is a good example of why it is wise to keep reading down an indented list. Many times, you find the exact, specific descriptions you are looking for. In the tabular list, turn to:

√4th 906 Late effects of injuries to skin and subcutaneous tissues

Read down and review your choices for the required fourth digit, and find

906.6 Late effect of burn of wrist and hand

The last part of our PaCE coding for late effects will be an E-code because this is an injury. This time, you are going to look up 'late effect' in the Index to External Causes. Find

Late effect of
  fire, accident caused by (accident classifiable to E890–E899) E929.4

In the tabular list, turn to:

√4th E929 Late effects of accidental injury

The *excludes* note does not include anything relating to Dr. Walker's care of Bruce so keep reading to find the required correct fourth digit.

«« KEYS TO CODING

Review the **ICD-9-CM Coding Guidelines, Section 1. Chapter 7d. Late Effects of cerebrovascular disease** for more input on identifying what to code and what not to code. Use this to support your reading here, and as a reminder booster later on.

«« KEYS TO CODING

Review the **ICD-9-CM Coding Guidelines, Section 1. Chapter 11j. Code 677. Late effect of complication of pregnancy** for more input on identifying what to code and what not to code. Use this to support your reading here, and as a reminder booster later on.

E929.4 Late effects of accident caused by fire

This is good work. You have now found the three codes you need to report the reasons for the care provided to Bruce:

709.2 Scar conditions and fibrosis of skin . . . adherent scar (skin)

906.6 Late effect of burn of wrist and hand

E929.4 Late effects of accident caused by fire

YOU CODE IT! CASE STUDY

Marion Rilea, a 71-year-old female, came to see Dr. Mills for continued treatment of the acute gastric ulcer in her stomach. The ulcer developed as a result of her taking aspirin for her arthritis, as instructed. Dr. Miller recommends surgery, and Marion agrees.

You Code It!

Go through the steps of coding, and determine the codes that should be reported for this encounter between Dr. Miller and Marion Rilea.

Step 1: Read the case completely.

Step 2: Abstract the notes: Which key words can you identify relating to why Dr. Miller cared for Marion?

____

Step 3: Query the provider, if necessary.

Step 4: Code the diagnosis or diagnoses.

____

Step 5: Code the procedure(s): Office visit

Step 6: Link the procedure codes to at least one diagnosis code to confirm medical necessity.

Step 7: Back code to double-check your choices.

BRIDGE TO ICD-10-CM »»

The guidelines for reporting late effects will remain the same in ICD-10-CM.

Answer

Did you find the correct codes?

531.30 Acute gastric ulcer, without mention of hemorrhage or perforation, without mention of obstruction

909.5 Late effect of adverse effect of drug, medical, or biological substance

BRIDGE TO ICD-10-CM 

Codes from the Y38 category are used to report injuries resulting from terrorist activities.

CODING INJURIES FROM TERRORIST EVENTS

Category E979.0–E979.9 are to be used when the cause of an injury has been deemed the result of an act of terrorism by the Federal Bureau of Investigation (FBI) or other appropriate agency of the U.S. federal government.

CHAPTER SUMMARY

This chapter is just an overview of what the following chapters will be reviewing, in detail, about coding diagnoses. As you look back over this chapter, you should notice one very important thing: The ICD-9-CM book will almost always guide you to the correct code. The alphabetic index will guide you to the correct page in the tabular list (volume 1), so you can read the notations and symbols, evaluate all the choices, and determine the best, most accurate code. If no codes seem to match the attending physician's notes, just go back and keep looking.

Two principles important to becoming a good coder:

1. Identify the key words in the physician's notes so that you can look up the best, most accurate code or codes.
2. In case of an injury, poisoning, or adverse effect, you will need to add an E code.

The ICD-9-CM book will guide you through the rest with its notations and instructions. The Official Coding Guidelines are always there, in the book for you to reference—no memorization! It all can point you in the right direction toward the best, most accurate code. Just look and read. And when the time comes, you will have no problem transitioning to ICD-10-CM.

9. Millie Andujar, a 43-year-old female, comes to Seaside Diagnostic Imaging for another mammogram because her mother died of breast cancer.

____

10. Edward Madison, an 81-year-old male, is brought to Dr. Abbott for a follow-up on the progress of the malignant melanoma on his forehead.

____

11. Lawrence Bowers, a 33-year-old male, comes to the emergency room for treatment of bilateral second-degree sunburn on his shoulder areas. Lawrence has been a firefighter for 10 years.

____

12. Salvatore Mulkey, a 2-year-old male, is brought to the ER by ambulance after his mother found him unconscious. Her bottle of ampicillin was found empty next to him.

____

13. Debra Gilliam, a 19-year-old female, was camping with her boyfriend when she was bitten by a tick. She began to feel sick and came to the doctor. After a thorough exam, Dr. Chung diagnoses her with Lyme disease.

____

14. Kathleen Wilcox, a 4-year-old female, is brought by her father to Dr. Bridges to remove a jellybean from Kathleen's nose.

____

15. Christopher Edison, a 1-year-old male, is brought in to Dr. Vasquez for Christopher's routine examination.

____

YOU CODE IT! Simulation

Chapter 2. Introduction to ICD-9-CM

On the following pages, you will see physicians' notes documenting encounters with patients at our textbook's health care facility, Taylor, Reader, & Associates. Carefully read through the notes, and find the best ICD-9-CM code or codes for each case. Include E codes as necessary.

TAYLOR, READER, & ASSOCIATES
A Complete Health Care Facility
975 CENTRAL AVENUE • SOMEWHERE, FL 32811 • 407-555-4321

PATIENT:	VAN DYKE, OLIVIA
ACCOUNT/EHR #:	VANDOL001
Date:	09/16/11
Attending Physician:	Suzanne R. Taylor, MD

S: Pt is a 25-year-old female who has had a sore throat for the past week. She states that she has felt feverish for the last two days, and had a temperature of 100.5 degrees last night.

O: Ht 5′5″ Wt. 159 lb. R 16. T 99. BP 110/85 Pharynx is inspected, and there is obvious purulent material in the left posterior pharynx. Neck: supple, no nodes. Chest: clear. COR: RRR without murmur.

A: Acute pharyngitis

P:
1. Send pt for test to rule/out Strep
2. Recommend patient gargle with warm salt water and use OTC lozenges to keep throat moist
3. Will write Rx once results of Strep test come back
4. Return in three weeks for follow-up

Suzanne R. Taylor, MD

SRT/pw D: 9/16/11 09:50:16 T: 9/18/11 12:55:01

Find the best, most appropriate ICD-9-CM code(s).

TAYLOR, READER, & ASSOCIATES
A Complete Health Care Facility
975 CENTRAL AVENUE • SOMEWHERE, FL 32811 • 407-555-4321

PATIENT: WILLIAMS, CONRAD
ACCOUNT/EHR #: WILLCO001
Date: 06/21/11

Attending Physician: Suzanne R. Taylor, MD

S: Pt is a 51-year-old male who I have not seen since his annual physical exam last September. He states that 5-6 weeks ago he noted some intermittent soft stool and decrease in the caliber of stools. He also noted some bleeding that discontinued four days ago. He denies any cramps or abdominal pain.

O: External examination of the anus revealed some external skin tags present in the left anterior position. Anal examination revealed an extremely tight anal sphincter. This was dilated manually to allow instrumentation with the anoscope, which was accomplished in a 360-degree orientation. There was some prominence of the crypts and some inflammation of the rectal mucosa, a portion of which was sent for biopsy. This was friable. In the left anterior position there was a fistula that was healing with some formation of a sentinel pile on the outside, which had been noticed on external examination.

A: Anal fissure, unusual position, nontraumatic

P: 1. Rule out inflammatory bowel disease with air contrast barium enema examination and reflux into terminal ileum.
2. Patient to return for sigmoidoscopy after BE.

Suzanne R. Taylor, MD

SRT/pw D: 06/21/11 09:50:16 T: 06/25/11 12:55:01

Find the best, most appropriate ICD-9-CM code(s).

TAYLOR, READER, & ASSOCIATES
A Complete Health Care Facility
975 CENTRAL AVENUE • SOMEWHERE, FL 32811 • 407-555-4321

PATIENT:	BEVINS, NANCY
ACCOUNT/EHR #:	BEVINA001
Date:	08/11/11
Attending Physician:	Willard B. Reader, MD

S: Pt is a 37-year-old female who comes in every six months for an abdominal scan. She had been diagnosed with bladder cancer three years ago. After a sequence of radiation and chemotherapy, she was pronounced malignant-free one year ago. Since that time, she comes in for a check every six months. Pt denies any signs or symptoms indicating a return of the malignancy.

O: Ht 5′3″ Wt. 119 lb. R 18. T 98.6. BP 120/95 Abdomen appears to be normal upon manual examination. Results of CT scan indicated no abnormalities.

A: Personal history of bladder cancer

P: Pt to return PRN

Willard B. Reader, MD

WBR/pw D: 08/11/11 09:50:16 T: 08/13/11 12:55:01

Find the best, most appropriate ICD-9-CM code(s).

____

____

____

TAYLOR, READER, & ASSOCIATES
A Complete Health Care Facility
975 CENTRAL AVENUE • SOMEWHERE, FL 32811 • 407-555-4321

PATIENT: ROMANO, JOSEPH
ACCOUNT/EHR #: ROMAJO001
Date: 07/11/11

Attending Physician: Suzanne R. Taylor, MD

S: Pt is a 25-year-old male who states that he cut the back of his right index finger while cutting up a chicken while at work. Pt works as a chef at a local restaurant. He cannot extend his finger since the accident, and he had some bleeding, which he stopped with pressure. Pt had a tetanus toxoid administered last year when he sustained a wound to the forearm while at work. He has no past history of serious illnesses, operations, or allergies. Social history and family history are noncontributory.

O: Examination reveals a 3-cm laceration, dorsum of right index finger, with laceration of extensor tendon, proximal to the interphalangeal joint. The patient cannot extend the finger; he can flex, adduct, and abduct the finger. Sensation at this time appears to be normal. Pt was prepped, and a digital nerve block using 1% Carbocaine was carried out. When the block was totally effective, the wound was explored. After thorough irrigation of the wound with normal saline, the joint capsule was repaired with two sutures of 5-0 Dexon. The tendon repair was then carried out using 4-0 nylon. Dressings were applied, and a splint was applied holding the interphalangeal joint in neutral position, in full extension but not hyperextension. The Pt tolerated the procedure well and left the surgical area in good condition.

A: 3-cm laceration, dorsum of right index finger, with laceration of extensor tendon

P:
1. Rx Percocet, q4h prn for pain
2. Rx Augmentin, 250 mg tid
3. Patient to return for follow-up in three days

Suzanne R. Taylor, MD

SRT/pw D: 07/11/11 09:50:16 T: 07/13/11 12:55:01

Find the best, most appropriate ICD-9-CM code(s).

____

____

____

Let's turn to the tabular list and find 332.0. But, remember, you always want to start reading at the three-digit category:

√4th 332 Parkinson's disease

EXCLUDES dementia with Parkinsonism (331.82)

Read the notations. The EXCLUDES notation does not apply to this case, so keep reading. The symbol next to the 332 directs you to keep reading to find the correct four-digit code. The fourth digit provides additional descriptors to the diagnosis of Parkinson's disease.

Compare the descriptions of the two choices:

332.0 Paralysis agitans

Parkinsonism or Parkinson's disease: NOS, idiopathic, primary

332.1 Secondary Parkinsonism

Parkinsonism due to drugs

The difference between the 332.0 and 332.1 means quite a lot to the patient, and to the health care professionals who are caring for Renee now and in the future. In addition, the third-party payer needs to know.

The details you will need in order to determine which code is correct should be found in the medical notes. Here, the notes state that Renee's Parkinson's disease is idiopathic. This is how you know that 332.0 is correct.

«« CODING TIP

If you had not read up to the three-digit code description, you might have missed the *excludes* notation. The notation and others like it are very important to your ability to code accurately. We will discuss more about notations in the next few pages.

FIVE-DIGIT CODES [Subclassifications]

When additional specific details are available, the ICD-9-CM diagnosis code may go to a fifth digit. Just like the fourth-digit symbol, the requirement of a fifth digit is indicated by a box with a check mark and a "5th" or other symbol to the left of the four-digit code: √5th. Again, this is not a suggestion or a request. When you see the symbol, you *must* continue reading until you find the appropriate five-digit code.

«« CODING TIP

The letter V in V codes counts as a digit.

The letter E in E codes does *not* count as a digit.

Example

√4th 923 Contusion of upper limb

√5th 923.0 Shoulder and upper arm

923.00 Shoulder region

923.01 Scapular region

923.02 Axillary region

Remember! The boxes that indicate a fourth or fifth digit are not suggestions. The boxes are telling you that the extra digit is *required*! They are helping to guide you to the best, most appropriate code.

LET'S CODE IT! SCENARIO

Eileen Sucher, a 15-year-old female, is seen by Dr. Mazar. After a thorough examination and talking with Eileen, Dr. Mazar diagnoses her with nonorganic bulimia.

Let's Code It!

Dr. Mazar has diagnosed Eileen with *nonorganic bulimia*. In the alphabetic index, find

Bulimia 783.6
  nervosa 307.51
  non-organic origin 307.51

Great, Bulimia, non-organic origin 307.51 appears to match the notes perfectly. But you never, never, never code from the alphabetic index, so let's go to the tabular list for code category 307:

√4th 307 Special symptoms or syndromes, not elsewhere classified
  √5th 307.5 Other and unspecified disorders of eating
    307.51 Bulimia nervosa; Overeating of non-organic origin

There are no guidelines or notations that apply to Dr. Mazar's notes or Eileen's case to alter the code, so it still matches Dr. Mazar's notes exactly. Good work!

On some pages in the ICD-9-CM volume 1, you will find the fourth or the fifth digit not by reading further down in the column but by reading up—toward the top of the column, the top of the page, or sometimes to the page beforehand—to a pink box. This saves space when the addition of this digit means the same additional information for many different codes.

LET'S CODE IT! SCENARIO

Roy Rollins, a 5-year-old male, was having severe trouble breathing, and his mother took him to see his pediatrician, Dr. Sacalolo. After an extensive examination, Dr. Sacalolo diagnosed Roy with extrinsic asthma with acute exacerbation.

Let's Code It!

BRIDGE TO ICD-10-CM 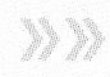

In an ICD-10-CM code, the seventh character will report how many times this patient has seen this provider for this specific condition. This is not required for all codes. The tabular list will identify when this is necessary to include.

Dr. Sacalolo's diagnosis of Roy's asthma was very specific: "extrinsic asthma with acute exacerbation." Turn to the alphabetic index and find *asthma:*

Asthma, asthmatic (bronchial) (catarrh) (spasmodic) 493.9

Go down the indented list to find

Asthma
  Extrinsic 493.0

Let's go to the tabular list and check out 493.0 Extrinsic asthma, starting, of course, at the three-digit category:

√4th 493 Asthma
  EXCLUDES wheezing NOS (786.07)

You know you need to keep reading to find that fourth digit. Look under the box.

> The following fifth-digit subclassification is for use with codes 493.0–493.2, 493.9:
> 0 Unspecified
> 1 With status asthmaticus
> 2 With (acute) exacerbation

√5th 493.0 Extrinsic asthma

√5th 493.1 Intrinsic asthma

√5th 493.2 Chronic obstructive asthma

√5th 493.8 Other forms of asthma

√5th 493.9 Asthma, unspecified

In all of the previous descriptions, the four-digit codes show boxes with check marks and "5th" next to them. However, when you keep reading, you can't find any codes with a fifth digit, can you? No. When that happens, you have to read up the column, to the box directly underneath the three-digit code 493 Asthma. Let's look at it carefully.

> The following fifth-digit sub-classification is for use with codes 493.0–493.2, 493.9:
> 0 Unspecified
> 1 With status asthmaticus
> 2 With (acute) exacerbation

Read the first sentence *inside* the box: "The following fifth-digit subclassification is for use with codes 493.0–493.2, 493.9." It means that the choices within the box are the choices for the fifth-digit that you must attach to the correct four-digit code (493.0, 493.1, 493.2, 493.9) found below. *Note:* 493.8 has its fifth-digit choices listed within the column right below the four-digit code.

«« KEYS TO CODING

Your process should go like this:

1. Start with the three-digit code.
2. Find the correct four-digit code.
3. Refer back to the box containing the fifth-digit code choices.
4. Choose the correct fifth-digit.
5. Attach the correct fifth-digit to the correct four-digit code to create a code with five digits.

Therefore, the most accurate code to report Roy's diagnosis is 493.02.

LET'S CODE IT! SCENARIO

Donna Arnold, a 23-year-old female, came to see Dr. Palducci for a checkup because she was diagnosed with subacute monocytic leukemia 5 years ago. Donna has been in remission for 6 months.

Let's Code It!

Dr. Palducci's notes state that Donna had a diagnosis of *subacute monocytic leukemia.* However, they also indicate that she has been in *remission.* What do you think? Looking in the alphabetic index, you don't find the word *remission.* With nothing else to look for, let's try *leukemia.* You find a very long list indented beneath it, but none of the entries has the word *remission.* So let's look for *monocytic* and then *subacute.*

Leukemia, leukemic

Monocytic (Schilling-type) (M9890/3) 206.9

Subacute (M9892/3) 206.2

(Note: You will learn about M codes in Chap. 5, "Coding Neoplasms." For now, don't worry about them. They are not used for reimbursement, only for research.)

Leukemia, monocytic, subacute 206.2 fits at least part of Dr. Palducci's notes. Let's check out the tabular listing for the complete description of code 206.2 . . . starting at the three-digit category:

√4th 206 Monocytic leukemia

INCLUDES leukemia: histiocytic, monoblastic, monocytoid

The following fifth-digit subclassification is for use with codes 206:
0 without mention of having achieved remission
1 in remission
2 in relapse

√5th 206.0 Acute

√5th 206.1 Chronic

√5th 206.2 Subacute

√5th 206.8 Other monocytic leukemia

√5th 206.9 Unspecified monocytic leukemia

Remember that Donna's diagnosis was subacute monocytic leukemia.

√4th 206 Monocytic leukemia

You must add a fourth-digit to supply the specific descriptor of subacute. Read down the column.

√5th 206.2 Monocytic leukemia, subacute

Now, you have the opportunity to tell the rest of the story. Remember that Donna is actually in remission. Read up to find the correct fifth digit that explains the remission:

206.21 Monocytic leukemia, subacute, in remission

Good job!

YOU CODE IT! CASE STUDY

Elvin Kilbridge, a 21-year-old male, was walking on the beach barefoot when he stepped on a rusty nail and cut the sole of his foot. He ignored it until the next day when the wound was red, swollen, and so painful it was difficult to walk. He went to see Dr. Gweinne, who cleaned out the open wound that had been complicated by sand and dirt. In addition, Dr. Gweinne gave Elvin a tetanus antitoxin injection to prevent him from contracting tetanus.

You Code It!

Go through the steps and determine the diagnosis code(s) that should be reported for this encounter between Dr. Gweinne and Elvin Kilbridge.

Step 1: Read the case completely.

Step 2: Abstract the notes: Which key words can you identify relating to why Dr. Gweinne cared for Elvin?

Step 3: Query the provider, if necessary.

Step 4: Code the diagnosis or diagnoses.

Step 5: Code the procedure(s): Debridement of wound, tetanus shot.

Step 6: Link the procedure codes to at least one diagnosis code to confirm medical necessity.

Step 7: Back code to double-check your choices.

Answer

Did you find the following diagnosis codes?

892.1 Open wound of foot except toe(s) alone, complicated

V07.2 Prophylactic immunotherapy

E920.8 Accidental injury (by) nail

E849.8 Place of occurrence, seashore

Great job!

ICD-10-CM uses a "placeholder character"—the letter X—when, for example, a code needs a sixth or seventh character, but has no applicable fifth character. This is done to keep the codes consistent.

NOTATIONS

You have already skimmed across some of the notations and guidelines found throughout the alphabetic index and tabular list. Now, let's go through all of them and develop a clear understanding of their meaning.

Includes and Excludes

As you have seen, the ICD-9-CM volume 1—tabular list may provide additional information with an *includes* or *excludes* notation. Below the description of the code, the notation will stipulate other variations of the condition and names of conditions that are either included or excluded.

INCLUDES

Sometimes, an INCLUDES notation is like looking in a medical dictionary to find alternate terms for the same or similar condition identified by the physician in his or her notes. (See Fig. 3-2.) Typically shown with a white box outlined in black around the word *includes*, the notation can help you confirm that you have the most accurate code available.

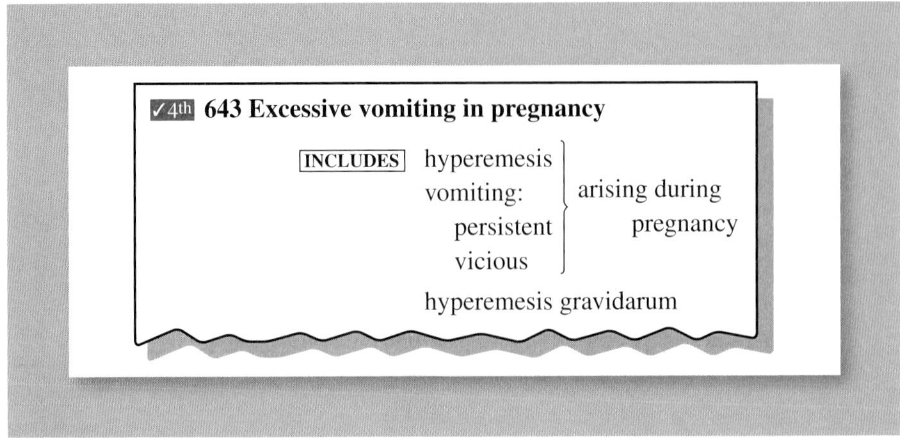
✓4th 643 Excessive vomiting in pregnancy

INCLUDES hyperemesis } arising during pregnancy
vomiting:
persistent
vicious
hyperemesis gravidarum

Figure 3-2 Example of an Includes Notation.

Example

020 Plague

INCLUDES infection byYersinia [Pasteurella] pestis

The alphabetic index may direct you to a code that does not specifically mention your key term in the tabular list's description. That is okay. It indicates that the key term shown in the alphabetic index is included within the description of the code.

EXCLUDES

A black box with the word *excludes* gives you the heads up that there are related or similar conditions that are *not* included in this code description and you need to keep reading. (See Fig. 3-3.) The good news is that, very often, the ICD-9-CM tabular list provides you with the correct code for these excluded conditions.

BRIDGE TO ICD-10-CM

ICD-10-CM uses virtually the same notations and conventions. One exception is the implementation of two EXCLUDES notations: Excludes1 and Excludes2 to differentiate the reasons why one particular code would not apply to certain diagnoses.

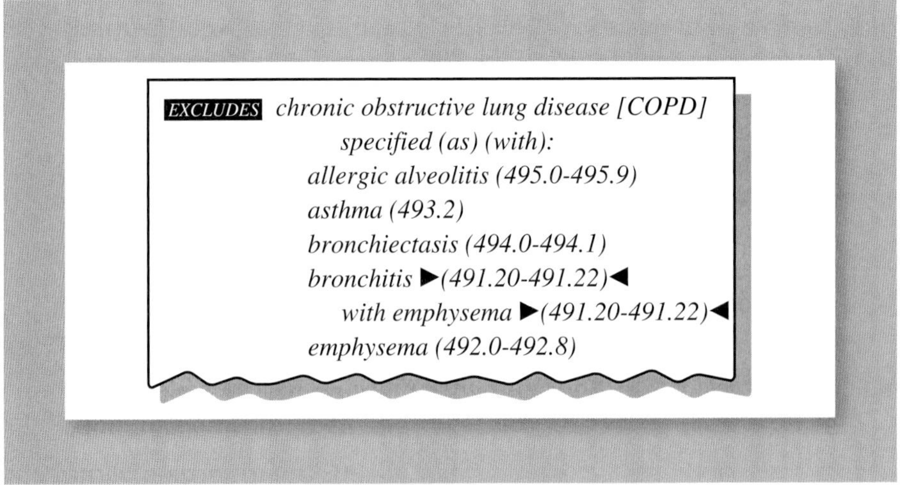
EXCLUDES *chronic obstructive lung disease [COPD]*
specified (as) (with):
allergic alveolitis (495.0-495.9)
asthma (493.2)
bronchiectasis (494.0-494.1)
bronchitis ►(491.20-491.22)◄
with emphysema ►(491.20-491.22)◄
emphysema (492.0-492.8)

Figure 3-3 Example of an Excludes Notation.

Example

748 Congenital anomalies of respiratory system

EXCLUDES congenital defect of diaphragm (756.6)

LET'S CODE IT! SCENARIO

Allen White, a 1-day-old male, was born prematurely. Blood tests were run, and Allen was found by Dr. Equillas to have abnormal red blood cells, causing anemia.

Let's Code It!

Dr. Equillas noted that Allen has *abnormal red blood cells.* In the alphabetic index, look up *abnormal* and read down the list to red blood cells.

Abnormal, red blood cells 790.09

If you go to the code description in the tabular list, you see

√4th 790 Nonspecific findings on examination of blood

EXCLUDES abnormality of;

Platelets (287.0-287.9)

Thrombocytes (287.0-287.9)

White blood cells (288.0-288.9)

√5th 790.0 Abnormality of red blood cells

790.01 Precipitous drop in hematocrit

790.09 Other abnormality of red blood cells

However, remember earlier you learned that you should start reading in the tabular list at the three-digit description just in case there are important guidelines or notations that may affect your code choice. Let's look up the column. This time, read this fourth-digit listing more carefully, especially the EXCLUDES note:

√5th 790.0 Abnormality of red blood cells

EXCLUDES *anemia*:

of premature infant (776.6)

Aha! So, now you need to turn to category 776 to confirm that this is the accurate code.

√4th 776 Hematological disorders of newborn

INCLUDES disorders specific to the newborn though possibly originating in utero

EXCLUDES fetal hematologic conditions (678.0)

776.0 Hemorrhagic disease of newborn

776.1 Transient neonatal thrombocytopenia

776.2 Disseminated intravascular coagulation in newborn

776.3 Other transient neonatal disorders of coagulation

776.4 Polycythemia neonatorum

776.5 Congenital anemia

776.6 Anemia of prematurity

Perhaps you chose "anemia" as the main term of the diagnosis and looked in the alphabetic index at *anemia*. That's reasonable. Let's go together to *anemia* in the alphabetic index:

Anemia 285.9

Let's go to the tabular list and see what you might find

√4th 285 Other and unspecified anemias

As you carefully read through the list of four-digit code choices, you will see nothing that either confirms or *excludes* the diagnosis of *anemia for this neonate. The code suggested by the alphabetic index does not appear to be wrong:*

285.9 Anemia, unspecified

However, professional coding specialists should only use an "unspecified" code as a last resort. How can you improve on this code? It seems direct and matches the notes. But is it specific enough?

Go back to the physician's notes to see if they provide any other words that might help you sift through the long list of descriptors indented below anemia in the alphabetic index: no abnormal, no infant. Looking at *fetus or newborn* does not bring you any closer. The notes do include the detail *premature*. The term premature is not shown in the list, but when you read it all, carefully, you can find it shown as *of prematurity*.

Anemia of prematurity 776.6

The scenario illustrates that there is more than one way to reach the correct code. The best thing to learn here is that you need to keep reading, keep looking, and keep thinking, and you will find the best, most accurate code. Determination . . . perseverance . . . is important.

YOU CODE IT! CASE STUDY

Anita Carnahan is a 27-year-old female who is 13 weeks pregnant. She goes to see her obstetrician, Dr. Hammond, because she has been vomiting the last few days. After a complete examination, Dr. Hammond diagnoses her with hyperemesis.

You Code It!

Go through the steps of coding, and determine the codes that should be reported for this encounter between Dr. Hammond and Anita Carnahan.

Step 1: Read the case completely.

Step 2: Abstract the notes: Which key words can you identify relating to why Dr. Hammond cared for Anita?

____

Step 3: Query the provider, if necessary.

Step 4: Code the diagnosis or diagnoses.

____

Step 5: Code the procedure(s): Office visit.

Step 6: Link the procedure codes to at least one diagnosis code to confirm medical necessity.

Step 7: Back code to double-check your choices.

Answer

Did you find the correct code?

643.03 Mild hyperemesis gravidarum, antepartum condition

Hyperemesis gravidarum, mild or unspecified, starting before the end of the 22nd week of gestation

Anita is only in her 13th week, so the code is correct. Good work!

Code First

Certain conditions and diseases can cause additional problems in the body. Individuals with diabetes are known to have problems with their eyes or circulation, just to name a few, as a direct result of having diabetes. Patients found to be HIV-positive are prone to such conditions as pneumonia, again, directly linked to the fact that they have human immunodeficiency virus infection. This is known as an **underlying condition.** The resulting condition (e.g., pneumonia) is called a **manifestation.**

The *code first* notation is a reminder that you are going to need another code to identify the underlying disease that caused this condition (see Fig. 3-4). This notation is also telling you in what order to report the two codes: the underlying condition first, followed by the code for the manifestation. Often, the notation will offer you a reference to the most common underlying diseases along with their codes! Cool!

Underlying condition

One disease that affects or encourages another condition.

Manifestation

A condition caused or developed from the existence of another condition.

Example

366.41 Diabetic cataract

Code first diabetes (249.5, 250.5)

366.42 Tetanic cataract

Code first underlying disease, as:

Calcinosis (275.4)

Hypoparathyroidism (252.1)

«« KEYS TO CODING

The underlying condition must come first, and then the manifestation develops from that. Think of the underlying condition as the trunk of a tree, and the manifestation as a branch that grows out from that trunk. If the tree trunk didn't exist, there would be no branch.

The description for code 366.41 tells you exactly which code to include on the claim form (although you still need to look this up in the

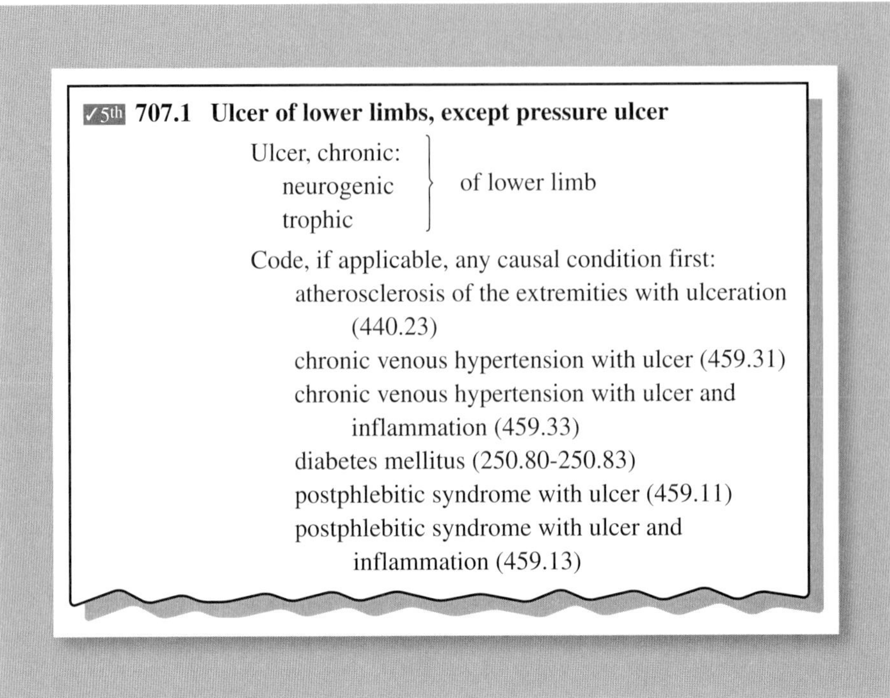
✓5th 707.1 **Ulcer of lower limbs, except pressure ulcer**

Ulcer, chronic:
neurogenic } of lower limb
trophic

Code, if applicable, any causal condition first:
atherosclerosis of the extremities with ulceration (440.23)
chronic venous hypertension with ulcer (459.31)
chronic venous hypertension with ulcer and inflammation (459.33)
diabetes mellitus (250.80-250.83)
postphlebitic syndrome with ulcer (459.11)
postphlebitic syndrome with ulcer and inflammation (459.13)

Figure 3-4 Example of Code First Notation.

tabular list to confirm that this is the most accurate code). When you look at the description for 366.42, you see that there are a couple of conditions that may cause a tetanic cataract, so the book lists some suggestions, along with their codes.

Use Additional Code

When you are reading the description of the underlying disease, this notation will direct you to look for and identify any of the manifestations or other conditions that may occur.

The tabular list will help you from both sides. Look at the notation under code 250.5. You see it suggests 366.41. In our example under code first, the notation under 366.41 directed you to 250.5. *But* not always! Herpes zoster is a known manifestation of AIDS (HIV positive) infection. You will see the *use additional code* notation under the code for AIDS (042), but there is no such notation under category 053 Herpes zoster. You must always be diligent and check the physician's notes carefully.

Example

250.5 Diabetes with ophthalmic manifestations

Use additional code to identify manifestation, as:

Diabetic:

Blindness (369.00–369.9)

Cataract (366.41)

595 Cystitis

Use additional code to identify organism, such as Escherichia coli [E. coli] (041.4)

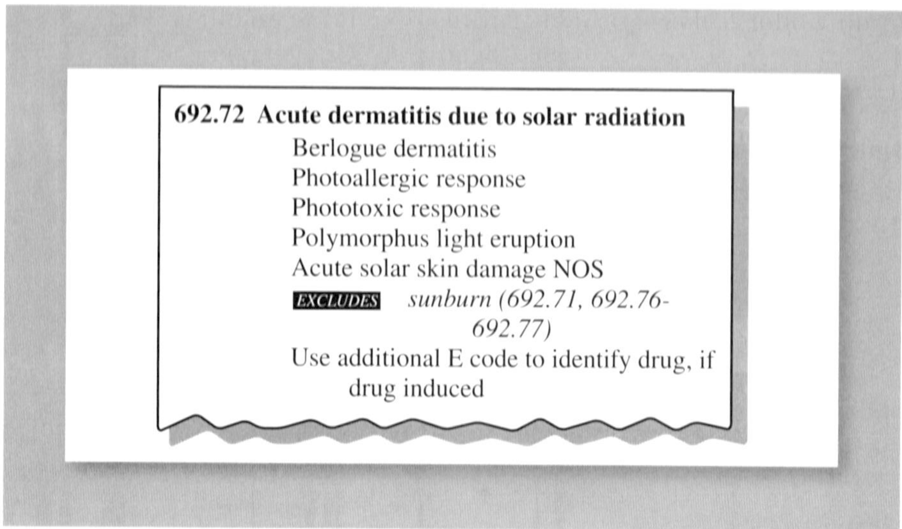
692.72 Acute dermatitis due to solar radiation
Berlogue dermatitis
Photoallergic response
Phototoxic response
Polymorphus light eruption
Acute solar skin damage NOS
EXCLUDES *sunburn (692.71, 692.76-692.77)*
Use additional E code to identify drug, if drug induced

Figure 3-5 Sometimes the ICD-9-CM Book Points You in a Specific Direction.

The *use additional code* notation means that the indicated additional code should be reported *after* the code that provides the notation (see Fig. 3-5).

Code, If Applicable

The *code, if applicable* notation is just like the *code first* note with some leeway. This is more of an alert to check the notes for an underlying condition or manifestation that may exist, which, if it is documented, you need to code separately. If there is no other condition involved, the code may be used as a principal, or first-listed, diagnosis code.

If the physician's notes state that the patient's leg ulcer was caused by atherosclerosis, then you would code 440.23, 707.10—in that order. If the physician's notes merely state that the patient had an ulcer on his leg, with an unknown cause, then you would report 707.10 alone.

Example

707.1 Ulcer of lower limbs, except pressure ulcer

Code, if applicable, any causal condition first:

Atherosclerosis of the extremities with ulceration (440.23)

Category Notes

Occasionally, you may see informational notes under the description of a three-digit code in the tabular list:

Example

041 Bacterial infection in conditions classified elsewhere and of unspecified site

Note: This category is provided to be used as an additional code to identify the bacterial agent; in disease classified elsewhere. This category will also be used to classify bacterial infections of unspecified nature or site.

CODING TIP

Sometimes notations appear under the three-digit code at the top of the category but are not repeated after each additional code in its section. This is another reason why it is important to read up to the three-digit code, even when the alphabetic index directs you to the perfect four- or five-digit code. You don't want to miss any important directives, such as an "includes," "excludes," "code first," or "code additional" notations.

And

The guidelines for the accurate usage of ICD-9-CM instruct you to interpret the use of the word *and* in a code description as *and/or*. Therefore, if the physician's notes only include one part but not the other, the code may still be correct.

Code 173.4 would be the correct choice if the physician documented malignancy of the patient's scalp, the skin of the patient's neck, or both the patient's scalp and neck skin.

KEYS TO CODING »»

Forgetting that, in ICD-9-CM, the word "and" really means "and/or" can throw a new coder off a correct code because the notes do not indicate both elements of the code description. Therefore, you need to make yourself a special note so you don't forget.

Example

173.4 Malignant neoplasm of skin; scalp and skin of neck

Other Notations

NEC

Not elsewhere classifiable (NEC)

Specifics that are not described in any other code in the book; also known as *not elsewhere classified.*

Not elsewhere classifiable, or classified (NEC), indicates that the physician provided additional details of the condition but the ICD-9-CM book did not include those extra details in any of the other codes in the book.

Example

259.4 Dwarfism, not elsewhere classified

Dermatomegaly NEC 701.8

Other Specified

Other specified

Additional information that the physician specified andisn't included in any other code description.

The phrase **other specified** means the same thing as NEC: The physician specified additional information that the ICD-9-CM book doesn't have in any of the other codes in the category.

Example

057.8 Other specified viral exanthemata

259.8 Other specified endocrine disorders

NOS

Not otherwise specified (NOS)

The absence of additional details documented in the notes.

Not otherwise specified (NOS) means that the physician did not document any additional details that are identified in any of the other available code descriptions.

Example

261 Nutritional marasmus, severe malnutrition NOS

780.39 Other convulsions, convulsive disorder NOS

Unspecified

Unspecified

The absence of additional specifics in the physician's documentation.

Unspecified has the same meaning as NOS: The physician was not specific in his or her notes. (See Fig. 3-6.) Its notations are examples of how the ICD-9-CM diagnosis book will guide you to the correct code, if you pay attention.

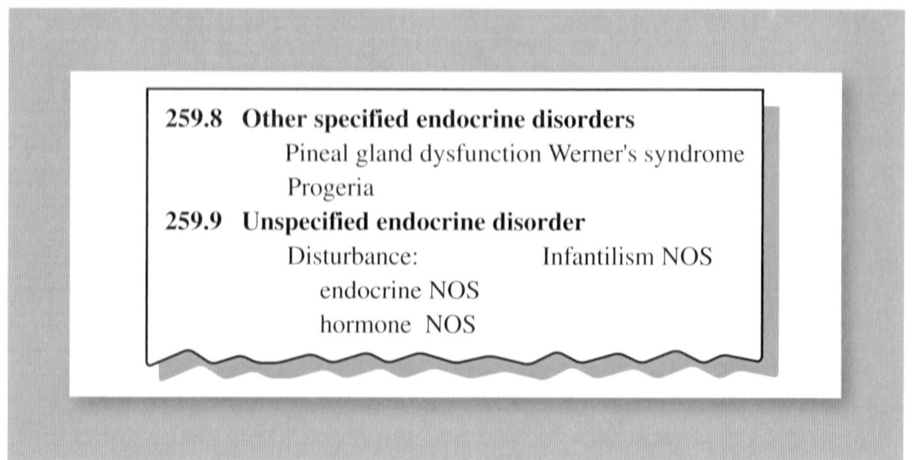

259.8 Other specified endocrine disorders
Pineal gland dysfunction Werner's syndrome
Progeria
259.9 Unspecified endocrine disorder
Disturbance: Infantilism NOS
endocrine NOS
hormone NOS

Figure 3-6 Example of Other Specified and Unspecified Code Descriptions.

«« KEYS TO CODING

Before choosing any code with NOS or Unspecified in the description, double check the notes and patient record to be certain you cannot find a more specific code. If not, then query the provider and ask for the additional details you may need to determine a more accurate code. An unspecified or NOS code should always be a last resort.

Example

259.9 Unspecified endocrine disorder

Paraganglioma, jugular, unspecified site 194.6

See

In the alphabetic index of ICD-9-CM, you may look up a term and notice that next to it, the book instructs you to ***see*** another term. This is an instruction in the index that the information you are looking for is listed under another term. In this example, you can see that the alphabetic index is sending you to a different spelling of this diagnostic term.

Example

Ankylostoma—*see* Ancylostoma

See Also

In other places in the alphabetic index, you may see that the instruction ***see also*** is next to the term you are investigating. Here, the ICD-9-CM index is explaining that additional details may be found under another term, as well as what you see here. In this example, you can see that several suggested codes follow the main term. The index is providing you with an alternate term that may show terms more accurate to the physician's documentation.

Example

Cardiomegaly—*see also* Hypertrophy, cardiac 429.3
- congenital 746.89
- glycogen 271.0
- hypertensive (see also Hypertension, heart) 402.90
- idiopathic 429.3

See Condition

The alphabetic index may also point you in a less detailed way when you look up a term and the notation tells you to *see condition*. This can be confusing. The index is not telling you to look up the term "condition." What it is instructing you to do is to find the term that describes the health-related situation involved with this word and look up that term.. You will see this most often next to the listing for an anatomical site.

Example

Heart–*see* condition

This instruction comes back to the reason you are looking for a code in the first place. Remember, you are looking for a code to explain why the physician cared for the patient during the encounter. Using our example, having a heart is not a reason for a physician to meet with a patient. Everyone has a heart. Therefore, the index is telling you to look, instead, for the term that describes the condition of this patient's heart—the problem or concern about his or her heart that brought the patient together with the physician at this time. So, instead of heart, cervix, or lung, you need to look up atrophy, fracture, or deformity.

As you go through the chapters in this book, you will learn more about determining the condition and the best way to look up terms in both the alphabetic index and the tabular list of ICD-9-CM.

Punctuation

Punctuation in ICD-9-CM adds information and helps you further in your quest for the best, most appropriate code.

[ ]

Found in the tabular list, *brackets* will show you alternate terms, alternate phrases, and/or synonyms to provide additional detail or explanation to the description. In our example below, the provider may have diagnosed the patient with either food poisoning due to *Clostridium perfringens* or *C. welchii.* In either case, 005.2 would be the correct code. The same for our second example: If the documentation reads either Diethylstilbestrol or DES, the code 760.76 is valid.

Example

005.2 Food poisoning due to Clostridium perfringens [C. welchii]

760.76 Diethylstilbestrol [DES]

[ ]

Italicized, or slanted, brackets, used in the alphabetic index, will surround additional code(s) (i.e., secondary codes) that *must* be included with the initial code. It is the alphabetic index's version of the *code first* and *use additional code* notations (see Fig. 3-7).

ulcer (skin) 250.8☑ *[707.9]*
lower extremity 250.8☑ *[707.10]*
ankle 250.8☑ *[707.13]*
calf 250.8☑ *[707.12]*
foot 250.8☑ *[707.15]*
heel 250.8☑ *[707.14]*
knee 250.8☑ *[707.19]*
specified site NEC 250.8☑ *[707.19]*
thigh 250.8☑ *[707.11]*
toes 250.8☑ *[707.15]*
specified site NEC 250.8☑ *[707.8]*
xanthoma 250.8☑ *[272.2]*

Figure 3-7 Alphabetic Listing Showing Required Secondary Code.

The italic brackets tell you that if the patient has been diagnosed with arteriosclerotic retinopathy, you have to use two codes: first, 440.8 for the underlying cause of the retinopathy (the arteriosclerosis) and second, 362.13 for the retinopathy itself.

Example

Retinopathy
Arteriosclerotic 440.8 *[362.13]*

( )

Parentheses show you additional descriptions, terms, or phrases that are also included in the description of the particular code. The additional terms are called **nonessential modifiers.** The modifiers can be used to provide additional definition but do not change the description of the condition. The additional terms are not required in the documentation, so if the provider did not use the additional term, the code description is still valid.

Nonessential modifiers
Descriptors that are not absolutely necessary to have been included in the physician's notes and are provided simply to further clarify a code description; optional terms.

Take a look at this first example, if the physician wrote the diagnosis as *lanugo* or *persistent lanugo*, code 757.4 would still apply.

In our second example, this code would be valid for a diagnosis written by the physician as varicella pneumonitis or varicella hemorrhagic pneumonitis.

Example

Lanugo (persistent) 757.4
052.1 Varicella (hemorrhagic) pneumonitis

the area around his right eye was swollen and the conjunctiva in the eye was red. After examining him, Dr. MacRhone took a head x-ray which confirmed a closed fracture of the left mandible. Kalem admitted that he got into a fight at school with two other kids.

Dr. MacRhone wired Kalem's left jaw and ordered him NPO except liquids for the next 3 weeks. He also ordered cold, wet compresses for his eye, 3 times a day, and wrote a prescription for some eye drops. Diagnosis was fracture of the left mandible, angle (closed), and black eye.

So, how many codes do you need?

You need as many codes as necessary to tell the ***whole story*** about WHY Kalem was cared for by Dr. MacRhone at this visit. Why did Dr. MacRhone examine Kalem, take the x-ray, and then wire his jaw shut? Because Kalem's jaw was fractured. The first code to use is 802.25 to relate this part of the story.

802.25 Fracture of the face bones, mandible, closed, angle of jaw

That's one part of the story. Is there anything else to relate about this reason WHY Dr. MacRhone did all those services for Kalem? Ask yourself, why did Dr. MacRhone examine Kalem and order cold compresses and eye drops for his eye? Because Kalem had a black eye. The second code to use is 921.0 to relate more of the story.

921.0 Black eye, not otherwise specified

Now, you also learned in Chapter 2 that, ***when a patient is injured (or poisoned)*** you must also relate HOW and WHERE the injury occurred. This is used not only for statistical purposes but also to confirm which third-party payer will be responsible for paying the medical expenses. HOW and WHERE is reported with E codes. Ask yourself, HOW did Kalem's jaw get fractured and his eye injured? Code E960.0 relates this part of the story.

E960.0 Unarmed fight or brawl

WHERE was Kalem when his jaw got fractured and his eye injured? Code E849.6 explains this detail.

E849.6 Place of occurrence, public building, school (state)(public)(private)

Now, you can see that, with these four codes, you and anyone reading these codes clearly can see that Dr. MacRhone cared for Kalem because he had a fractured jaw and a black eye and that the fractured jaw was the result of a fight at school. Without ALL FOUR codes, you don't have the ***whole story.*** So, for every case, every encounter, every scenario, you are responsible for telling *the WHOLE STORY about the encounter.*

Code Sequencing

Principal diagnosis

The condition that is the primary, or main, reason for the encounter.

When more than one diagnosis code is required to tell the whole story of the encounter accurately, you then must determine in which order the codes should be listed. The code reporting the most important reason for the encounter is called the **principal diagnosis.**

Sometimes the ICD-9-CM book will tell you which code should come first and which should come second with the *code first* and *use additional code* notations. Remember, an *E-code* can never be the principal, or first-listed, diagnosis.

Example

Roman Fletcher was diagnosed with a type I diabetic cataract. You will find the notations directing you how to sequence these two codes.

√5th 250.5 Diabetes with ophthalmic manifestations

Use additional code to identify manifestation

366.41 Diabetic cataract

Code first diabetes (249.5, 250.5)

In cases when there are multiple confirmed diagnoses identified, the guidelines instruct you to list the codes in order of severity from the most severe to the least severe. Take a look at the example below about Wade Padgett. For Wade's encounter, a fracture is more severe than a dislocation. Therefore, you would show the codes in the following order:

815.03 Fracture of metacarpal bone(s), closed, shaft

831.01 Dislocation, shoulder, closed, anterior dislocation of humerus

Example

Wade Padgett came to see Dr. Stein after falling off his bicycle. After a thorough examination, Dr. Stein diagnosed Wade with a closed fracture of the metacarpal shaft and an anterior dislocation of his humerus.

CODING TIP

Remember, an *E-code* could never be the principal, or first-listed, diagnosis.

CODING TIP

If two (or more) diagnoses are of equal severity, then it will not matter in which order you list them. The code for the issue stated as the primary reason for the visit, then, would be coded first.

Acute and Chronic Conditions

If one patient has one health concern diagnosed by the physician as being both acute (severe) and chronic (ongoing) and the condition offers you separate codes for the two descriptors, you should report the code for the acute condition first, as directed by the guidelines. Remember from your medical terminology lessons, acute is more serious than chronic.

YOU CODE IT! CASE STUDY

Varna Jackson has acute and chronic lymphoid leukemia, now in remission. She is seeing Dr. Roosevelt today for a checkup of this condition.

You Code It!

Can you find the correct codes for Varna's visit with Dr. Roosevelt?

Step 1: Read the case completely.

Step 2: Abstract the notes: Which key words can you identify relating to why Dr. Roosevelt cared for Varna?

____

Step 3: Query the provider, if necessary.

Step 4: Code the diagnosis or diagnoses.

Step 5: Code the procedure(s): Office visit.

Step 6: Link the procedure codes to at least one diagnosis code to confirm medical necessity.

Step 7: Back code to double-check your choices.

Answer

Did you find the correct codes?

204.01 Lymphoid leukemia, acute, in remission

204.11 Lymphoid leukemia, chronic, in remission

Great job!

Two or More Conditions—Only One Confirmed Diagnosis

There may be cases where the physician documents treatment of two (or more) complaints and only one is identified by a confirmed diagnosis.

LET'S CODE IT! SCENARIO

Louise Jorgensen, a 61-year-old female, came to see Dr. Mulkey. Earlier in the day, she was lightheaded and a little dizzy. In addition, she complained that her heart was beating so wildly that she thought she may have had a heart attack. Due to her previous diagnosis of type I diabetes, Dr. Mulkey ordered a blood glucose test. He also performed an EKG to check her heart. After getting the results of the tests, Dr. Mulkey determined that Louise's lightheadedness and dizziness were a result of her glucose being too high. He spoke with Louise about how to bring her diabetes under control. He also told her that her EKG was negative and that there were no signs of a heart attack.

Let's Code It!

Dr. Mulkey confirmed that Louise's *type I diabetes mellitus* was *uncontrolled.* (This is indicated by his discussion with her on how to bring it under control.) Turn to the alphabetic index and find:

Diabetes 250.0

Turn to the tabular listing, and see:

√4th 250 Diabetes mellitus

√5th 250.0 Diabetes mellitus without mention of complication

You can see that code 250.0 is correct and needs a fifth digit. Look up to the box, and determine the correct fifth digit.

250.03 Diabetes mellitus without mention of complication, type I, uncontrolled

Uncontrolled type 1 diabetes mellitus seems to be the only confirmed diagnosis in Dr. Mulkey's notes. However, the doctor performed an EKG. A diagnosis for diabetes does not provide any medical rationale for doing an EKG. In addition, the test was negative and, therefore, provided no diagnosis. So you still need a diagnosis code to report the medical necessity for running the EKG. Why did Dr. Mulkey perform the EKG? Because Louise complained of a *rapid heartbeat*. The alphabetic index suggests

Rapid, heart (beat) 785.0

The tabular list confirms

√4th 785 Symptoms involving cardiovascular system

EXCLUDES heart failure NOS (428.9)

785.0 Tachycardia, unspecified

For the encounter, you have one confirmed diagnosis (the diabetes) and one symptom (rapid heartbeat). The guidelines state that a confirmed diagnosis should precede a sign or symptom, so you will list the diabetes code first and then the tachycardia.

«« CODING TIP

Louise Jorgensen's case illustrates that sometimes asking yourself, "*Why* did the physician provide a specific test, treatment, or service," can help you find the necessary diagnostic key words for an encounter.

«« KEYS TO CODING

An electrocardiogram may be referred to as either an ECG or an EKG. *Tachycardia* is the medical term for rapid heartbeat.

Differential Diagnoses

In the case where a provider indicates a differential diagnosis by using the word *versus* or *or* between two diagnostic statements, you need to code both as if they were confirmed, and either may be listed first.

YOU CODE IT! CASE STUDY

Colin Oliver, a 63-year-old male complaining of chest pain and shortness of breath, was seen by his family physician. Dr. Budman admitted him into the hospital with a differential diagnosis of congestive heart failure versus pleural effusion with respiratory distress.

You Code It!

Review the notes of the encounter between Dr. Budman and Colin Oliver, and find the applicable diagnosis code(s).

Step 1: Read the case completely.

Step 2: Abstract the notes: Which key words can you identify relating to why Dr. Budman cared for Colin?

____

Step 3: Query the provider, if necessary.

Step 4: Code the diagnosis or diagnoses.

____

Preoperative Evaluations

Whenever a patient is scheduled for a surgical procedure (on a non-emergency basis), there are typical tests that must be done to ensure that the patient is healthy enough to have the operation. Cardiovascular, respiratory, and other examinations are often done within a couple of days prior to the date of surgery. Often these tests do not necessarily relate directly to the diagnostic reason the surgery will be performed. Therefore, they will need a different diagnosis code to report medical necessity.

Coding those encounters carries a specific guideline. In such cases, the principal, or first-listed, diagnosis code will be from the following category:

V72.8*x* Other specified examinations

Follow that code with the code or codes that identify the condition(s) documented as the reason for the upcoming surgical procedure.

Example

Tameka was diagnosed with carpal tunnel syndrome in her right wrist. Dr. Rothenstein recommended a surgical solution. Because of her history of atrial fibrillation, Tameka was required to get approval from her cardiologist before she could have the procedure.

354.0 Carpal tunnel syndrome is the code that will be used to report the medical necessity for the surgery on Tameka's wrist. However, it will not support the examination performed by her cardiologist. Think about it . . . who would agree to pay for a cardiologist to examine a patient with a diagnosis of carpal tunnel syndrome? The cardiologist is not qualified to do the job that is better suited for an orthopedist.

V72.81 Preoperative cardiovascular examination will support the cardiologist's time and expertise to clear Tameka for the procedure on her wrist.

KEYS TO CODING »»

Review the **ICD-9-CM Coding Guidelines, Section II. Selection of Principal Diagnosis** and **Section III. Reporting Additional Diagnoses** for more input on identifying what to code, what not to code, and in what order to put multiple codes. Use this to support your reading here, and as a reminder booster later on.

Preoperative/Postoperative Diagnoses

You may have already noticed that procedure and operative reports usually include both a preoperative diagnosis and a postoperative diagnosis. For cases where the two statements differ, the guidelines state that you should code the postoperative diagnosis because it is expected that it is the more accurate of the two.

CHAPTER SUMMARY

ICD-9-CM volumes 1 and 2 are formatted to guide you toward the best, most accurate code. Notations, symbols, and punctuation help coders follow guidelines and ensure that codes are complete in their descriptions of why the health care provider cared for the patient during this encounter. Three-, four-, and five-digit codes are offered so the coder can use the proper level of specificity to report the medically necessary rational for the procedures, services, and treatments provided.

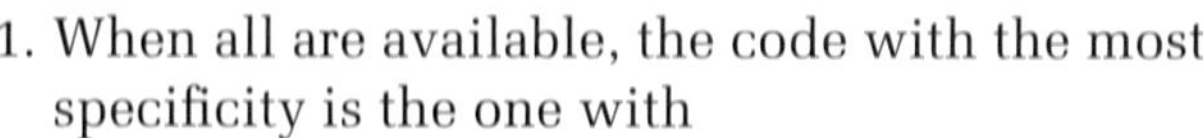

Chapter 3 Review

General Guidelines and Notations

1. When all are available, the code with the most specificity is the one with
   a. Two digits.
   b. Three digits.
   c. Four digits.
   d. Five digits.

2. NOS means
   a. The hospital didn't provide more details.
   b. The physician didn't provide more details.
   c. The ICD-9-CM didn't provide a code with more details.
   d. The patient didn't provide more details.

3. Coding directly from the alphabetic index is permitted
   a. Never.
   b. When the index shows only one code choice.
   c. For annual physicals.
   d. For patients covered by Medicare.

4. A descriptor presented within parentheses is
   a. A mandatory part of the code description.
   b. An optional part of the code description.
   c. A previously deleted code description.
   d. A manifestation.

5. NEC means
   a. The hospital didn't provide more details.
   b. The physician didn't provide more details.
   c. The ICD-9-CM didn't provide a code with more details.
   d. The patient didn't provide more details.

6. An underlying condition
   a. Encourages another condition.
   b. Causes another condition.
   c. Is the result of another condition.
   d. Is a late effect of another condition.

7. A nonessential modifier is a word or phrase that does all except
   a. Further describe the condition.
   b. Invalidate the code.
   c. Provide alternate phrasing or terms.
   d. Provide an optional description.

8. When one code describes two concurrent conditions, it is known as a(n)
   a. Preventive code.
   b. History code.
   c. Combination code.
   d. Procedure code.

9. Diagnosis codes are important because they
   a. Describe why the provider treated the patient.
   b. Identify medical necessity for procedures and services.
   c. (*a*) and (*b*) only.
   d. None of the above.

10. When ICD-9-CM identifies that an additional digit is available for a particular code,
    a. The additional digit is required.
    b. The additional digit is optional.
    c. The code with the smaller number of digits is invalid.
    d. Both (*a*) and (*c*).

YOU CODE IT! Practice

CHAPTER 3. General Guidelines and Notations

1. Helen Whitworth, an 18-year-old female, came to see Dr. Hunter after falling off a ladder at home and twisting her left ankle. Dr. Hunter confirmed that her ankle was sprained and wrapped it with an Ace bandage.

____

2. Gary Beatty went to see Dr. Meredith with a complaint of shortness of breath and chest pain. Dr. Meredith diagnosed him with congestive heart failure.

____

3. Patrick Glass, a 59-year-old male, was seen by Dr. Grayson because Patrick was very upset and agitated. After a complete psychological evaluation, Dr. Grayson diagnosed Patrick with severe major depressive disorder with psychotic features.

____

4. Beatrice Hayward, a 29-year-old female, is a professional water skier and comes to see Dr. Maudi with a recurrent dislocation of her right shoulder.

____

5. Rudy Shaw, a 63-year-old male, comes to see Dr. Witsil for the results of his cervical lymph node biopsy. Dr. Witsil informs Rudy that the test confirmed Hodgkin's sarcoma disease.

____

6. Dennis Curran, a 35-year-old male, attended a beach party and barbecue where he had hot dogs and potato salad. Several hours later, he began vomiting and having severe diarrhea. The next morning, he went to see Dr. Haberstock, who diagnosed him with dehydration caused by *Salmonella* infection.

____

7. Charlene Goodwin, a 73-year-old female, is diagnosed with left arm paralysis (her dominant side), a late effect of poliomyelitis, which she had when she was a child.

____

8. Cecil Williams, a 7-year-old male, came in to see Dr. Beasley for a therapeutic bronchoscopy due to the doctor's diagnosis of cystic fibrosis.

____

9. Norman Siegel, a 3-year-old male, was brought into the clinic and seen by Dr. Norris. After a complete examination, Dr. Norris diagnosed Norman with severe malnutrition.

____

10. Gayle Sentine, a 9-year-old female, is brought in to Dr. Matlock because she is having trouble in school. Dr. Matlock, after a thorough examination and testing, diagnoses her with attention deficit disorder with hyperactivity.

____

11. Carlos Siplin, an 81-year-old male, was unable to speak. Dr. Permane performed a laryngoscopy and determined a diagnosis of complete bilateral paralysis of Carlos's vocal cords.

____

12. Craig Liefer, a 49-year-old male, was diagnosed with Lou Gehrig's disease and came to the testing center for an EMG series.

____

13. After having a grand mal seizure, Louise Garrett, a 39-year-old female, was taken to the emergency room by her husband, and Dr. Sherman diagnosed her with intractable epilepsy.

____

14. Eliot Cox, a 4-year-old male, was brought to his pediatrician, Dr. Germain, because of a cough and fever. After a complete examination, Dr. Germain confirmed Eliot had an upper respiratory infection with bilateral acute conjunctivitis.

____

15. Roger Simpkin, a 43-year-old male, was diagnosed with adenoma of the prostate and came into the ambulatory surgery center (ASC) to have a prostatectomy performed.

____

YOU CODE IT! ICD-9-CM Simulation

CHAPTER 3. General Guidelines and Notations

On the following pages, you will see physicians' notes documenting encounters with patients at our textbooks' health care facility, Taylor, Reader, & Associates. Carefully read through the notes, and find the best ICD-9-CM diagnosis code or codes for each case.

TAYLOR, READER, & ASSOCIATES
A Complete Health Care Facility
975 CENTRAL AVENUE • SOMEWHERE, FL 32811 • 407-555-4321

PATIENT: FALLON, WILLA
ACCOUNT/EHR #: FALLWI001
Date: 07/16/11

Attending Physician: Suzanne R. Taylor, MD

S: This Pt is a 26-year-old female who I have not seen since last September when she came in for her annual physical. She presents today with burning upon urination and lower back pain. She stated that the symptoms began 2—3 days ago. She had been on vacation in Mexico and arrived back home yesterday.

O: Ht 5′ 7″ Wt. 169 lb. R 19. HEENT: unremarkable. Abdomen is tender. I ordered an automated urinalysis with microscopy, which was analyzed in our laboratory on the second floor. After the UA showed the presence of white blood cells in the urine, I ordered a culture and sensitivity test, which was positive for *E. coli*.

A: Cystitis cystica due to *E. coli*

P: 1. Rx. Broad-spectrum antibiotics
2. Return prn

Suzanne R. Taylor, MD

SRT/pw D: 7/16/11 09:50:16 T: 7/18/11 12:55:01

Find the best, most appropriate ICD-9-CM code(s).

TAYLOR, READER, & ASSOCIATES
A Complete Health Care Facility
975 CENTRAL AVENUE • SOMEWHERE, FL 32811 • 407-555-4321

PATIENT: MARSHALL, BARRY
ACCOUNT/EHR #: MARSBA001
Date: 11/09/11

Attending Physician: Willard B. Reader, MD

S: Pt is a 51-year-old male who comes in concerned about a sore he noticed on his left temple, directly at the hairline. He states that his mother died 6 years ago from melanoma, and his brother was diagnosed with precancerous cells of the epidermis. Pt states he is the captain of a beach volleyball team, and volunteers at the local YMCA as a water aerobics instructor. He says that he tries to be diligent about sunscreen, but sometimes he forgets.

O: Ht 5′ 11″ Wt. 189 lb. R 20. T 98.6. BP 120/95 Cultures of lesion were taken and sent to our in-house lab. The pathology report confirms the lesion is malignant. I discussed options with the patient and recommended surgical removal of the lesion as soon as possible.

A: Malignant melanoma of skin of scalp

P: Pt to call to make appointment for surgical procedure.

Willard B. Reader, MD

WBR/pw D: 11/09/11 09:50:16 T: 11/13/11 12:55:01

Find the best, most appropriate ICD-9-CM code(s).

TAYLOR, READER, & ASSOCIATES
A Complete Health Care Facility
975 CENTRAL AVENUE • SOMEWHERE, FL 32811 • 407-555-4321

PATIENT: GARISON, BENJAMIN
ACCOUNT/EHR #: GARIBE001
Date: 09/16/11

Attending Physician: Suzanne R. Taylor, MD

S: This Pt is a 5-month-old male brought in by his father because of severe rash on Benjamin's buttocks.

O: Ht 35″ Wt. 19 lb. T 98.6 Pt appears in minor distress; however, examination shows nothing out of the ordinary.

A: Diaper rash

P: 1. Rx A&D ointment to be applied after each diaper change
2. Return prn

Suzanne R. Taylor, MD

SRT/pw D: 9/16/11 09:50:16 T: 9/18/11 12:55:01

Find the best, most appropriate ICD-9-CM code(s).

___

___

___

TAYLOR, READER, & ASSOCIATES
A Complete Health Care Facility
975 CENTRAL AVENUE • SOMEWHERE, FL 32811 • 407-555-4321

PATIENT: BENTON, EARL
ACCOUNT/EHR #: BENTEA001
Date: 12/01/11

Attending Physician: Willard B. Reader, MD

S: Pt is a 44-year-old male who comes in with severe pain in the lower right quadrant of his abdomen. He states that the pain is sharp and shoots across his belly from right to left. Patient also states that he has been somewhat nauseated over the last 2 days.

O: Ht 5′ 9″ Wt. 177 lb. R 21. T 101.6. BP 130/95 Abdomen appears to be tender upon manual examination. Comprehensive metabolic blood test, general health panel blood workup, and an MRA, abdomen, angiography are taken. Results of all tests confirm diagnosis of appendicitis.

A: Acute appendicitis, w/o peritonitis

P: Pt to go to hospital immediately to be admitted for appendectomy

---

Willard B. Reader, MD

WBR/pw D: 12/01/11 09:50:16 T: 12/01/11 12:55:01

Find the best, most appropriate ICD-9-CM code(s).

____

____

____

While problems with circulation can affect a patient of any age, older individuals are more susceptible to such conditions. This is because as the body ages, the strength and elasticity of blood vessels decrease and become less efficient. In addition, long-term improper nutrition and lack of cardiovascular exercise take their toll and contribute to the circulatory system's inability to do its job (see Fig. 4-1).

KEYS TO CODING »»

Cardio = heart; vascular = veins and arteries

HEART FAILURE

A diagnosis of heart failure is serious; however, this does not mean the heart has totally 'failed' to function. Also known as congestive heart failure (CHF), this condition identifies that the individual's heart is unable to pump a sufficient quantity of blood throughout the body. This can cause fluid to back up into the lungs, resulting in respiratory problems such as shortness of breath and fatigue. In addition, fluid might build up in the lower extremities causing edema (swelling) in the feet, ankles, and

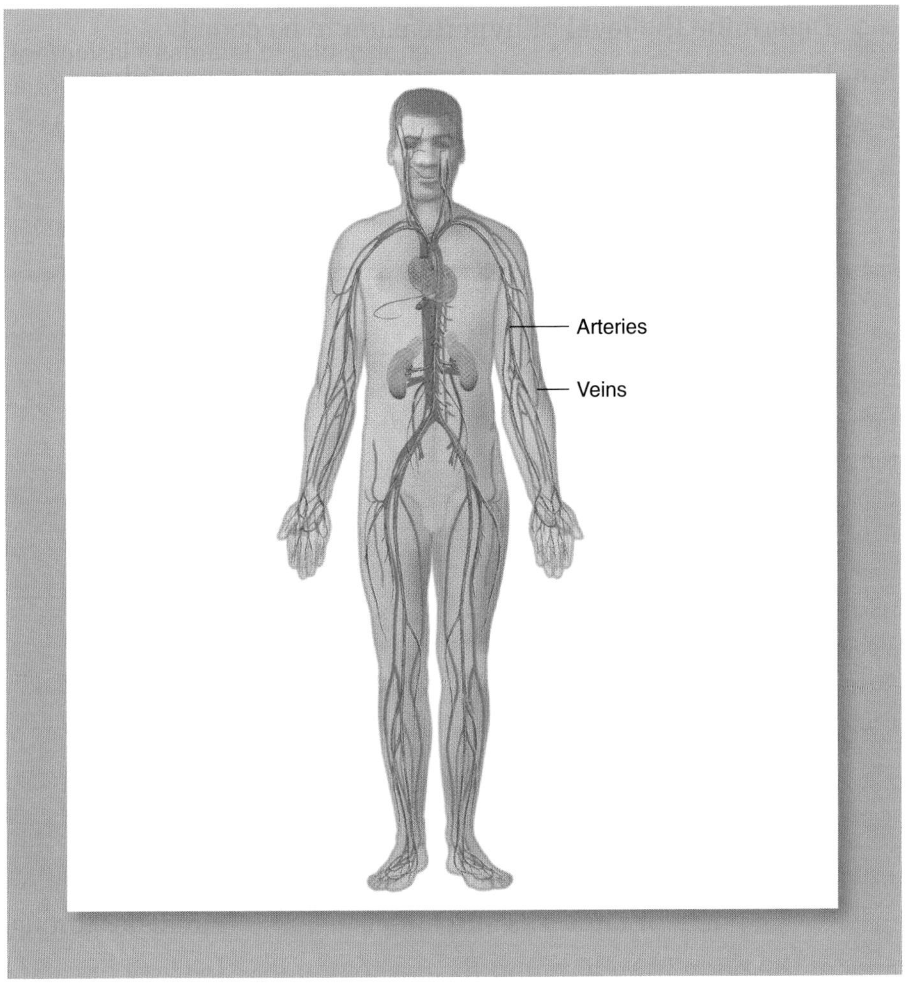

Figure 4-1 The Blood System Transports Life-Sustaining Nutrients to All Parts of the Body.

legs. Patients with CHF might have so much difficulty with edema that they may have pain and trouble walking.

According to the National Heart, Lung, and Blood Institute, approximately 5 million people in the United States have been diagnosed with heart failure and this has contributed to the death of as many as 30,000 of these patients each year.

Left heart failure, also known as pulmonary edema or cardiac asthma, indicates an insufficiency of the heart's left ventricle. This malfunction results in the accumulation of fluid in the lungs. When this happens, patients can develop respiratory problems as well.

Right heart failure, secondary to left heart failure, is diagnosed when the heart cannot pump and circulate the blood needed throughout the body. Patients can develop hypertension, congestion, edema, and fluid collection in the lungs.

Systolic heart failure occurs when the contractions of the ventricles are too weak to push the blood through the heart.

Diastolic heart failure is the result of a ventricle of the heart being unable to fill as it should. Combined systolic and diastolic heart failure means that the function of the heart is weak and it is unable to process blood properly through the heart.

Patients with heart failure may also have hypertension. You will learn about determining the diagnosis codes for this condition later in this chapter.

««« KEYS TO CODING

To determine the diagnosis code for heart failure, you need to know:

- The type of heart failure
- Whether it is acute or chronic

««« KEYS TO CODING

When a condition, such as right heart failure, causes the patient to develop another condition, such as **hypertension**, that may be referred to as a secondary condition. For example, if Mary developed hypertension due to her right heart failure, you would report the hypertension as **secondary hypertension**. More details on hypertension are presented later in this chapter.

YOU CODE IT! CASE STUDY

Ellyn Carrera, an 81-year-old female, came to see her cardiologist, Dr. Odem, to follow up on her CHF. Swelling in her legs has improved but she continues to have shortness of breath with mild exertion. No syncope at this time. Dx: Chronic diastolic congestive heart failure.

You Code It!

Look at Dr. Odem's notes for Ellyn Carrera, and find the most accurate diagnosis code(s). When you are done, check your codes with those that follow.

Step 1: Read the case completely.

Step 2: Abstract the notes: Which key words can you identify relating to why Dr. Odem spent time caring for Ellyn?

____

Step 3: Query the provider, if necessary.

Step 4: Code the diagnosis or diagnoses.

____

Step 5: Code the procedure(s): Office visit, ECG

Step 6: Link the procedure codes to at least one diagnosis code to confirm medical necessity.

Step 7: Back code to double-check your choices.

Answer

Did you find the following diagnosis code?

428.32 Chronic diastolic heart failure

Good job!

Myocardial Infarction (MI)

Malfunction of the heart due to necrosis or deterioration of a portion of the heart muscle; also known as a heart attack.

Infarction

Tissue or muscle that has deteriorated or died (necrotic).

KEYS TO CODING »»

To determine the diagnosis code for a diagnosis of MI, you will need to know

- What specific part of the heart was affected by the infarction?
- Has this patient been treated for this occurrence before?

KEYS TO CODING »»

Review the **ICD-9-CM Coding Guidelines, Section I.c.7. Diseases of Circulatory System,** subsection **e. Acute myocardial infarction (AMI)** for more input on identifying what to code, what not to code, and in what order to put multiple codes. Use this to support your reading here and as a reminder booster later on.

Myocardial Infarction

When a part of the heart muscle deteriorates, or actually dies, it can no longer function properly. This malfunction within a person's heart, known as a **myocardial infarction (MI)**, will cause persistent pain in the chest, left arm, jaw, and neck; fatigue; nausea; vomiting; and shortness of breath. This diagnosis can be confirmed by an electrocardiogram (ECG), blood tests measuring the serial serum enzyme levels, and/or an echocardiogram.

Examples

410.01 Acute myocardial infarction of the anterolateral wall, initial episode of care

410.32 Acute myocardial infarction of the inferoposterior wall, subsequent episode of care

When reporting an MI, the episode of care, either initial or subsequent, is not determined by how many times this provider or facility has cared for this patient but by the timing of the care. Initial episode of care would be described as the time during which the patient has presented to a health care provider with complaints of signs and symptoms through this treatment sequence, even if the patient was transferred from one location to another.

Subsequent episode of care would describe the treatment of the patient after this first episode, such as admission to the hospital.

Let's look at an example scenario:

Jason is sitting in the stands watching his son play softball when all of a sudden he feels this horrible pain in his chest. He is having difficulty taking a breath and the pain is radiating down his left arm. He arrives at the emergency department (ED) via ambulance and the physicians and nurses work on him, taking blood and administering an ECG. It is determined that Jason has had an ST elevation myocardial infarction (STEMI) of the inferolateral wall. Once he is stabilized, Jason is admitted into the hospital and transferred to the intensive care unit (ICU).

410.21 Acute myocardial infarction of the inferolateral wall, initial episode of care

After Jason is discharged from the hospital he goes to his cardiologist's office for a follow-up appointment. In the office, an ECG and an echo are taken and the doctor talks with Jason about his diet, activity level, and other related issues.

410.22 Acute myocardial infarction of the inferolateral wall, subsequent episode of care

Disease of Veins

A great deal of attention has been paid recently to the concern of **thrombosis**. These clots block the blood flow, causing venous insufficiency and affecting the ability for oxygen to get to the tissues throughout the body. A lack of, or reduction, of blood flow can cause edema, congestion, necrosis, and pain. In addition, there is the danger that the blood clot can break loose and travel within the veins and arteries, causing damage to internal organs, blocking oxygen from the lungs (pulmonary embolism), or blocking blood flow through the heart.

Thrombosis

The formation of a blood clot in a blood vessel (plural = thrombi)

Reporting this diagnosis will require you to know a few specifics to determine the diagnosis code:

- Is the condition identified as acute or chronic?
- Where (the specific anatomical site) has the thrombus been located?

Examples

453.51 Chronic venous embolism and thrombosis of deep vessels of proximal lower extremity

453.81 Acute venous embolism and thrombosis of superficial veins of upper extremity

HYPOTENSION AND HYPERTENSION

Hypotension is the condition by which a patient has lower than normal blood pressure. Low blood pressure indicates an inadequate flow of blood and, therefore, inadequate oxygen to the brain, heart, and other vital organs. Light-headedness and dizziness can occur in a person with hypotension.

Some medications, such as antianxiety drugs and diuretics, can cause hypotension, as can alcohol and narcotics. Conditions such as advanced diabetes, dehydration, or arrhythmia can also result in a patient suffering from hypotension.

Hypertension is a condition that millions of people must deal with every day and is a major cause of death. There are estimates that as many as 60 million Americans have hypertension, but only about one-third have been officially diagnosed and are getting treatment. It is also expected that as many as 50% of all people over age 60 are included in these numbers. (See Table 4-1.)

Hypertension

High blood pressure, usually a chronic condition; often identified by a systolic blood pressure above 140 mm/Hg and/or a diastolic blood pressure above 90 mm/Hg.

TABLE 4-1 Blood Pressure Levels

<90/60	Hypotension
90–120/60–80	Normal
120–139/80–89	Prehypertension
140–159/90–99	Hypertension Stage 1
160–179/100–119	Hypertension Stage 2
180–209/110–119	Hypertension Stage 3
210/120+	Hypertension Stage 4

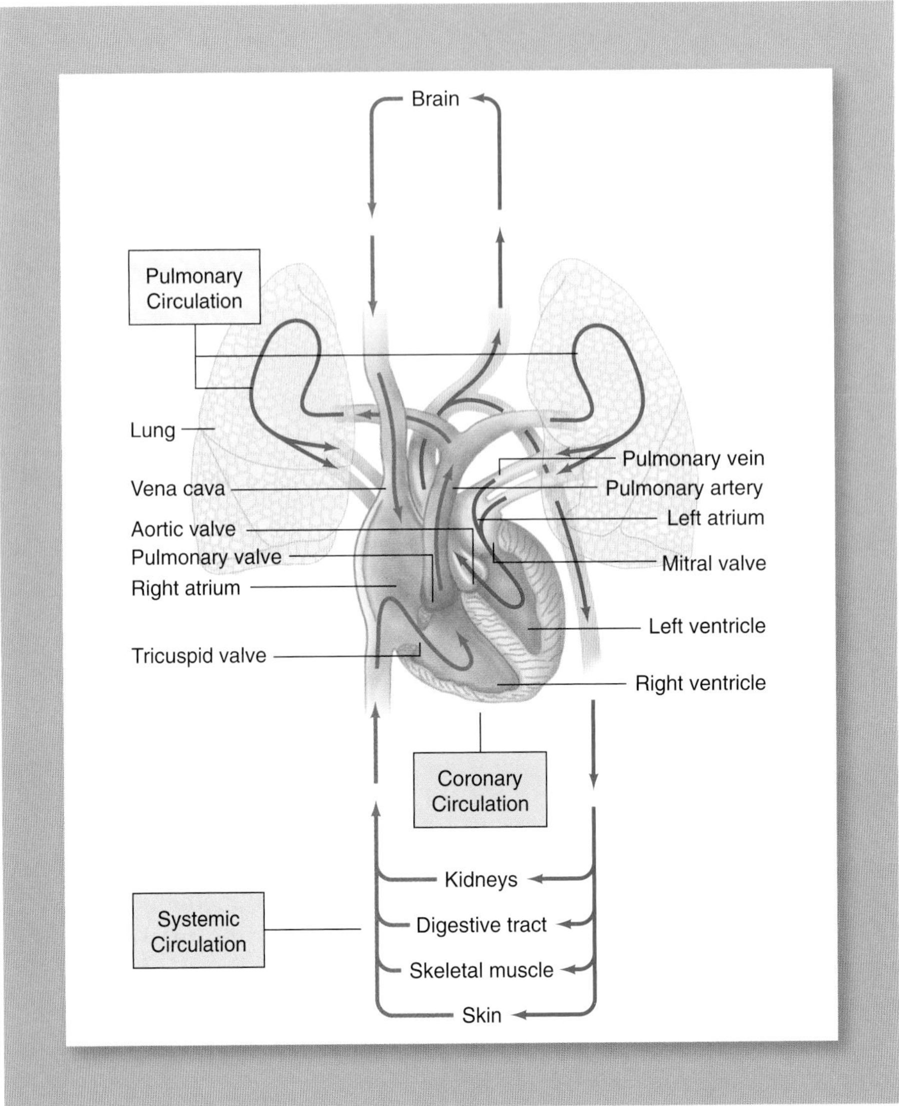

Figure 4-2 The Heart Pumps Blood throughout the Cardiovascular System via the Blood Vessels, Arteries, and Veins.

Statistics show that hypertension has caused 35,000 deaths and was a contributing factor in 180,000 deaths each year. The risk of heart disease is increased 300% by hypertension, and the risk of stroke is increased 700%. Research proves that African Americans are at a much higher risk of hypertension, and its effects, than any other racial or ethnic group.

HYPERTENSION VS. ELEVATED BLOOD PRESSURE

Elevated blood pressure

An occurrence of high blood pressure; an isolated or infrequent reading of a systolic blood pressure above 140 mm/Hg and/or a diastolic blood pressure above 90 mm/Hg.

As coders, the first rule when coding hypertension is that the attending physician must specifically state the diagnosis of *hypertension.* The patient may simply have **elevated blood pressure** (code 796.2) rather than the actual chronic disorder of hypertension.

Among the many causes of hypertension are the following:

- An underlying disorder such as renal disease or Cushing syndrome
- Chronic emotional stress

- A sedentary lifestyle
- Excessive diet of sodium
- Family history of hypertension
- Postmenopausal state
- Advancing age
- Excessive use of alcohol
- Obesity
- African-American ancestry

««« KEYS TO CODING

Review the **ICD-9-CM Coding Guidelines, Section I. Chapter 7a11. Elevated blood pressure** for more input on identifying what to code, what not to code, and in what order to put multiple codes. Use this to support your reading here, and as a reminder booster later on.

CONTROLLED VS. UNCONTROLLED HYPERTENSION

Code selection is not affected by whether a patient's condition is described as **controlled hypertension** or **uncontrolled hypertension** in the physician's notes. You should choose the appropriate code from the range 401–405.

Controlled hypertension

Hypertension that is successfully being treated.

Uncontrolled hypertension

Hypertension that is either untreated or not responding to therapy.

THE HYPERTENSION TABLE

Turn to the listing for hypertension in the alphabetic index. Rather than the usual, indented listing, you will see a four-column table (see Fig. 4-3).

The first column on the left is the main listing, shown in the usual, indented listing fashion and identifying the many descriptors that go along with a diagnosis of hypertension. Your first step in coding a diagnosis of hypertension is to find the type of hypertension, as described by the physician, in the first column. Then read across the three columns to the right to find the suggested code. The three columns are titled malignant, benign, and unspecified. Now, let's investigate what the headings mean.

««« BRIDGE TO ICD-10-CM

At this time, it appears that the ICD-10-CM will keep the alphabetic index listing of hypertension terms in regular column format, just like all the other diagnoses. There will be no table format.

Malignant Hypertension

Malignant hypertension is a rather unusual diagnosis that signifies extremely high blood pressure that is accompanied by papilledema (swelling of the optic nerve behind the eye). Often, the condition is also associated with other organ damage, such as heart failure, kidney failure, and hypertensive encephalopathy. Only about 5% of patients who have been diagnosed with hypertension have malignant hypertension.

Malignant hypertension

Hypertension accompanied by optic nerve swelling and other serious manifestations.

Benign hypertension

Hypertension kept under control with diet and medication.

Benign Hypertension

A more common case of high blood pressure is **benign hypertension**. It is typically brought under control with medication and diet. Benign hypertension can be reasonably stable for years.

««« CODING TIP

Even though 95% of hypertension cases are benign, you cannot assume. Only code benign or malignant when the physician specifically uses either word in the notes. If the physician does not use either word, you must code the hypertension as unspecified.

Unspecified Hypertension

Choose codes from the unspecified hypertension column when the physician's notes do not specifically identify the patient's hypertension as either malignant or benign. Before using an unspecified code, it is

Answer

Did you find the following diagnosis codes?

404.91 Hypertensive heart and chronic kidney disease, unspecified, with heart failure and with chronic kidney disease stage I through stage IV, or unspecified

428.0 Congestive heart failure, unspecified

585.1 Chronic kidney disease, stage I

SECONDARY HYPERTENSION

Secondary hypertension

The condition of hypertension caused by another condition or illness.

Up to this point, you have learned about all the manifestations of, and the conditions that can be caused by, hypertension. However, other conditions and illnesses can cause an individual to develop hypertension. This is called **secondary hypertension** because it is generated after, or secondarily to, another disease.

Hypertension is coded as secondary when the physician uses terms such as "due to" an underlying disease or "resulting from" another condition, or other descriptors that point to another disease or condition. In such cases, you will need two codes:

1. The underlying condition
2. The type of hypertension (405.*xx*)

The order in which you will list the two codes is determined by the answer to the question, "Why did the physician care for this patient today?"

KEYS TO CODING »»

Review the **ICD-9-CM Coding Guidelines, Section I. chapter 7a7. Hypertension, secondary** for more input on identifying what to code, what not to code, and in what order to put multiple codes. Use this to support your reading here, and as a reminder booster later on.

LET'S CODE IT! SCENARIO

Samantha Dennis, a 63-year-old female, came to see Dr. Wiley in his office. She was having headaches and bouts of dizziness. After a physical examination, a urinalysis, and blood work, he diagnosed her with benign hypertension. Dr. Wiley's notes stated that her hypertension was the result of her existing diagnosis of Cushing's disease.

Let's Code It!

Dr. Wiley diagnosed Samantha with *benign hypertension due to Cushing's disease.* It means that Cushing's disease caused Samantha's hypertension. First, go to the alphabetic index, and look under *hypertension.* Look down the indented column until you see "due to" (which is the same as "result of" stated in the physician's notes). Now, look at the indented listing under "due to" until you reach "Cushing's disease." Now that you found the description, according to the physician's notes, look across the table to the right to find the suggested diagnosis code. Looking back at the physician's notes, you see that the diagnosis was benign. Therefore, we are going to go all the way across and use

Hypertension, due to Cushing's disease, benign 405.19

Now, let's turn to the tabular list and begin reading at the three-digit code:

√4th 405 Secondary hypertension

There are no notations here so read down the column to review the choices for the required fourth digit.

√5th 405.0 Malignant secondary hypertension

√5th 405.1 Benign secondary hypertension

√5th 405.9 Unspecified secondary hypertension

Look back at the notes. Dr. Wiley determined Samantha had benign hypertension, so look carefully at

√5th 405.1 Benign secondary hypertension

There are two choices for the mandatory fifth-digit

405.11 Renovascular benign secondary hypertension

405.19 Other benign secondary hypertension

The term "renovascular" refers specifically to the veins of the kidneys. There is no mention of this detail in Dr. Wiley's notes, so you can report 405.19 with confidence that it is correct.

That looks good. However, even though there is no notation, don't you think something is missing? That's right—a code for the Cushing's disease. In the alphabetic index, you find the following under *Disease*

Cushing's (pituitary basophilism) 255.0

In the tabular list find

√4th 255 Disorders of adrenal glands

Take a look at the INCLUDES notation. You are in the right place. You can see that this code requires a fourth digit, so continue reading down the column to

255.0 Cushing's syndrome

There are two notations here. The first states:

"Use additional E code to identify cause, if drug-induced"

The documentation does not indicate any drug-related issue with this diagnosis, so you will not need the E code.

Next, there is an EXCLUDES note:

EXCLUDES congenital adrenal hyperplasia (255.2)

Just because Samantha is 63 years old does not mean this isn't a congenital condition. However, Dr. Wiley provides no documentation stating that her Cushing's disease is congenital, so this EXCLUDES note does not apply to this patient for this encounter.

The claim form you complete for Samantha's encounter with Dr. Wiley today will show both 255.0 and 405.19.

In what order should these codes be listed? Samantha's claim will list the hypertension first (405.19) because it was the reason for her visit with Dr. Wiley.

HYPERTENSION AND PREGNANCY

When a pregnant woman has a diagnosis of hypertension, it is not necessary to limit your code choices to the 401–405 range.

A woman with an existing diagnosis of hypertension who then becomes pregnant will continue to have the appropriate code from the 401–405 range reported. This code reports this situation clearly.

Gestational hypertension

Hypertension that develops during pregnancy and typically goes away once the pregnancy has ended.

However, if the hypertension is diagnosed as **gestational hypertension** or transient hypertension, you will not use a 401–405 code. Instead, use code 642.3x, *Transient hypertension of pregnancy.* This is not unusual and generally means that the hypertension will go away after the baby is born.

Should the woman's diagnosed hypertension cause problems directly related to the pregnancy or complicating the pregnancy, you will choose the best, most appropriate code from category 642, *Hypertension complicating pregnancy, childbirth, and the puerperium.*

LET'S CODE IT! SCENARIO

Carla Jennings, a 23-year-old female, is 5 months pregnant. Dr. Jacoby diagnoses her with hypertension with severe edema. He is concerned about the effect of this condition on her pregnancy and writes a prescription.

Let's Code It!

Carla Jennings has *hypertension with severe edema.* Her hypertensive condition is complicating her pregnancy. Turn to the hypertension table in the alphabetic index, and begin to look down the column of adjectives below the primary term *hypertension.* You see

Hypertension
  Complicating pregnancy, childbirth, or the puerperium
    With
      Edema (mild)
        Severe 642.5

That matches Dr. Jacoby's notes perfectly. Now, you must turn to the tabular list to confirm the code. Of course, you will begin reading at the three-digit code:

√4th 642 Hypertension complicating pregnancy, childbirth, and the puerperium

There are no notations so read down the column to review the choices for the required fourth-digit. The code that matches Dr. Jacoby's notes is

√5th 642.5 Severe pre-eclampsia

Hypertension in pregnancy, childbirth, or the puerperium, not specified as pre-existing, with either albuminuria or edema, or both; specified as severe

In this subsection of the ICD-9-CM tabular list, the fifth-digit choices are not located below the four-digit code. You will need to turn to the previous page to find the box containing the fifth-digit options that go with code 642 (within the range of 640–648). Carla is in her fifth month, so this is an antepartum condition or complication, and she has not delivered the baby during the encounter. It points us to the correct fifth digit of 3.

The code to be used for this visit between Dr. Jacoby and Carla Jennings is 642.53.

HYPERTENSIVE RETINOPATHY

Retinopathy is a degenerative disease of the eye, most specifically the retina. The condition can be caused by diabetes, hypertension, and other circumstances. In those cases when the patient is diagnosed with hypertensive retinopathy, or retinopathy due to hypertension, you will need two codes to thoroughly report the patient's condition.

Your first code is 362.11 Hypertensive retinopathy. Then you will need an additional code to identify the type of hypertension that caused the retinopathy. Choose that code from the 401–405 range.

«« KEYS TO CODING

Review the **ICD-9-CM Coding Guidelines, Section 1, chapter 7a6 Hypertensive retinopathy** for more input on identifying what to code, what not to code, and in what order to put multiple codes. Use this to support your reading here, and as a reminder booster later on.

HYPERTENSIVE CEREBROVASCULAR DISEASE

Patients with cerebrovascular disease due to hypertension will have two codes assigned. The first code will report the cerebrovascular disease, a code from the 430–438 range. The second code will identify the hypertension, using the appropriate code from the 401–405 range. Both the guidelines and a notation under the category heading shown directly above code 430 remind you of the necessity for a second code. You will easily see that the notation also instructs you as to the order in which to place the codes:

Use additional code to identify presence of hypertension.

«« KEYS TO CODING

Review the **ICD-9-CM Coding Guidelines, Section 1, chapter 7b. Cerebral infarction/stroke/ cerebrovascular accident (CVA); and c. Postoperative cerebrovascular accident** for more input on identifying what to code, what not to code, and in what order to put multiple codes. Use this to support your reading here, and as a reminder booster later on.

YOU CODE IT! CASE STUDY

Heather Harper, a 47-year-old female, came to see Dr. Azevedo because she was experiencing headaches and problems with her vision. Heather was diagnosed with essential benign hypertension 3 years ago. After a thorough physical examination and further questioning about her visual disturbances, Dr. Azevedo ordered a CT scan of her head and a few other tests. The test results indicated that Heather had hypertensive encephalopathy.

You Code It!

Carefully review Dr. Azevedo's notes on his visit with Heather, along with the test results. Abstract the notes; find the best, most appropriate diagnosis codes; then look to check the codes you have found.

KEYS TO CODING »»

There is a note in the tabular list, directly under code 438 that reads:

"Note: This category is to be used to indicate conditions in 430-437 as the cause of late effects . . ."

This can be confusing to understand. This means that you read in the patient's chart that he or she was previously diagnosed with a condition that was originally reported with any of the codes in the range 430-437. During this visit, the doctor documents that the patient currently has a neurologic deficit, such as paralysis or dysphasia, as a result of that earlier condition. With both of these facts, you will use a code from category 438 to report the new condition–the neurologic deficit.

Step 1: Read the case completely.

Step 2: Abstract the notes: Which key words can you identify relating to why Dr. Azevedo spent time caring for Heather?

____

Step 3: Query the provider, if necessary.

Step 4: Code the diagnosis or diagnoses.

____

Step 5: Code the procedure(s): Office visit; CT scan, head; query physician about "other tests."

Step 6: Link the procedure codes to at least one diagnosis code to confirm medical necessity.

Step 7: Back code to double-check your choices.

Answer

Did you find the following diagnosis codes?

437.2 Hypertensive encephalopathy

401.1 Essential hypertension, benign

Good job!

Late Effects of Cerebrovascular Disease

The late effects of cerebrovascular disease are coded differently than other late effects, as you learned in Chap. 2.

ICD-9-CM provides a series of combination codes in category 438 Late effects of cerebrovascular disease. It is not unusual for patients who are status-post CVA to suffer with neurologic deficits that last past the initial onset of the condition. In these cases, the physician must connect the dots and specifically identify the current condition as a late effect of the cerebrovascular issue.

Should the patient be diagnosed both with neurologic deficits from a previous cerebrovascular condition AND have a current **cerebrovascular accident (CVA)**, you are permitted to use both a code from the 430 to 437 range *and* code 438.

Cerebrovascular accident (CVA)

Rupture of a blood vessel in the brain; also known as *stroke*.

When there are no neurologic deficits present and the patient has a personal history of cerebrovascular disease, use code V12.59 Personal history of other diseases of the circulatory system and *not* code 438. Remember, you will code that history only when it has been documented that the physician addressed the condition during the current encounter.

LET'S CODE IT! SCENARIO

Priscilla Lewis goes to see Dr. Belman. She was diagnosed with a cerebral embolism 3 months ago that has now been resolved. She explains that she has been having difficulty putting words together to make a sentence and it seems to be getting worse. After examination, he diagnoses her with post-cerebral embolic dysphasia.

Let's Code It!

Priscilla has been diagnosed with post-cerebral embolic dysphasia. This is one way the physician may state that the dysphasia is a late effect of the cerebral embolism she had before.

Turn to the ICD-9-CM alphabetic index and look up the term *dysphasia*. There is one code suggested—784.59. In the tabular list (volume 1), find the beginning of this code category:

√4th 784 Symptoms involving head and neck

A problem speaking occurs in this anatomical area, so that is OK, so far. There is nothing in the EXCLUDES note that relates to this patient, and the symbol to the left of 784 tells you that a fourth digit is required, so read down the column. The best choice is

√5th 784.5 Other speech disturbance

Having difficulty speaking is a speech disturbance, and this is where the alphabetic index pointed you, so look closely at this code. Below this code is another EXCLUDES note which tells you this code EXCLUDES a diagnosis of a speech disorder resulting from a late effect of cerebrovascular accident and directs you to the codes within the range 438.10–438.19.

Go back to the physician's notes (the scenario). They don't state Priscilla had a CVA; they state she had a cerebral embolism. Is this the same thing or unrelated to this notation?

A cerebral embolism is a type of CVA. Therefore, this EXCLUDES note applies to this encounter, and you must turn to code 438 to find the correct code to report Priscilla's diagnosis.

√4th 438 Late effects of cerebrovascular disease

The notation directly under 438 Late effects of cerebrovascular disease confirms that you are in the right place, now. Read down and review the choices for the required fourth digit.

√5th 438.1 Speech and language deficits

This fourth digit is the most accurate, so read down the column to review the choices for the mandatory fifth digit.

438.12 Dysphasia, late effect of cerebrovascular disease

«« KEYS TO CODING

Review the **ICD-9-CM Coding Guidelines, Section I.c.7. d. Late Effects of Cerebrovascular disease** for more input on identifying what to code, what not to code, and in what order to put multiple codes. Use this to support your reading here, and as a reminder booster later on.

«« KEYS TO CODING

Read carefully! "Dysphasia" (with an "s") means impaired speech, and "dysphagia" (with a "g") means difficulty swallowing. Another word that is close is "dysplasia" which means abnormal cell growth. Big difference!

«« KEYS TO CODING

When you look it up, you will see that a cerebral embolism is reported with code 434.10–clearly in the range of 430-437. This means you will report Priscilla's dysphasia from a code in the 438 category.

STROKE AND CVA

Although hypertension is not always specified in the diagnosis, and therefore not coded separately, cerebral infarction and stroke/CVA conditions are included in this section.

While not technically the same condition, the terms stroke and CVA are frequently used interchangeably to indicate a cerebral infarction. When given no other specifics in the physician's notes, these conditions are all coded using 434.91 Cerebral artery occlusion, unspecified, with cerebral infarction.

Be careful to read the exclusion for a CVA under code 436 Acute but ill-defined cerebrovascular disease. If the physician diagnoses the patient with a stroke or CVA, do not use that code.

It can happen that a cerebrovascular hemorrhage or infarction is brought about by a medical procedure, most typically surgery. When the procedure is plainly identified as the cause of the CVA, you have to use two codes.

The first code will be 997.02 Iatrogenic cerebrovascular infarction or hemorrhage, complications affecting specified body systems.

As noted below code 997, you will need an additional code to identify the exact complication. The second code will identify the exact nature of the CVA, so you should use a code from 430–434, as appropriate, according to the notes.

YOU CODE IT! CASE STUDY

Andrew Hogan, a 77-year-old male, was brought into the recovery room after having a craniectomy for the drainage of an intracranial abscess. Dr. Greenwald's notes indicate that Andrew had a postoperative intracranial hemorrhage with a subdural hematoma.

You Code It!

Look at Dr. Greenwald's notes for Andrew Hogan, and find the best, most appropriate code or codes. When you are done, check your codes with those shown below.

Step 1: Read the case completely.

Step 2: Abstract the notes: Which key words can you identify relating to why Dr. Greenwald spent time caring for Andrew Hogan?

Step 3: Query the provider, if necessary.

Step 4: Code the diagnosis or diagnoses.

Step 5: Code the procedure(s): Craniectomy.

Step 6: Link the procedure codes to at least one diagnosis code to confirm medical necessity.

Step 7: Back code to double-check your choices.

Answer

Did you find the following diagnosis codes?

997.02 Iatrogenic cerebrovascular infarction or hemorrhage; postoperative stroke

432.1 Subdural hemorrhage; subdural hematoma nontraumatic

Good job!

CHAPTER SUMMARY

As you learned throughout this chapter, cardiovascular conditions are often treated by a cardiologist. The manifestations of heart failure and heart disease can affect the patient anywhere in the body from the brain to the feet.

Hypertension is a condition that you may encounter as a professional coder while working for a family physician, an internist, a gerontologist, or a cardiologist. It can be a very dangerous condition and can cause many comorbidities and manifestations. As complex as the condition is, so is the coding of the diagnosis. As with all other situations, it must be diagnosed and documented by the attending physician. Read the notes carefully, and query the physician when necessary to get all the specifics you need to code accurately.

BRIDGE TO ICD-10-CM

Not much will change in this section when you transition to the new code set.

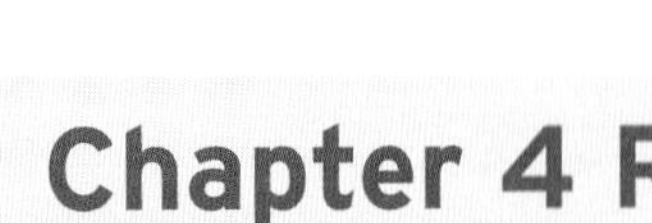

Chapter 4 Review

Coding Circulatory Conditions

1. Hypertension is a
   a. Genetic condition.
   b. Contagious condition.
   c. Chronic condition.
   d. Terminal condition.

2. When the patient's records indicate a current blood pressure reading of 150/100 and no diagnosis is related to that factor, you should
   a. Code elevated blood pressure.
   b. Query the physician.
   c. Code hypertension.
   d. Code history of hypertension.

3. Benign hypertension can usually be controlled with
   a. Proper diet.
   b. Certain medications.
   c. Surgery.
   d. Both (*a*) and (*b*).

4. A diagnosis of uncontrolled hypertension versus controlled hypertension
   a. Does not change the code.
   b. Requires a fifth digit.
   c. Uses a code from the 405 category.
   d. Is indicated with a second code.

5. Essential hypertension is included in the code description for
   a. High blood pressure.
   b. Primary hypertension.
   c. Hypertensive vascular disease.
   d. All of these.

6. The diagnostic statement states, "Heart condition due to hypertension." You will report
   a. One code.
   b. Two codes.
   c. Three codes.
   d. Four codes.

7. A diagnosis of secondary hypertension means you will code
   a. The underlying condition only.
   b. The hypertension only.
   c. The underlying condition code and the hypertension code.
   d. The hypertension code first and then the underlying condition code.

8. When a pregnant woman is diagnosed with hypertension, you must determine
   a. If it is gestational hypertension.
   b. If it is an infarction.
   c. If it is transient hypertension.
   d. If it is familial.

9. A patient with no neurologic deficits and who had a previous diagnosis of cerebrovascular disease (which has since resolved) should be reported with a code from
   a. the 430–437 range.
   b. the 438 code category.
   c. V12.59.
   d. None of the above.

10. A diagnosis of hypertension
    a. Occurs with other conditions only.
    b. Will often affect the treatment of almost any other condition.
    c. Always is coded with other conditions.
    d. Is temporary.

YOU CODE IT! Practice

Chapter 4: Coding Circulatory Conditions

1. Sarah Linscott, a 37-year-old female, was diagnosed with benign hypertension due to a brain tumor.

    ____

2. David Nguyen, a 53-year-old male, is diagnosed with unspecified hypertension due to renal artery stenosis.

    ____

3. Dr. Sirianni diagnosed Gordon Baxa with secondary malignant hypertension due to Cushing's disease.

    ____

4. Robert Hall, a 61-year-old male, was diagnosed with accelerated hypertension.

    ____

5. Pauline Robinson, a 27-year-old obese female, was diagnosed with intermittent vascular hypertensive disease.

    ____

6. Glenn Livingston, a 79-year-old male, was diagnosed with heart failure due to benign hypertension.

    ____

7. Vanessa Dostoimov, a 67-year-old female, was diagnosed with hypertrophy of the heart due to malignant hypertension.

    ____

8. Angelo Vila, a 75-year-old male, was diagnosed with angina decubitus with hypertension.

    ____

9. Kathy Griffo, a 41-year-old obese female, was diagnosed with hyperpiesia.

    ____

TAYLOR, READER, & ASSOCIATES
A Complete Health Care Facility
975 CENTRAL AVENUE • SOMEWHERE, FL 32811 • 407-555-4321

PATIENT: JACKELLSOHN, BRANDON
ACCOUNT/EHR #: JACKBR002
Date: 11/04/11

ADMITTING DIAGNOSES: Deep venous thrombosis (DVT) right leg
Urinary tract infection (UTI)
Parkinson's disease

FINAL DIAGNOSES: Acute DVT, right
UTI
Parkinson's disease

HOSPITAL COURSE: The patient had presented to the office with pain in right leg, discomfort, and also some foul-smelling urine. He was evaluated and Doppler studies of the leg confirmed DVT suggestive of infection. The patient was started on Levaquin and Lovenox subcu 1 mg per kg twice a day, and in 2 days the patient was symptomatic with both his urinary symptoms and with pain in the calf leg. His physical examination revealed his vital signs stable. He is afebrile. Lungs clear. Heart rhythm regular.

Neurologic examination: Tremors and rigidity secondary to Parkinson's disease. Rest is unremarkable. His Doppler studies were positive for right popliteal vein thrombosis and some flow abnormalities in superficial femoral vein. He did have a pelvic sonogram suggesting an enlarged prostate and questionable intraluminal. Kidney showed normal right kidneys. Simple cyst lower pole of left kidney. His symptoms improved.

PT, INR on the day of discharge was 14.4 and 1.1 His UA was positive for blood, negative for leukocyte esterase, nitrites, and WBC. His CHEM-7 showed sodium of 140, potassium 4.1, chloride 102, CO2 31, sugar 112, BUN 15 and creatinine 0.9. WBC 5,300, H&H 15.5 and 45.8. Platelets 116,000. He was discharged home.

DISPOSITION: Arrange for home health

Arrange for follow-up with his primary physician in 1 week. He will need patient evaluation for repeat urine and possible urology consultation for prostate and questionable bladder mass.

Suzanne R. Taylor, MD

SRT/pw D: 11/04/11 09:50:16 T: 11/07/11 12:55:01

Find the best, most appropriate ICD-9-CM code(s).

____

____

____

TAYLOR, READER, & ASSOCIATES
A Complete Health Care Facility
975 CENTRAL AVENUE • SOMEWHERE, FL 32811 • 407-555-4321

PATIENT: FRONNETH, VALERIE
ACCOUNT/EHR #: FRONVA001
Date: 08/21/11

Attending Physician: Willard B. Reader, MD

S: Pt is a 61-year-old female who comes in today complaining of syncope, angina, and dyspnea. She states that the symptoms began approximately 5 days ago. Pt has essential hypertension, diagnosed 2 years ago. She has been successful in keeping the hypertension under control with diet and exercise.

O: Ht 5′7″ Wt. 173 lb. R 18. T 98.6. BP 155/95 Blood tests, UA, CBC, and EKG are ordered. Results indicate the development of renal sclerosis (stage V) with benign hypertension. Evidence also shows left ventricular failure and acute systolic heart failure.

A: Renal sclerosis with benign hypertension; left ventricular failure and acute systolic heart failure

P: 1. Pt to return PRN
2. Referral for renal dialysis evaluation

Willard B. Reader, MD

WBR/pw D: 08/21/11 09:50:16 T: 08/23/11 12:55:01

Find the best, most appropriate ICD-9-CM code(s).

TAYLOR, READER, & ASSOCIATES
A Complete Health Care Facility
975 CENTRAL AVENUE • SOMEWHERE, FL 32811 • 407-555-4321

PATIENT: HARRIS, FELIX
ACCOUNT/EHR #: HARRFE001
Date: 08/23/11

Attending Physician: Willard B. Reader, MD

S: Pt is a 57-year-old male coming in to discuss the results of testing done 2 days ago at our imaging center.

O: Ht 5′7″ Wt. 173 lb. R 18. T 98.6. BP 155/95 I explain to the patient and his wife that the test results show a narrowing of the basilar, carotid, and vertebral arteries on his left side. Stricture of these arteries branching into the brain are shown to be the cause of the symptoms he discussed with me at our last encounter including headaches, dizziness, and reduced mental acuity. Currently, there is no cerebral infarction. We discussed a variety of treatment options and they both agreed to a referral for a surgical consult to investigate the insertion of a shunt.

A: Stenosis of precerebral arteries, including the basilar, carotid, and vertebral arteries.

P: 1. Pt to return PRN
2. Referral for surgical consult for shunt placement

Willard B. Reader, MD

WBR/pw D: 08/23/11 09:50:16 T: 08/28/11 12:55:01

Find the best, most appropriate ICD-9-CM code(s).

TAYLOR, READER, & ASSOCIATES
A Complete Health Care Facility
975 CENTRAL AVENUE • SOMEWHERE, FL 32811 • 407-555-4321

PATIENT: SCHOLAL, AMIR
ACCOUNT/EHR #: SCHOAM001
Date: 08/03/11

Attending Physician: Willard B. Reader, MD

Pt is a 59-year-old male who entered the hospital because of weakness, dry mouth, no energy. The patient claimed that he has been very weak, drinking water, but has not been passing enough water. His blood pressure was elevated and he has been having pain in the left side of the face.

PMH: The patient has a history of rheumatic fever as a child. In 2008, he had a segment of coccyx removed. He had bladder suspension operation in 1995 and has a history of arrhythmias.

The patient has been placed in the past on Norpace and Pronestyl. He was changed to Tenormin. The patient has had trouble with some swelling of the ankles.

The electrocardiogram shows a sinus rhythm with premature ventricular contractions.

FH: The family history is contributory by longevity. Father died of stroke. There is a lot of cancer in the family.

CURRENT MEDICATIONS: Inderal; Ativan; Zestril

ALLERGIES: NKA

FINAL DIAGNOSES:

1. Acute myocardial infarction
2. Systemic arterial hypertension
3. Cardiomegaly without other signs of CHF
4. Cardiac arrhythmia

Willard B. Reader, MD

WBR/pw D: 08/03/11 09:50:16 T: 08/05/11 12:55:01

Find the best, most appropriate ICD-9-CM code(s).

5 Coding Neoplasms

KEY TERMS

Benign
Carcinoma
Functional activity
Histology
Malignant
Mass
Metastasize
Morphology
Neoplasm
Overlapping boundaries

LEARNING OUTCOMES

5.1 Explain the difference between benign and malignant.
5.2 Identify the various types of neoplasms.
5.3 Determine the proper sequencing of coding multiple neoplasms.
5.4 Distinguish between primary and secondary malignancies.
5.5 Use morphology codes correctly.
5.6 Apply the guidelines for coding admissions for the treatment of complications.

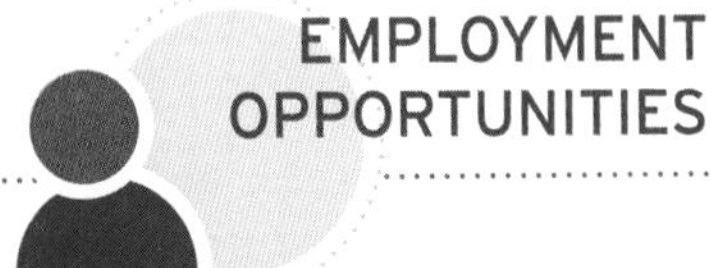

EMPLOYMENT OPPORTUNITIES

Hospitals
Doctors' offices
Nursing homes/assisted living
Clinics
Rehabilitative centers
Home health care providers
Hospice
Pharmaceutical companies
Pharmacies
Medical supply companies
Diagnostic imaging
Laboratories
Insurance companies
HMOs
Self-insured companies
Government agencies
Software manufacturers
Clearinghouses
Patient advocacy groups
Auditing organizations
Law firms

Neoplasm
Abnormal tissue growth; tumor.

When normal cells mutate, they may create a **neoplasm**, also known as a tumor. Even though the health care industry is making tremendous strides in the battle against cancer (malignant neoplasms), there will still be many opportunities for you to code a patient with this diagnosis.

NEOPLASMS

Before you can properly code a neoplasm, you need to understand that a neoplasm is an abnormal tissue growth, or a tumor.

In some cases, you will see the term **mass** used to describe a patient's condition. Mass is *not* the same as a neoplasm. More often, mass is used to identify a cyst or other thickening of tissue. You will find the term *mass* has its own listing in the alphabetic index of ICD-9-CM.

While many people think that neoplasm and cancer are synonymous, they are not. Cancer is the common term for **carcinoma** (see Fig. 5-1).

Neoplasms might be **malignant** or **benign** or have aspects of both characteristics. In diagnoses, neoplasms are also defined by individual name. The physician's notes may state one of the following:

Mass

Abnormal collection of tissue.

Carcinoma

A malignant neoplasm or cancerous tumor.

Malignant

Invasive and destructive characteristic of a neoplasm; possibly causing damage or death.

Benign

Nonmalignant characteristic of a neoplasm; not infectious or spreading.

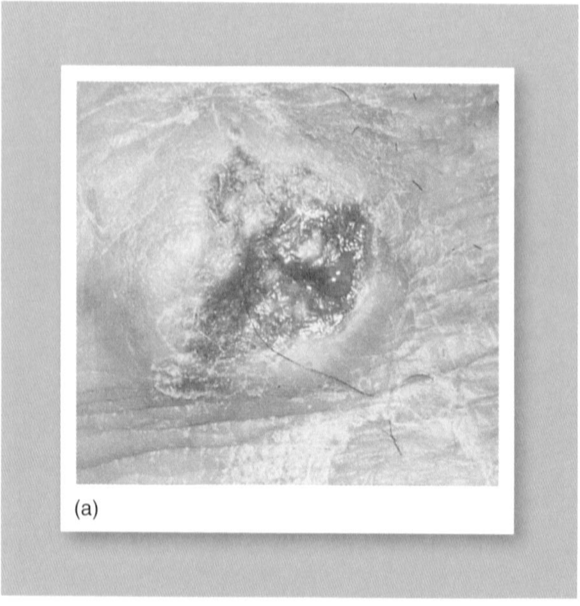

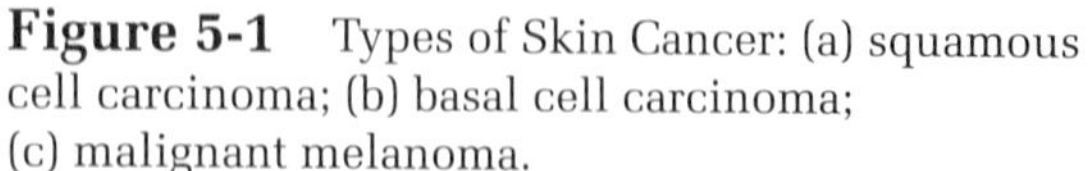

Figure 5-1 Types of Skin Cancer: (a) squamous cell carcinoma; (b) basal cell carcinoma; (c) malignant melanoma.

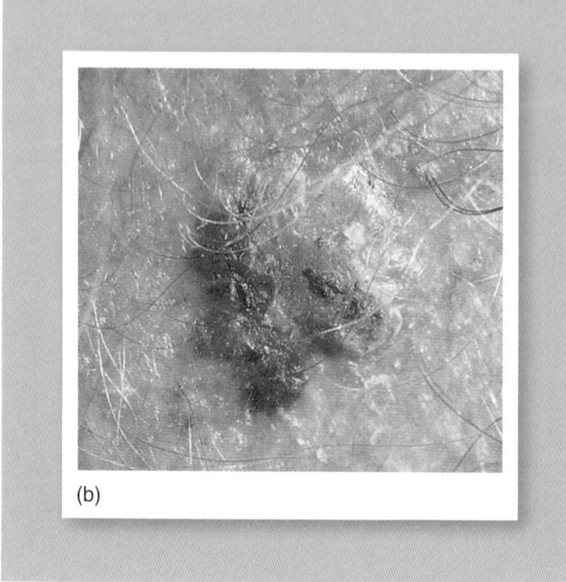

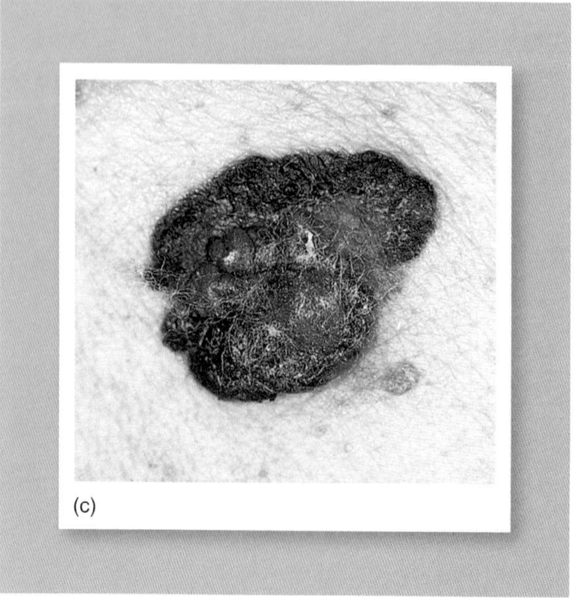

KEYS TO CODING »»

In medical terminology, the suffix -oma means tumor.

- Adenoma
- Melanoma
- Leukemia
- Papilloma

When you see terms like those in the previous list, it is better to look for that specific term in the alphabetic index first, before looking under the term *neoplasm*. One of the most important reasons for doing so is to find additional information to help you code more accurately.

LET'S CODE IT! SCENARIO

Earl Show, a 46-year-old male, comes to see Dr. Lee to get the results of his tests. Dr. Lee explains that Earl has an adenoma of the thyroid. Dr. Lee spends 30 minutes discussing treatment options.

Let's Code It!

CODING TIP »»

Always begin with the terms the physician writes in his or her notes. Then, only when that does not bring you to an accurate code, you can look up alternate terms. This rule of thumb will save you a lot of time.

Dr. Lee has diagnosed Earl with an *adenoma of the thyroid.* You have been working with Dr. Lee as his coder for a while, so you know that an adenoma is a neoplasm, but what kind of neoplasm is it—benign or malignant? To help you determine this, instead of going to neoplasm, let's see if there is a list in the alphabetic index under adenoma. When you find adenoma, the book refers you to

See Neoplasm, by site, benign

This tells you an adenoma is a benign tumor. Or you can continue down this list to the indented term thyroid, and find

Adenoma, thyroid 226

Turn to the tabular list and read the complete description of code 226:

226 Benign neoplasm of thyroid glands

That matches Dr. Lee's diagnosis. Good job!

KEYS TO CODING »»

To determine the code to report a neoplasm, you need to know

- Where in the body (specifically which anatomical site) is the neoplasm located?
- Is the neoplasm benign, malignant, in situ, or uncertain? Uncertain is a pathological determination and is NOT the same as unspecified.
- If the neoplasm is malignant, is this the first diagnosis of malignancy for this patient? If so, this is the primary site. If not, this is a secondary malignancy because it metastasized from the primary.

THE NEOPLASM TABLE

Another way to look up a diagnosis of a tumor in the ICD-9-CM book is to follow the alphabetic index's notation to turn to neoplasm in the alphabetic index. Here, you see a table, similar in structure to the Hypertension Table you read about in Chap. 4.

In the first column of this table, neoplasms are listed by anatomical site (the part of the body where the tumor is located) in alphabetical order. To the right of the first column, you see six columns across: Primary (malignant), Secondary (malignant), Ca in situ (malignant), Benign, Uncertain behavior, and Unspecified. Let's review each of these titles (see Fig. 5-2).

Neoplasm, bone **Index to Diseases**

Neoplasm, neoplastic — *continued*	Malignant: Primary	Malignant: Secondary	Malignant: Ca in situ	Benign	Uncertain Behavior	Unspecified
bone — *continued*						
atlas	170.2	198.5	—	213.2	238.0	239.2
axis	170.2	198.5	—	213.2	238.0	239.2
back NEC	170.2	198.5	—	213.2	238.0	239.2
calcaneus	170.8	198.5	—	213.8	238.0	239.2
calvarium	170.0	198.5	—	213.0	238.0	239.2
carpus (any)	170.5	198.5	—	213.5	238.0	239.2
cartilage NEC	170.9	198.5	—	213.9	238.0	239.2
clavicle	170.3	198.5	—	213.3	238.0	239.2
clivus	170.0	198.5	—	213.0	238.0	239.2
coccygeal vertebra	170.6	198.5	—	213.6	238.0	239.2
coccyx	170.6	198.5	—	213.6	238.0	239.2
costal cartilage	170.3	198.5	—	213.3	238.0	239.2
costovertebral joint	170.3	198.5	—	213.3	238.0	239.2
cranial	170.0	198.5	—	213.0	238.0	239.2
cuboid	170.8	198.5	—	213.8	238.0	239.2
cuneiform	170.9	198.5	—	213.9	238.0	239.2
ankle	170.8	198.5	—	213.8	238.0	239.2
wrist	170.5	198.5	—	213.5	238.0	239.2
digital	170.9	198.5	—	213.9	238.0	239.2
finger	170.5	198.5	—	213.5	238.0	239.2
toe	170.8	198.5	—	213.8	238.0	239.2
elbow	170.4	198.5	—	213.4	238.0	239.2
ethmoid (labyrinth)	170.0	198.5	—	213.0	238.0	239.2
face	170.0	198.5	—	213.0	238.0	239.2
lower jaw	170.1	198.5	—	213.1	238.0	239.2
femur (any part)	170.7	198.5	—	213.7	238.0	239.2
fibula (any part)	170.7	198.5	—	213.7	233.0	239.2
finger (any)	170.5	198.5	—	213.5	238.0	239.2
foot	170.8	198.5	—	213.8	238.0	239.2
forearm	170.4	198.5	—	213.4	238.0	239.2
frontal	170.0	198.5	—	213.0	238.0	239.2
hand	170.5	198.5	—	213.5	238.0	239.2
heel	170.8	198.5	—	213.8	238.0	239.2
hip	170.6	198.5	—	213.6	238.0	239.2
humerus (any part)	170.4	198.5	—	213.4	238.0	239.2
hyoid	170.0	198.5	—	213.0	238.0	239.2
ilium	170.6	198.5	—	213.6	238.0	239.2
innominate	170.6	198.5	—	213.6	238.0	239.2
intervertebral cartilage or disc	170.2	198.5	—	213.2	238.0	239.2
ischium	170.6	198.5	—	213.6	238.0	239.2
jaw (lower)	170.1	198.5	—	213.1	238.0	239.2
upper	170.0	198.5	—	213.0	238.0	239.2
knee	170.7	198.5	—	213.7	238.0	239.2
leg NEC	170.7	198.5	—	213.7	238.0	239.2
limb NEC	170.9	198.5	—	213.9	238.0	239.2
lower (long bones)	170.7	198.5	—	213.7	238.0	239.2
short bones	170.8	198.5	—	213.8	238.0	239.2
upper (long bones)	170.4	198.5	—	213.4	238.0	239.2
short bones	170.5	198.5	—	213.5	238.0	239.2
long	170.9	198.5	—	213.9	238.0	239.2
lower limbs NEC	170.7	198.5	—	213.7	238.0	239.2
upper limbs NEC	170.4	198.5	—	213.4	238.0	239.2
malar	170.0	198.5	—	213.0	238.0	239.2
mandible	170.1	198.5	—	213.1	238.0	239.2
marrow NEC	202.9 ✓	198.5	—	—	—	238.7
mastoid	170.0	198.5	—	213.0	238.0	239.2
maxilla, maxillary (superior)	170.0	198.5	—	213.0	238.0	239.2
inferior	170.1	198.5	—	213.1	238.0	239.2
metacarpus (any)	170.5	198.5	—	213.5	238.0	239.2
metatarsus (any)	170.8	198.5	—	213.8	238.0	239 2
navicular (ankle)	170.8	198.5	—	213.8	238.0	239.2
hand	170.5	198.5	—	213.5	238.0	239.2
nose, nasal	170.0	198.5	—	213.0	238.0	239.2
occipital	170.0	198.5	—	213.0	238.0	239.2
orbit	170.0	198.5	—	213.0	238.0	239.2
parietal	170.0	198.5	—	213.0	238.0	239.2
patella	170.8	198.5	—	213.8	238.0	239.2
pelvic	170.6	198.5	—	213.6	238.0	239.2
phalanges	170.9	198.5	—	213.9	238.0	239.2
foot	170.8	198.5	—	213.8	238.0	239.2
hand	170.5	198.5	—	213.5	238.0	239.2
pubic	170.6	198.5	—	213.6	238.0	239.2
radius (any part)	170.4	198.5	—	213.4	238.0	239.2
rib	170.3	198.5	—	213.3	238.0	239.2
sacral vertebra	170.6	198.5	—	213.6	238.0	239.2

Neoplasm, neoplastic — *continued*	Malignant: Primary	Malignant: Secondary	Malignant: Ca in situ	Benign	Uncertain Behavior	Unspecified
bone — *continued*						
sacrum	170.6	198.5	—	213.6	238.0	239.2
scaphoid (of hand)	170.5	198.5	—	213.5	238.0	239.2
of ankle	170.8	198.5	—	213.8	238.0	239.2
scapula (any part)	170.4	198.5	—	213.4	238.0	239.2
sella turcica	170.0	198.5	—	213.0	238.0	239.2
short	170.9	198.5	—	213.9	238.0	239.2
lower limb	170.8	198.5	—	213.8	238.0	239.2
upper limb	170.5	198.5	—	213.5	238.0	239.2
shoulder	170.4	198.5	—	213.4	238.0	239.2
skeleton, skeletal NEC	170.9	198.5	—	213.9	238.0	239.2
skull	170.0	198.5	—	213.0	238.0	239.2
sphenoid	170.0	198.5	—	213.0	238.0	239.2
spine, spinal (column)	170.2	198.5	—	213.2	238.0	239.2
coccyx	170.6	198.5	—	213.6	238.0	239.2
sacrum	170.6	198.5	—	213.6	238.0	239.2
sternum	170.3	198.5	—	213.3	238.0	239.2
tarsus (any)	170.8	198.5	—	213.8	238.0	239.2
temporal	170.0	198.5	—	213.0	238.0	239.2
thumb	170.5	198.5	—	213.5	238.0	239.2
tibia (any part)	170.7	198.5	—	213.7	238.0	239.2
toe (any)	170.8	198.5	—	213.8	238.0	239.2
trapezium	170.5	198.5	—	213.5	238.0	239.2
trapezoid	170.5	198.5	—	213.5	238.0	239.2
turbinate	170.0	198.5	—	213.0	238.0	239.2
ulna (any part)	170.4	198.5	—	213.4	238.0	239.2
unciform	170.5	198.5	—	213.5	238.0	239.2
vertebra (column)	170.2	198.5	—	213.2	238.0	239.2
coccyx	170.6	198.5	—	213.6	238.0	239.2
sacrum	170.6	198.5	—	213.6	238.0	239.2
vomer	170.0	198.5	—	213.0	238.0	239.2
wrist	170.5	198.5	—	213.5	238.0	239.2
xiphoid process	170.3	198.5	—	213.3	238.0	239.2
zygomatic	170.0	198.5	—	213.0	238.0	239.2
book-leaf (mouth)	145.8	198.89	230.0	210.4	235.1	239.0
bowel—see Neoplasm, intestine						
brachial plexus	171.2	198.89	—	215.2	238.1	239.2
brain NEC	191.9	198.3	—	225.0	237.5	239.6
basal ganglia	191.0	198.3	—	225.0	237.5	239.6
cerebellopontine angle	191.6	198.3	—	225.0	237.5	239.6
cerebellum NOS	191.6	198.3	—	225.0	237.5	239.6
cerebrum	191.0	198.3	—	225.0	237.5	239.6
choroid plexus	191.5	198.3	—	225.0	237.5	239.6
contiguous sites	191.8	—	—	—	—	—
corpus callosum	191.8	198.3	—	225.0	237.5	239.6
corpus striatum	191.0	198.3	—	225.0	237.5	239.6
cortex (cerebral)	191.0	198.3	—	225.0	237.5	239.6
frontal lobe	191.1	198.3	—	225.0	237.5	239.6
globus pallidus	191.0	198.3	—	225.0	237.5	239.6
hippocampus	191.2	198.3	—	225.0	237.5	239.6
hypothalamus	191.0	198.3	—	225.0	237.5	239.6
internal capsule	191.0	198.3	—	225.0	237.5	239.6
medulla oblongata	191.7	198.3	—	225.0	237.5	239.6
meninges	192.1	198.4	—	225.2	237.6	239.7
midbrain	191.7	198.3	—	225.0	237.5	239.6
occipital lobe	191.4	198.3	—	225.0	237.5	239.6
parietal lobe	191.3	198.3	—	225.0	237.5	239.6
peduncle	191.7	198.3	—	225.0	237.5	239.6
pons	191.7	198.3	—	225.0	237.5	239.6
stem	191.7	198.3	—	225.0	237.5	239.6
tapetum	191.8	198.3	—	225.0	237.5	239.6
temporal lobe	191.2	198.3	—	225.0	237.5	239.6
thalamus	191.0	198.3	—	225.0	237.5	239.6
uncus	191.2	198.3	—	225.0	237.5	239.6
ventricle (floor)	191.5	198.3	—	225.0	237.5	239.6
branchial (cleft) (vestiges)	146.8	198.89	230.0	210.6	235.1	239.0
breast (connective tissue) (female) (glandular tissue) (soft parts)	174.9	198.81	233.0	217	238.3	239.3
areola	174.0	198.81	233.0	217	238.3	239.3
male	175.0	198.81	233.0	217	238.3	239.3
axillary tail	174.6	198.81	233.0	217	238.3	239.3
central portion	174.1	198.81	233.0	217	238.3	239.3
contiguous sites	174.8	—	—	—	—	—
ectopic sites	174.8	198.81	233.0	217	238.3	239.3
inner	174.8	198.81	233.0	217	238.3	239.3
lower	174.8	198.81	233.0	217	238.3	239.3

Figure 5-2 The Neoplasm Table, in Part.

BRIDGE TO ICD-10-CM

ICD-10-CM will also contain a Neoplasm Table with the same column headings.

Metastasize

To proliferate, reproduce, or spread.

Primary (Malignant)

The term *primary* indicates the anatomical site (the place in the body) where the malignant neoplasm was first seen and identified. If the physician's notes do not specify primary or secondary, then the site mentioned is primary.

Secondary (Malignant)

The term *secondary* identifies the anatomical site to which the malignancy **metastasized.** One very strange thing about cancerous cells is that they travel through the body and do not necessarily spread to adjoining body parts. Cancer can be identified in the breast as the primary site and metastasize to the liver without actually interacting with anything in between. Notes will state that a site is "secondary to" (*primary site*), "metastasized from" (*primary site*), or (*primary site*) "metastasized to" (*secondary site*).

The terms *disseminated cancer, generalized cancer,* or *widely metastatic* would indicate that the malignancy has infiltrated the body throughout and affects all or most of the patient's anatomy. That would be coded as a malignant neoplasm without specification of site (code 199.0). In such cases, it is not that the physician forgot to specify the site. It is that there are too many sites to list.

Ca In Situ (Malignant)

The term *Ca in situ* indicates that the tumor has undergone malignant changes but is still limited to the site where it originated (i.e., it has not spread). Ca is short for carcinoma, and you can remember *situ* as in the word *situated.* So think of it as a cancerous tumor that is staying in place.

Benign

As you learned earlier, the term *benign* means there is no indication of invasion of adjacent cells. Generally, benign means not cancerous.

Uncertain Behavior

The classification *uncertain behavior* indicates that the pathologist is not able to specifically determine whether a tumor is benign or malignant because indicators of both are present.

Unspecified

Choose codes in the Unspecified column when the physician's notes do not include any specific information regarding the nature of the tumor. Before choosing a code from the column, please query the physician and make certain that a laboratory report is not available or on its way with the information you need.

LET'S CODE IT! SCENARIO

Stephen Mathis is a 44-year-old male who is seen by his regular primary care physician, Dr. Fornari. After the imaging and laboratory test results come back, Stephen is diagnosed with a benign neoplasm of the ascending colon.

Let's Code It!

Dr. Fornari diagnosed Stephen with *a benign neoplasm of the ascending colon.* Turn to the Neoplasm Table in the alphabetic index. Go down the list of anatomical sites until you reach *colon.* There is a notation that directs you to *See also Neoplasm, intestine, large.* Indented under *colon* are the words *and rectum.* Go back to Dr. Fornari's notes, his diagnosis does not include the rectum, so follow the book's advice and turn to the listing for *intestine, large,* and find out what is shown there.

Continue through the list until you get to *intestine, intestinal.* Beneath the term *intestine,* you will find the word *large* indented. Indented under *large* is *colon.* Indented under *colon,* you see *ascending.* This matches Dr. Fornari's diagnosis of Stephen's neoplasm exactly! Now, go across the table to the right to the Benign column. Here, the code 211.3 is suggested. Remember the rule, never, never code from the alphabetic index, and that includes the Neoplasm Table, so turn to the tabular list to confirm this suggested code. Start reading at the three-digit number.

√4th 211 Benign neoplasm of other parts of digestive system

The colon (large intestine) is a part of the digestive system, so you know you are in the right place. The *excludes* note does not relate to this patient's diagnosis for this encounter, so continue reading down the column to review all of the choices for the required fourth digit.

211.3 Benign neoplasm of colon

The ascending colon is actually the portion of the large intestine that goes from the cecum to the transverse colon. The additional descriptors listed under code 211.3 include the terms *cecum* and *large intestine NOS.* Good coding!

FUNCTIONAL ACTIVITY

Certain neoplasms require an additional code to report **functional activity**. Take a look at the beginning of the tabular list, chapter 2, Neoplasms (directly above code 140). There are several notes here to help you find the most accurate neoplasm code. Take a look at number 2 Functional activity. This note states, "An additional code from chapter 3 may be used to identify such functional activity associated with any neoplasm." Chapter 3 of the ICD-9-CM tabular list is titled: Endocrine, Nutritional, and Metabolic Disease, and Immunity Disorders (240–279). Beneath the heading for chapter 3 (directly above code 240) reminds you of this detail:

"Note: All neoplasms, whether functionally active or not, are classified in Chapter 2. Codes in Chapter 3 (i.e., 242.8, 246.0, 251–253, 255–259) may be used to identify such functional activity associated with any neoplasm, or by ectopic endocrine tissue."

What the note means is that if a patient has been diagnosed with a neoplasm affecting the individual's glandular function, you have to identify the functional activity (of the gland) with an additional code.

For example, take a look beneath code 183.0 Ovarian cancer (malignant neoplasm of the ovary). There is a notation that says:

"Use additional code to identify any functional activity"

Functional activity

Glandular secretion in abnormal quantity.

This note regarding functional activity also appears under the following terms:

Benign neoplasm of ovary
Malignant neoplasm of endocrine glands
Benign neoplasm of endocrine glands
Malignant neoplasm of islets of Langerhans
Benign neoplasm of islets of Langerhans
Malignant neoplasm of the testis
Benign neoplasm of the testis
Malignant neoplasm of thyroid glands
Benign neoplasm of thyroid glands

Example

Catecholamine-producing malignant pheochromocytoma of throid
- 193 Malignant neoplasm of thyroid gland
- 255.6 Medulloadrenal hyperfunction

Ovarian carcinoma with hyperestrogenism
- 183.0 Malignant neoplasm of ovary
- 256.0 Hyperestrogenism

Basophil adenoma of pituitary with Cushing's disease
- 227.3 Benign neoplasm of pituitary gland
- 255.0 Cushing's syndrome

LET'S CODE IT! SCENARIO

Taylor Chattman, a 37-year-old male, came to see Dr. Bornstein for a checkup. He was diagnosed with functioning thyroid carcinoma. Dr. Bornstein reviews with Taylor the results of his latest thyroid scan, TSH and TRH stimulation tests, and an ultrasonogram and informs him that he has developed hyperthyroidism.

Let's Code It!

Dr. Bornstein has diagnosed Taylor with *functioning thyroid carcinoma* and *hyperthyroidism.* The hyperthyroidism is the functional activity of the thyroid carcinoma. Turn to the alphabetic index and look for

Carcinoma – see also Neoplasm, by site, malignant

Look down the list. Neither the term *functioning* nor the term *thyroid* is shown here, so you will need to turn to the Neoplasm Table and find

Neoplasm, thyroid, malignant, primary 193

Let's go to the tabular list, to confirm

193 Malignant neoplasm of thyroid gland

Use additional code to identify any functional activity

This code is correct and the ICD-9-CM book is telling you that you need an additional code to report the functional activity. The only other detail Dr. Bornstein included in her diagnostic statement is hyperthyroidism. Turn back to the alphabetic index, and look up hyperthyroidism:

Hyperthyroidism (latent) (preadult) (recurrent) (without goiter) 242.9

Turn to the tabular list to confirm this suggested code.

√4th 242 Thyrotoxicosis with or without goiter

The *excludes* note mentions nothing that relates to this encounter for our patient, so read down the column to review the choices for the required fourth digit.

√5th 242.9 Thyrotoxicosis without mention of goiter or other cause; Hyperthyroidism NOS

This matches the notes, so you are in the correct place. The symbol to the left of the code tells you that a fifth digit is required. There is nothing beneath this code, so you will need to read up the column until you find the box, directly below code 242 that provides your choices.

242.90 Thyrotoxicosis without mention of goiter or other cause, hyperthyroidism NOS, without mention of thyrotoxic crisis or storm

Did you notice that this code is located in chapter 3 and is describing the functional activity of the neoplasm? Great! The two diagnosis codes for Taylor's claim are 193 and 242.90.

OVERLAPPING BOUNDARIES

The nature of a malignant neoplasm includes its potential to spread to adjoining tissue. As you learned earlier in this chapter, you code malignancies by their anatomical site in the order in which the malignancy developed: primary and secondary. However, there are cases where the condition of the patient involves more than one code subcategory. Neoplasms with **overlapping boundaries,** also known as **contiguous,** may blur the anatomical descriptors. Included in the description of code 147.8 is the following notation:

Overlapping boundaries

Multiple sites of carcinoma without identifiable borders.

Example

Arnaud Plummer was diagnosed with malignant neoplasm of the nasopharynx, posterior and lateral walls. You don't have to rely on the following two codes:

147.1 Malignant neoplasm of nasopharynx, posterior wall

147.2 Malignant neoplasm of nasopharynx, lateral wall

Instead, you can use a single code:

147.8 Malignant neoplasm of nasopharynx, other specified sites

Malignant neoplasm of contiguous or overlapping sites of nasopharynx whose point of origin cannot be determined

You will find that just about every subcategory throughout the neoplasm section has a code with this notation. For cases in which the physician cannot identify a specific site, usually because the malignancy has metastasized so dramatically, the code subcategory 195 enables you to report the malignancy identifying only the section of the patient's body, such as head, abdomen, or lower limb.

√4th 195 Malignant neoplasm of other and ill-defined sites

BRIDGE TO ICD-10-CM

You will follow these same exact steps when ICD-10-CM is implemented. This process will not change. Only the way the codes look will change.

NEOPLASMS AND MORPHOLOGY CODES (M Codes)

In addition to the code for a neoplasm, the alphabetic index may also include an M code. The M stands for **morphology,** and the M code identifies the behavior and **histology** of the neoplasm.

Morphology

The study of the configuration or structure of living organisms.

Histology

The study of the microscopic composition of tissues.

Example

Craniopharyngioma (M9350/1) 237.0

M codes are not shown in the tabular list of the ICD-9-CM. Instead, they are listed in numerical order in Appendix A, "Morphology of Neoplasms," located directly after the E code tabular list. These codes are also available as a separate book, the *International Classification of Diseases for Oncology* (ICD-O). Morphology codes are not structured like the other diagnosis codes. The codes always begin with the letter M, which is followed by four digits, a slash (/), and a single digit. The neoplasm's histology is described by the first four digits of the M code.

Example

Craniopharyngioma **M9350/**1

Some of the M code categories include:

M800 Neoplasms NOS

M809–M811 Basal cell neoplasms

M880 Soft tissue tumors and sarcomas NOS

Example

Craniopharyngioma M9350**/1**

The single number, shown after the slash of the M code, describes the behavior of the neoplasm. The numbers represent

/0 Benign

/1 Uncertain behavior whether benign or malignant; borderline malignancy

/2 Carcinoma in situ; intraepithelial; noninfiltrating; noninvasive

/3 Malignant, primary site

/6 Malignant, metastatic site; secondary site

/9 Malignant, uncertain whether primary or metastatic site

In our example, the behavior of this neoplasm is *uncertain behavior*, as indicated by the number 1 after the slash. When you reference the ICD-9-CM code for this diagnosis, craniopharyngioma, you will see that the code description is in agreement.

237.0 Neoplasm of uncertain behavior of the pituitary gland and craniopharyngeal duct

M codes are used for providing specific data about the site (topography) and the histology (morphology) of the affected tissue to tumor and cancer registries. Pathologists may also use the codes to provide more detail about a particular tissue sample. Normally, M codes are not used for reimbursement and are not placed on insurance claim forms.

CODING SEQUENCES

When you are coding encounters with a patient diagnosed with a neoplasm, our basic rule still applies. The principal diagnosis code should answer the question, "Why did the health care professional care for this patient today?"

When multiple issues are addressed during the visit, you report the primary site of malignancy first, followed by any secondary sites, in order of severity, and then anatomy (most severe first, top of the body first). As you know, however, every rule has an exception. When only the secondary site and not the primary site of a neoplasm is treated, you should list the secondary neoplasm first, followed by the code for the primary site.

«« KEYS TO CODING

Review the **ICD-9-CM Coding Guidelines, Section I.c.2 Neoplasms,** subsection **c. Coding and sequencing of complications** for more input on identifying what to code, what not to code, and in what order to put multiple codes. Use this to support your reading here, and as a reminder booster later on.

LET'S CODE IT! SCENARIO

Sean O'Boyle, a 30-year-old male, presents today with concerns of a recurrent incident of cancer. He was diagnosed with osteogenic sarcoma of the left femur 3 years ago and went through a treatment sequence of surgery and chemotherapy. After reviewing his symptoms and running a battery of tests, Dr. Hostetler confirms the presence of chondrosarcoma of the ribs, secondary to osteogenic sarcoma. Dr. Hostetler discusses his recommendation of a surgical resection of the ribs, to be followed by radiation and chemotherapy treatments. Dr. Hostetler paid no attention to the previous diagnosis of osteogenic sarcoma.

Let's Code It!

Dr. Hostetler diagnosed Sean with *chondrosarcoma of the ribs, secondary to osteogenic sarcoma.* As you learned earlier in this chapter, it means that the primary site of the neoplasm is the osteogenic sarcoma, a malignant bone cancer most often in the ends of the long bones. Dr. Hostetler's notes specify the femur–a long bone in the thigh. In addition, the secondary site is documented as a chondrosarcoma of the ribs. A chondrosarcoma is a malignancy that forms in cartilage cells. Let's find the codes.

In the alphabetic index, next to the list for *osteosarcoma* (the combined form of osteogenic sarcoma), the notation states, *See Neoplasm, bone, malignant.* Now, turn to the Neoplasm Table in the alphabetic index and find *neoplasm, bone.* Beneath it, indented, find the anatomical site of Sean's osteosarcoma—his left *femur.* Look across the line to the Malignant, primary column. The code 170.7 is suggested. Let's turn to the tabular list to confirm the code:

√4th 170 Malignant neoplasm of bone and articular cartilage

This time, you have *excludes* notes above and below this code to read. None of these diagnoses relate to this case, so read down the column to review the choices for the required fourth digit.

170.7 Malignant neoplasm of long bones of lower limb, femur

Now, you need to find the code for the second issue. Under *chondrosarcoma,* in the alphabetic index, the notation states, *See also Neoplasm, cartilage, malignant.* At the Neoplasm Table, find *cartilage,* and then look for the anatomical part in which Sean was found to have chondrosarcoma—his ribs. Move across the line to Malignant, secondary column this time, and find the suggested code 198.5. Confirm the code by looking at the complete code description in the tabular list:

√4th 198 Secondary malignant neoplasm of other specified sites

There are a couple of *excludes* notes but they don't relate to this case, so read down the column and review all of the choices for the required fourth digit.

198.5 Secondary malignant neoplasm, bone and bone marrow

Good work! You have found both diagnostic codes for Sean's encounter with Dr. Hostetler. However, you still must determine the order in which to list the two codes. When you go back to the notes for the visit, you read that Dr. Hostetler specifically mentions that *no attention to the previous diagnosis of osteogenic sarcoma* was provided. Our rule is that the first-listed code should identify the main reason why Sean came to see Dr. Hostetler. This rule is in sync with the exception to the neoplasm rule that tells you to code the condition that was the focus of treatment first. So the correct order of the codes is 198.5 followed by 170.7. You are doing a great job!

KEYS TO CODING »»

Review the **ICD-9-CM Coding Guidelines, Section I. c2b Treatment of secondary site** for more input on identifying what to code, what not to code, and in what order to put multiple codes. Use this to support your reading here, and as a reminder booster later on.

EXCISED MALIGNANCIES

Thanks to modern medical science and technology, health care professionals are more successful than ever at getting rid of certain neoplasms (tumors), often by excising them, or cutting them out. When that happens, the patient no longer has the site of the malignancy and, therefore, can no longer have that condition. At that time, the code will change from a malignancy code (140–239.9) to a personal history of a malignancy code (V10.*xx*).

Example

Mary Alice Arkin was diagnosed with a malignant neoplasm of the central portion of the breast. The diagnosis code was:

174.1 Malignant neoplasm of the female breast, central portion

She underwent a mastectomy, a surgical procedure to remove her breast. Once the anatomical site (her breast) that contained the malignant neoplasm was removed, she no longer had the disease. From this point on, the diagnosis code is:

V10.3 Personal history of malignant neoplasm, breast

Suppose a patient has a primary site of malignancy and the disease has already metastasized to a second location; if the primary site is removed, the secondary malignancy is still coded as secondary but listed first. Confusing? Let's look at an example.

Example

Joshua Miller was diagnosed with prostate cancer. It spread to his liver before he was able to have surgery. The diagnosis codes, in this sequence, are

185 Malignant neoplasm of the prostate

197.7 Secondary malignant neoplasm of liver, specified as secondary

Dr. Farina removes Joshua's prostate successfully. The new codes are:

197.7 Secondary malignant neoplasm of liver, specified as secondary

V10.46 Personal history of malignant neoplasm, prostate

Once Joshua has the site of his primary malignancy removed, his prostate condition becomes "history." His secondary malignancy in the liver moves up in order, but it will always be the *second* site at which Joshua developed a malignancy.

«« KEYS TO CODING

Review the **ICD-9-CM Coding Guidelines, Section I.c.2 Neoplasms,** subsection **d. Primary malignancy previously excised** for more input on identifying what to code, what not to code, and in what order to put multiple codes. Use this to support your reading here, and as a reminder booster later on.

YOU CODE IT! CASE STUDY

Randolph Holloway, a 47-year-old male, came to see Dr. Johnson, his dermatologist, for an annual checkup. Two years ago, Dr. Johnson removed a malignant melanoma from Randolph's left forearm. The malignancy was totally removed, but he comes to see his physician for a checkup once a year.

You Code It!

Go through the steps of coding, and determine the diagnosis code or codes that should be reported for this encounter between Dr. Johnson and Randolph Holloway.

Step 1: Read the case completely.

Step 2: Abstract the notes: Which key words can you identify relating to why Dr. Johnson cared for Randolph?

____

Step 3: Query the provider, if necessary.

Step 4: Code the diagnosis or diagnoses.

Step 5: Code the procedure(s): Annual dermatological evaluation.

Step 6: Link the procedure codes to at least one diagnosis code to confirm medical necessity.

Step 7: Back code to double-check your choices.

Answer

Did you find the following diagnosis code?

V10.82 Personal history of malignant melanoma of skin

Good job!

KEYS TO CODING »»

Professional coding specialists must be cautious when determining the difference between a patient in remission and a patient with a personal history of a condition, such as leukemia. If the documentation is not absolutely clear on this, the physician must be queried. There is a big difference between these two diagnostic identifications.

BRIDGE TO ICD-10-CM 

These guidelines remain the same with the ICD-10-CM code set.

REMISSION

Remission is a period of time during which symptoms of a disease subside. While this is a term that may be used by nonprofessionals in connection with a malignancy, it is actually clinically limited. You will find that, when coding a malignancy such as leukemia, multiple myeloma, and immunoproliferative neoplasms, there is a fifth-digit option to report that the patient is in remission.

PROPHYLACTIC ORGAN REMOVAL

Advances in science have given us genetic predisposition testing and other identification exams. The information, along with personal and family histories, enables patients and health care professionals to predict an individual's risk for cancer and other diseases more accurately. Studies show, for example, that a woman that has inherited a mutation in BRCA1 or BRCA2 gene faces a dramatically higher risk for developing breast cancer by age 65. A strong family history of colon cancer may lead an individual to be tested for a variant in the APC gene. There are many others that can now be tested.

Prophylactic, or preventive, surgery can reduce the risk by as much as 90%. In the case of breast cancer, it would mean having a double mastectomy (the surgical removal of both breasts) while they are still healthy and without any signs or symptoms of carcinoma.

As a coder, the question becomes, How do you code a diagnosis for a surgical procedure on a healthy anatomical site? Of course, you will use a V code: V50.4*x* Prophylactic organ removal.

For those patients who have had genetic testing with a confirmed abnormal gene, you will also use a second code from category V84.*xx*, Genetic susceptibility to disease.

If the reason for the preventive surgery is due to a family history of cancer, you will add another code from the V16 category.

YOU CODE IT! CASE STUDY

Janis Olivette, a 29-year-old female, was admitted today for the prophylactic removal of her breasts. Her grandmother, mother, and sister have all had breast cancer, so she had genetic testing performed, indicating that she did have a genetic susceptibility to breast cancer. She elected to have the surgery instead of taking chances with her health.

You Code It!

Go through the steps of coding, and determine the diagnosis code or codes that should be reported for Janis Olivette's surgery.

Step 1: Read the case completely.

Step 2: Abstract the notes: Which key words can you identify relating to why Janis was admitted into the hospital?

____

Step 3: Query the provider, if necessary.

Step 4: Code the diagnosis or diagnoses.

____

Step 5: Code the procedure(s): Double mastectomy.

Step 6: Link the procedure codes to at least one diagnosis code to confirm medical necessity.

Step 7: Back code to double-check your choices.

Answer

Did you find the following diagnosis codes?

V50.41 Prophylactic removal of breast

V84.01 Genetic susceptibility to malignant neoplasm of breast

V16.3 Family history of malignant neoplasm, breast

Good job!

CHEMOTHERAPY AND RADIATION THERAPY

Patients diagnosed with a malignancy often undergo chemotherapy and/or radiation therapy. During the course of treatment, the patient may be admitted into the hospital for the treatment and then discharged. When the only treatment or service provided for the patient during this stay at the hospital is the administration of the chemotherapy or radiation, then, you will code the chemotherapy (V58.11) or radiotherapy (V58.0) first and then the malignancy or malignancies being treated.

Example

Douglas Brunner is admitted into the hospital for administration of chemotherapy for malignant neoplasm of the pharynx.

V58.11 Encounter for antineoplastic chemotherapy

149.0 Malignant neoplasm of pharynx, unspecified

In some cases, a patient is admitted into the hospital for surgical treatment of a malignancy with the plan to have chemotherapy or radiation follow immediately (during the same admission). In such cases, the standard coding rule will hold true. Why did the patient come to the hospital? To have a malignancy treated. How was this treated? First, surgery and then chemotherapy or radiation. Therefore, the code for the malignancy will be listed first, followed by the code for the chemotherapy or radiation.

Example

Glynnis Gallimore is admitted to the hospital for the surgical removal of the navicular of her right ankle. Dr. Faison scheduled Glynnis to begin radiation treatments after the surgery has been successfully completed.

170.8 Malignant neoplasm of short bones of lower limb

V58.0 Encounter for radiotherapy

KEYS TO CODING »»

Review the **ICD-9-CM Coding Guidelines, Section I.c.2. Neoplasms,** subsection **e. Admissions/Encounters involving chemotherapy, immunotherapy and radiation therapy** for more input on identifying what to code, what not to code, and in what order to put multiple codes. Use this to support your reading here, and as a reminder booster later on.

Should the patient develop complications as a result of the chemotherapy or radiotherapy while still in the hospital and getting treatment, you will still code the V58.*xx* code first and follow that with the appropriate code or codes for the symptoms, such as uncontrolled nausea and vomiting or dehydration. The code for the malignancy being treated by the radiation or chemotherapy should be listed after that.

ADMISSIONS FOR TREATMENT OF COMPLICATIONS

Treatment for malignancies can wreak havoc on a patient's body. Complications of either the malignancy itself, surgical treatment of the malignancy, or chemotherapy/radiation treatments, may need attention. In those cases, when the patient is treated for the complication, such as anemia or dehydration, the code for the complication should be listed first, followed by the code for the malignancy.

However, if the admission is for treatment of the malignancy and complications are *also* treated, then you must code the malignancy first, followed by the code or codes for the complications.

BRIDGE TO ICD-10-CM »»

These same guidelines will continue with ICD-10-CM.

KEYS TO CODING »»

To determine the correct code for an admission of a patient with a complication and a malignancy, you must identify whether both conditions were treated or only the complication. This will affect the sequencing of the codes.

Example

Lorina Lardner was admitted to the hospital for surgical treatment of a melanoma on her upper lip. While Lorina was there, Dr. Bowen treated her anemia, which she developed as a result of the chemotherapy.

173.0 Malignant neoplasm of skin, skin of lip

285.3 Antineoplastic chemotherapy induced anemia

YOU CODE IT! CASE STUDY

Kirby Graham has been receiving chemotherapy treatments for the last 6 weeks. He was diagnosed with malignant neoplasm of the pyloric canal three months ago. After Kirby began showing signs of dehydration, Dr. Rodriguez admitted him into the hospital for intravenous rehydration. He was discharged the next day.

You Code It!

Read Dr. Rodriguez's notes on his encounter with Kirby Graham, and find the best, most appropriate diagnosis code or codes.

Step 1: Read the case completely.

Step 2: Abstract the notes: Which key words can you identify relating to why Dr. Rodriguez cared for Kirby?

____

Step 3: Query the provider, if necessary.

Step 4: Code the diagnosis or diagnoses.

____

Step 5: Code the procedure(s): Intravenous rehydration.

Step 6: Link the procedure codes to at least one diagnosis code to confirm medical necessity.

Step 7: Back code to double-check your choices.

Answer

Did you find the following diagnosis codes?

276.51 Volume depletion, dehydration

151.1 Malignant neoplasm of the stomach, pylorus

Good job!

BRIDGE TO ICD-10-CM

ICD-10-CM guidelines include an exception for coding the treatment of anemia specifically when associated with a neoplasm. Guidelines for Chapter 2, subsection L.4. Encounter for complication associated with a neoplasm state that anemia is an exception that will require the malignancy code to be first-listed, followed by the code D63.0 Anemia in neoplastic disease, when only the anemia is treated.

CHAPTER SUMMARY

In this chapter, you learned how to identify the key words in physicians' notes and lab reports that can guide you toward the most accurate code. You learned the differences in the types of neoplasms, the proper sequencing of codes, and how to use morphology codes. In addition, you reviewed the correct way to code a patient's admission for various treatments and the services rendered for complications of those treatments.

There have been, and continue to be, incredible advancements made in the treatments of all types of neoplasms, as well as modifications to sociological behaviors to help prevent the development of those insidious health concerns. As a professional coding specialist, your ability to properly code the diagnostic tests and procedures used in the care of individuals can open many job opportunities for you.

Chapter 5 Review
Coding Neoplasms

1. A neoplasm is the same as a
   a. Tumor.
   b. Cancer.
   c. Malignancy.
   d. Metastasis.

2. Different types of neoplasms include all except
   a. Adenoma.
   b. Melanoma.
   c. Carcinoma.
   d. Chemotherapy.

3. The column title of the Neoplasm Table that does not identify a malignancy is
   a. Primary.
   b. Benign.
   c. Ca in situ.
   d. Secondary.

4. Morphology codes are used
   a. For reimbursement.
   b. To describe treatment.
   c. To describe the behavior and histology of the neoplasm.
   d. For identification of manifestations.

5. At subsequent encounters after the surgical removal of a neoplasm, the diagnosis code changes to a(n)
   a. V code.
   b. E code.
   c. Late effects code.
   d. Comorbidity code.

6. When a patient is admitted for chemotherapy to treat a malignant neoplasm and that is the extent of treatment, the first code listed is the code for
   a. The primary malignancy.
   b. The secondary malignancy.
   c. The chemotherapy.
   d. Observation in a hospital.

7. When a patient is treated for a complication, such as anemia or dehydration, the code for this complication should be listed
   a. After the primary malignancy.
   b. First.
   c. After the chemotherapy or radiation code.
   d. As an E code.

8. Metastasized means
   a. Spread.
   b. Noncancerous.
   c. Malignant.
   d. Measured.

9. The term *disseminated cancer* has the same meaning as
   a. Widely metastatic.
   b. Ca in situ.
   c. Uncertain behavior.
   d. Unspecified.

10. When coding a neoplasm, you must know
    a. The anatomical site.
    b. Whether it is primary or secondary.
    c. Whether it is benign or malignant.
    d. All of these.

YOU CODE IT! Practice

Chapter 5. Coding Neoplasms

1. Scott Mercado was diagnosed with a malignancy of his pancreatic duct.

    ____

2. Dorinna Ziegler was diagnosed with bronchial adenoma.

    ____

3. Jonathan Jones, a 47-year-old male, was diagnosed with a malignant neoplasm of cerebral meninges metastasized from the breast.

    ____

4. Tina Baker was diagnosed with carcinoma in situ of the eye.

    ____

5. Glenn Shutts was diagnosed with subacute lymphoid leukemia now in remission.

    ____

6. Dr. Shaughnessy diagnosed Harriet Hubbell with a nonspecific tumor of the hilus lung.

    ____

7. Jeffrey Sharp was diagnosed with a malignant lymphosarcoma.

    ____

8. Susan Kasbeer was told she had a carcinoma in situ of the vermilion border of her lip.

    ____

9. Thomas Kelly was diagnosed with a subcutaneous lipoma of the face.

    ____

10. Marissa Kirby was diagnosed with ovarian cancer.

    ____

11. Greg Phillips was told he had a benign neoplasm of the occipital bone.

    ____

TAYLOR, READER, & ASSOCIATES
A Complete Health Care Facility
975 CENTRAL AVENUE • SOMEWHERE, FL 32811 • 407-555-4321

PATIENT: CANNELLO, MORGAN
ACCOUNT/EHR #: CANNMO001

Date: 08/11/11

Attending Physician: Willard B. Reader, MD

Pt is a 45-year-old female with terminal carcinoma of the breast, metastatic to the liver and the brain. She was admitted today with dehydration, due to the program of chemotherapy she has been on. Rehydrated 3 hours with IV infusion and discharged with no treatment given to the cancer.

Willard B. Reader, MD

WBR/pw D: 08/11/11 09:50:16 T: 08/13/11 12:55:01

Find the best, most appropriate ICD-9-CM codes.

ADVERSE REACTION

When health care providers determine that a pharmaceutical substance may improve an individual's health status, they will typically prescribe that medication for **therapeutic** use. A patient is diagnosed with an adverse effect, or reaction, when all of the following occurs:

- A health care professional correctly prescribes a drug for a patient.
- The correct patient receives the correct drug.
- The correct dosage is given to the patient (or taken by the patient). The correct dosage includes the correct amount in the correct frequency.
- The correct route of administration is used.

Example

Dr. Tennyson prescribes 10 mg of Lexapro, bid, po, for Terence Romulles for anxiety.

- *Lexapro* is the brand name of an anti-anxiety medication
- *10 mg* is the amount of the dosage
- *bid* is the abbreviation for 'twice a day'-the frequency of the dosage
- *po* is the abbreviation for 'by mouth'-the route of administration

-AND-

- The patient has an unexpected bad reaction to that drug. Perhaps there was no way to know the patient was allergic to the drug, but the patient broke out in a rash, had difficulty breathing, or lost consciousness.

Unpredictable reactions can be due to genetic factors, other diseases or allergies, the method of administration of the drug (subcutaneous, intravenous, inhalation, intramuscular, etc.), and other issues.

When an adverse reaction has occurred, you will need a minimum of *two codes*.

E = *effect.* The code or codes will report exactly what reaction or reactions the patient had to the substance, such as a rash, vomiting, or unconsciousness. It might be a confirmed diagnosis of the problem or the signs and/or symptoms experienced by the patient as a result of taking the medicine.

E = *E code.* The E code will explain that the patient took the drug for *therapeutic use.* You can find this code in the Table of Drugs and Chemicals in the column under the heading "Therapeutic Use." More about this is covered later in the chapter.

Example

Giana Roman took her prescription for the antibiotic exactly as the doctor and the pharmacist instructed. She broke out in a rash because it turned out she was allergic to the antibiotic and no one knew. The "effect" is the rash, and the E code explains "therapeutic use of antibiotic."

Poisoned

A condition produced by a substance that harms or causes death.

Adverse effect

An unexpected, bad result; also known as an adverse reaction.

Toxic effect

Poisonous substance causing a health-related reaction.

Therapeutic

Intended to restore good health or reduce the effect of disease or negative condition.

«« KEYS TO CODING

Remember, you have more information at your fingertips within the ICD-9-CM book, referring specifically to **ICD-9-CM Coding Guidelines, Section 1, chapter 17 (800-999),** subsection **e. Adverse effects, poisoning and toxic effects** for more input on identifying what to code, what not to code, and in what order to put multiple codes. Use this to support your reading here, and as a reminder booster later on.

«« BRIDGE TO ICD-10-CM

The guidelines for coding injury and poisoning can be found in **ICD-10-CM Coding Guidelines, Section 1, chapter 19 (S00-T88),** subsection **e. Adverse effects, poisoning, underdosing, and toxic effects.**

«« KEYS TO CODING

You may need more than one code to report the negative *effect* this medication has had on the patient. Remember, you need to tell the *whole story* of what went wrong for this patient when taking this prescribed medication as ordered.

POISONING

Most people think of poisoning as something from a great detective novel or movie. However, poisoning can happen under many different circumstances. In reality, when a person comes in contact with a chemical or drug (not prescribed by a physician or not taken as prescribed) and a health problem results, it is called a *poisoning*. The substance can be ingested, inhaled, absorbed through the skin, injected, or taken by some other method.

Of course, you will need to name the substance that poisoned the patient, just as you did with an adverse reaction.

Next, you will need to discover the circumstances under which this patient came to be poisoned. Was it . . .

- *An accident?* Things happen, such as a child finding a bottle of medication and thinking it's candy, an error in dosage, the wrong patient receiving the medication, or an over-the-counter drug unknowingly taken with a prescription.
- *A suicide attempt?* Sadly, a person might take an overdose with the intention of trying to harm himself or herself.
- *An assault?* An assault occurs when someone tries to cause intentional harm to someone else. It sounds like a scene from that detective movie, but it does happen in real life.

When a poisoning occurs, you will need a minimum of three codes: Think of the little saying: *P.E.E.* for poison.

P = *poison.* The first-listed code will report the poisoning by the specific substance, from the code range 960–979.9. The Table of Drugs and Chemicals will help you find the right code. The table is covered later in this chapter.

E = *effect.* The next code(s) will indicate exactly the bad reaction the patient had to the substance, such as a rash, vomiting, or unconsciousness. It might be a confirmed diagnosis or the signs and/or symptoms the patient is having as a result of this event.

E = *E code.* The final code or codes will explain *how,* or the **intent** of how, the patient came to be poisoned.

Was it an . . .

Accident? Did the individual take the drug by mistake? Or possibly take too much or too little by mistake?

Attempted suicide? Did the individual take the drug, or the wrong amount of the drug, on purpose with the intent of causing himself or herself harm?

Assault? Did someone else give the drug to the patient, or the wrong quantity of the drug, with the intent of causing harm?

Undetermined? You may use undetermined in cases in which it is impossible to determine the intent. For example, if the patient is brought into the emergency department (ED) unconscious, you might have to wait until they regain consciousness or until an investigation has been completed to find out if it was an accident,

CODING TIP »»

There is no *P* in adverse effect... a reminder that no poisoning code is used.

KEYS TO CODING »»

Review the **ICD-9-CM Coding Guidelines, Section I. chapter 17. Injury and Poisoning (800-999),** subsection **e. Adverse effects, poisoning, and toxic effects, part 1 Adverse effect** for more input on identifying what to code, what not to code, and in what order to put multiple codes. Use this to support your reading here, and as a reminder booster later on.

CODING TIP »»

Think P.E.E. for Poison.

P = poison code

E = effect code

E = E code

Intent

The reason behind the cause of the incident.

KEYS TO CODING »»

You may need more than one code to tell the *whole story* about how this poisoning has affected the patient.

assault, or attempted suicide. NEVER ASSUME. Therefore, undetermined would be the correct code.

Again, the Table of Drugs and Chemicals will help you find the most accurate E code.

TOXIC EFFECT

Toxic substances may be ingested (such as food), inhaled (such as asbestos), or something an individual may come in contact with (such as acid). Think *T.E.E.* for toxic.

T = *toxic.* The first-listed code will report the specific toxic substance (poison), from the code range 980 through 989.9.

E = *effect.* The next code(s) will indicate exactly what reaction the patient had to the substance, such as a rash, vomiting, or unconsciousness.

E = *E code.* The final code or codes will provide the explanation of how the patient came to have the toxic reaction, such as accident, attempted suicide, or assault.

Example

Arsenic poisoning is the result of interaction with the toxic substance arsenic, which can cause stomach pain. It can happen, for example, when arsenic leaches into groundwater and taints water wells.

toxic substance = arsenic; effect = stomach pain; E code = environmental factors/accidental.

PATIENT NONCOMPLIANCE

Sometimes, a patient has an adverse effect because he or she did not take the medication as ordered by the physician . . . or didn't take the drugs at all. When an incorrect dosage (known as underdosing) is the will of the patient, rather than an error on the part of a health care professional, this is considered noncompliance and is reported with code

V15.81 Noncompliance with medical treatment

Example

George Henry was diagnosed with schizophrenia and given a prescription by Dr. Meuller for lithium. His mom takes him back to the doctor because George refused to take the medication. She is hoping that Dr. Meuller can convince him to take his medicine. The diagnosis codes for this encounter will include V15.81 Noncompliance with medical treatment in addition to the diagnosis code for George's schizophrenia 295.02 Schizophrenia simplex, chronic.

««« KEYS TO CODING

Review the **ICD-9-CM Coding Guidelines, Section I. chapter 17. Injury and Poisoning (800-999),** subsection **e. Adverse effects, poisoning, and toxic effects, part 2 Poisoning** for more input on identifying what to code, what not to code, and in what order to put multiple codes. Use this to support your reading here, and as a reminder booster later on.

««« BRIDGE TO ICD-10-CM

The ICD-10-CM guidelines reduce the number of codes you will need to report some conditions. "Codes in categories T36-T65 are combination codes that include the substances related to adverse effects, poisonings, toxic effects and underdosing, as well as the external cause. No additional external cause code is required for poisonings, toxic effects, adverse effects and underdosing codes."

««« KEYS TO CODING

You may need more than one code to tell the *whole story* about how this poisoning has affected the patient.

««« KEYS TO CODING

Review the **ICD-9-CM Coding Guidelines, Section I. chapter 17. Injury and Poisoning (800-999),** subsection **e. Adverse effects, poisoning, and toxic effects, part 3 Toxic effects** for more input on identifying what to code, what not to code, and in what order to put multiple codes. Use this to support your reading here, and as a reminder booster later on.

THE TABLE OF DRUGS AND CHEMICALS

BRIDGE TO ICD-10-CM

Most of the codes in this section require a seventh character to identify the encounter with the provider for this concern as:

A for initial encounter

D for subsequent encounter

Z for aftercare

S for the care of sequela or late effects

Drugs

Substances, natural or combined, created to treat or prevent illness or disease. Examples include aspirin, Lipitor, and Prozac.

Chemicals

Substances used in, or made by, the process of chemistry. Examples include benzene, turpentine, and bleach.

Directly located after the alphabetical listing in volume 2 is section 2, the Table of **Drugs** and **Chemicals** (see Fig. 6-1). The Table of Drugs and Chemicals is used when a drug or chemical caused an adverse reaction, has poisoned the patient, or caused a toxic effect. Similar to the Hypertension Table and the Neoplasm Table, the Table of Drugs and Chemicals is in columns.

(Note: Different published versions of the ICD-9-CM book may place sections in a different order. Therefore, volume 2 section 2 may be in a different location in your book.)

Drug and Chemical Names

The first column of the table lists the names of drugs and chemicals, in alphabetic order. The list includes prescription medications, over-the-counter medications, household and industrial chemicals, and many other items with a chemical basis. Aspirin, indigestion relief medication, drugstore brand allergy relievers, alcohol (for drinking or sterilization), window cleaner, battery acid, and lots of other similar substances are all included, as well as those medications prescribed by a physician.

		External Cause (E Code)					
	Poisoning	Accident	Therapeutic Use	Suicide Attempt	Assault	Undetermined
1-propanol	980.3	E860.4	—	E950.9	E962.1	E980.9
2-propanol	980.2	E860.3	—	E950.9	E962.1	E980.9
2,4-D (dichlorophenoxyacetic acid)	989.4	E863.5	—	E950.6	E962.1	E980.7
2,4-toluene diisocyanate	983.0	E864.0	—	E950.7	E962.1	E980.6
2,4,5-T (trichlorophenoxyacetic acid)	989.2	E863.5	—	E950.6	E962.1	E980.7
14-hydroxydihydromorphinone	965.09	E850.2	E935.2	E950.0	E962.0	E980.0
ABOB	961.7	E857	E931.7	E950.4	E962.0	E980.4
Abrus (seed)	988.2	E865.3	—	E950.9	E962.1	E980.9
Absinthe	980.0	E860.1	—	E950.9	E962.1	E980.9
beverage	980.0	E860.0	—	E950.9	E962.1	E980.9
Acenocoumarin, **acenocoumarol**	964.2	E858.2	E934.2	E950.4	E962.0	E980.4
Acepromazine	969.1	E853.0	E939.1	E950.3	E962.0	E980.3
Acetal	982.8	E862.4	—	E950.9	E962.1	E980.9
Acetaldehyde (vapor)	987.8	E869.8	—	E952.8	E962.2	E982.8
liquid	989.89	E866.8	—	E950.9	E962.1	E980.9
Acetaminophen	965.4	E850.4	E935.4	E950.0	E962.0	E980.0
Acetaminosalol	965.1	E850.3	E935.3	E950.0	E962.0	E980.0
Acetanilid(e)	965.4	E850.4	E935.4	E950.0	E962.0	E980.0
Acetarsol, acetarsone	961.1	E857	E931.1	E950.4	E962.0	E980.4
Acetazolamide	974.2	E858.5	E944.2	E950.4	E962.0	E980.4
Acetic						
acid	983.1	E864.1	—	E950.7	E962.1	E980.6
with sodium acetate (ointment)	976.3	E858.7	E946.3	E950.4	E962.0	E980.4
irrigating solution	974.5	E858.5	E944.5	E950.4	E962.0	E980.4
lotion	976.2	E858.7	E946.2	E950.4	E962.0	E980.4
anhydride	983.1	E864.1	—	E950.7	E962.1	E980.6
ether (vapor)	982.8	E862.4	—	E950.9	E962.1	E980.9
Acetohexamide	962.3	E858.0	E932.3	E950.4	E962.0	E980.4
Acetomenaphthone	964.3	E858.2	E934.3	E950.4	E962.0	E980.4
Acetomorphine	965.01	E850.0	E935.0	E950.0	E962.0	E980.0
Acetone (oils) (vapor)	982.8	E862.4	—	E950.9	E962.1	E980.9
Acetophenazine (maleate)	969.1	E853.0	E939.1	E950.3	E962.0	E980.3
Acetophenetidin	965.4	E850.4	E935.4	E950.0	E962.0	E980.0
Acetophenone	982.0	E862.4	—	E950.9	E962.1	E980.9

		External Cause (E Code)				
	Poisoning	Accident	Therapeutic Use	Suicide Attempt	Assault	Undetermined
Acetorphine	965.09	E850.2	E935.2	E950.0	E962.0	E980.0
Acetosulfone (sodium)	961.8	E857	E931.8	E950.4	E962.0	E980.4
Acetrizoate (sodium)	977.8	E858.8	E947.8	E950.4	E962.0	E980.4
Acetylcarbromal	967.3	E852.2	E937.3	E950.2	E962.0	E980.2
Acetylcholine (chloride)	971.0	E855.3	E941.0	E950.4	E962.0	E980.4
Acetylcysteine	975.5	E858.6	E945.5	E950.4	E962.0	E980.4
Acetyldigitoxin	972.1	E858.3	E942.1	E950.4	E962.0	E980.4
Acetyldihydrocodeine	965.09	E850.2	E935.2	E950.0	E962.0	E980.0
Acetyldihydrocodeinone	965.09	E850.2	E935.2	E950.0	E962.0	E980.0
Acetylene (gas) (industrial)	987.1	E868.1	—	E951.8	E962.2	E981.8
incomplete combustion of — *see* Carbon monoxide, fuel, utility						
tetrachloride (vapor)	982.3	E862.4	—	E950.9	E962.1	E980.9
Acetyliodosalicylic acid	965.1	E850.3	E935.3	E950.0	E962.0	E980.0
Acetylphenylhydrazine	965.8	E850.8	E935.8	E950.0	E962.0	E980.0
Acetylsalicylic acid	965.1	E850.3	E935.3	E950.0	E962.0	E980.0
Achromycin	960.4	E856	E930.4	E950.4	E962.0	E980.4
ophthalmic preparation	976.5	E858.7	E946.5	E950.4	E962.0	E980.4
topical NEC	976.0	E858.7	E946.0	E950.4	E962.0	E980.4
Acidifying agents	963.2	E858.1	E933.2	E950.4	E962.0	E980.4
Acids (corrosive) **NEC**	983.1	E864.1	—	E950.7	E962.1	E980.6
Aconite (wild)	988.2	E865.4	—	E950.9	E962.1	E980.9
Aconitine (liniment)	976.8	E858.7	E946.8	E950.4	E962.0	E980.4
Aconitum ferox	988.2	E865.4	—	E950.9	E962.1	E980.9
Acridine	983.0	E864.0	—	E950.7	E962.1	E980.6
vapor	987.8	E869.8	—	E952.8	E962.2	E982.8
Acriflavine	961.9	E857	E931.9	E950.4	E962.0	E980.4
Acrisorcin	976.0	E858.7	E946.0	E950.4	E962.0	E980.4
Acrolein (gas)	987.8	E869.8	—	E952.8	E962.2	E982.8
liquid	989.89	E866.8	—	E950.9	E962.1	E980.9
Actaea spicata	988.2	E865.4	—	E950.9	E962.1	E980.9
Acterol	961.5	E857	E931.5	E950.4	E962.0	E980.4
ACTH	962.4	E858.0	E932.4	E950.4	E962.0	E980.4
Acthar	962.4	E858.O	E932.4	E950.4	E962.0	E980.4
Actinomycin (C) (D)	960.7	E856	E930.7	E950.4	E962.0	E980.4
Adalin (acetyl)	967.3	E852.2	E937.3	E950.2	E962.0	E980.2
Adenosine (phosphate)	977.8	E858.8	E947.8	E950.4	E962.0	E980.4
Adhesives	989.89	E866.6	—	E950.9	E962.1	E980.9

Figure 6-1 The Table of Drugs and Chemicals.

Once you have determined whether this is an adverse reaction or a poisoning, you next need to find what substance caused the problem. Then, find that substance in the alphabetic list in the first column of the table.

Sometimes, it is easy to find. For example, Giselle had a bad reaction to Nytol. Even though this is a brand name of an over-the-counter sleep medication, you will find it easily in the list of substances on the Table of Drugs and Chemicals first column.

Other times, it may not be this easy, and the name, whether brand name, generic name, or chemical name, that is documented in the physician's notes may not be in the table. If you don't find it, you may have to do some research. Some of the drugs and chemicals are listed by their brand or common names, such as Metamucil or Nytol. Others are shown by their chemical or generic names, such as barbiturates (sedatives). If you are not certain, consult a ***Physician's Desk Reference* (PDR),** a series of books that lists all the approved drugs, herbal remedies, and over-the-counter medications by brand name, chemical name, generic name, and drug category.

Example

Vesicare–the brand name

Solifenacin succinate–the generic or chemical name

Muscarinic receptor antagonist–the drug category

Anticholinergen–general drug category

In the listing from the PDR, you can see Vesicare is shown as the trade or brand name. The generic or chemical name is shown: solifenacin succinate. If a physician prescribed it for a patient, who then had an adverse reaction or took an overdose, you would most likely see one or the other of those names in the notes.

However, you will find neither of these listed in the Table of Drugs and Chemicals. The next piece of information given to you by the PDR is in the description of the drug: muscarinic receptor antagonist. Unfortunately, there is nothing in the table under *muscarinic* either. Because the patient had either an adverse reaction or taken an overdose, take a look at the following paragraphs from the PDR:

> ADVERSE REACTIONS
>
> . . . Expected side effects of antimuscarinic agents . . .
>
> OVERDOSAGE
>
> . . . Overdosage with Vesicare can potentially result in severe *anticholinergic* effects . . .

The two paragraphs provide us with two new descriptors for the drug: antimuscarinic and anticholinergic. Both of them are shown in the Table of Drugs and Chemicals and, interestingly, lead you to the same codes.

Poisoning

As you learned earlier in this chapter, once you find the correct substance, you will then need to determine whether it was a poisoning/toxic effect or an adverse effect. In cases of poisoning or toxic effect, look at the

«« KEYS TO CODING

If the patient did not get the correct dosage and this circumstance had an adverse effect on him or her, you need to know *why* the correct dosage was not administered.
If it was an error, report as an accident.
If it was intentional by the patient because he or she did not want to take the medication, report as noncompliance.

***Physician's Desk Reference* (PDR)**

A series of reference books identifying all aspects of prescription and over-the-counter medications, as well as herbal remedies.

«« BRIDGE TO ICD-10-CM

In ICD-10-CM, noncompliance is reported with Z91 codes (Z91.12-, Z91.13-) or complication of care codes (Y63.61, Y63.8-Y63.9) plus an underdosing code to indicate intent, if known.

«« KEYS TO CODING

You do not code from the Table of Drugs and Chemicals when a physician writes a prescription or when a patient picks up an order at the pharmacy, only when a "problem" is being attended to by the health care professional.

«« CODING TIP

Never, never, never code from the alphabetic index–including the Table of Drugs and Chemicals! *Always* confirm the code's accuracy in the tabular list.

code presented in the first column to the right of the substance—the column titled *Poisoning*. The column will suggest the code to use when the patient has been poisoned, or had a toxic effect, to the substance on that line. It will be your first-listed, or principal, diagnosis code: the P in your three poisoning codes (P.E.E.) or the T in your three toxic effect codes (T.E.E.).

The next five columns to the right will direct you to the E code you need to report the intent of the poisoning, adverse reaction, or toxic effect.

BRIDGE TO ICD-10-CM »»

In the Table of Drugs and Chemicals in ICD-10-CM, the first column, listing all of the drugs and chemicals by name, is titled *SUBSTANCE*.

KEYS TO CODING »»

Reminder: Never report a poisoning code for a reaction to a medication that was taken as prescribed by the physician [an adverse reaction].

Accident

The second column is titled *Accident* and lists suggested E codes to be included when the poisoning or toxic effect was caused by an accidental overdose, accidentally taking the wrong substance, or accidents that happened during the use of drugs and chemical substances. Basically, it means that the ingestion or exposure to the drug or quantity of drug that caused the problem was unintentional.

LET'S CODE IT! SCENARIO

Jesse Winthrop found an unmarked barrel in the back of the warehouse where he works. He opened the top and leaned over to see what was inside. Vapors from the benzene solvent being stored in that barrel overcame Jesse. He passed out and lost consciousness for about one minute. He was taken to the doctor immediately. He had a toxic effect from accidentally inhaling the benzene.

Let's Code It!

Jesse had *a toxic effect from inhaling the benzene.* The notes also state that Jesse *lost consciousness for about one minute.* You learned that you need at least three codes: toxic effect = T.E.E.

The first code identifies the chemical or substance. In Jesse's case, it was the vapor from a barrel of benzene solvent. Turn to the alphabetic index's Table of Drugs and Chemicals. Look down the first column and find *benzene, solvent, vapor.*

Benzene (acetyl) (dimethyl) (methyl) (solvent) (vapor)

Look across to the first column, under the heading *Poisoning* and find the suggested code.

Benzene (acetyl) (dimethyl) (methyl) (solvent) (vapor) 982.0

In the tabular list, confirm the accuracy of the code with the complete description. Start at the three-digit number and be certain to check any notations or directives.

√4th 982 Toxic effect of solvents other than petroleum-based

There are no notations or directives, so keep reading down the column and review all of the choices for the required 4th digit.

982.0 Toxic effect of solvents, benzene and homologues

BRIDGE TO ICD-10-CM »»

In ICD-10-CM, the first code column is titled '*Poisoning Accidental* (unintentional)." This and the titles of the other columns reflect the combination codes in this section, eliminating the need for an additional code to explain the intent of the event.

Great! You now have the first-listed code for Jesse's encounter. The next code reports the *effect* that the benzene vapors had on Jesse. The notes state he was unconscious. In the main section of the alphabetic index, find:

Unconscious, unconsciousness 780.09

Turn to the three-digit code in the tabular list:

√4th 780 General symptoms

There are no notations or EXCLUDES lists, so continue reading down the column to review your choices for the required fourth digit.

√5th 780.0 Alteration of consciousness

Read the EXCLUDES note beneath this code description carefully. This code subcategory excludes alteration of consciousness when caused by a physical injury or coma caused by an underlying condition. These don't relate to Jesse's condition, so keep reading to review your choices for the required fifth digit.

780.09 Other alteration of consciousness, unconsciousness

Excellent! Was this the only effect the benzene vapor had on Jesse? According to the notes, yes. Therefore, you must move on to find the last code, the E code to explain how Jesse came to be poisoned by the benzene. Go back to the Table of Drugs and Chemicals, and check the listing for:

Benzene (acetyl) (dimethyl) (methyl) (solvent) (vapor)

The notes state that this was an accident. So, move across the line to the second column, titled *Accident,* and find:

Benzene (acetyl) (dimethyl) (solvent) (vapor) E862.4

Go to the tabular list to confirm the code. Begin reading at the top of the code category

√4th E862 Accidental poisoning by petroleum products, other solvents and their vapors, not elsewhere classified

Notice that there are no EXCLUDES or INCLUDES notes. Read down the column and review the choices for the required fourth digit.

E862.4 Accidental poisoning by petroleum products, other solvents, and their vapors, other specified solvents, Benzene

So Jesse's accidental poisoning is reported with three codes: 982.0, 780.09, and E862.4.

You may remember from Chap. 2 that you also need another E code to report where the accident occurred. In the Index to External Causes, turn to

Place of occurrence of accident – see Accident (to), occurring (at)(in)

The notes state that Jesse was working in a warehouse when this accident happened, so turn back to the list under Accident in this index, and you will find

Accident, occurring (at)(in)

«« KEYS TO CODING

If you look at the code directly above code 982 you can see, 981 Toxic effect of petroleum products, Benzine, you might ask, "Why is this not the correct code?" Look carefully at the spelling.

benzINE = code 981

benzENE = code 982.0

The notes state Jesse was affected by benzENE, so 982.0 is correct. This is a good illustration of why professional coding specialists must read very carefully.

Read all the way down to

Accident, occurring (at)(in), warehouse E849.3

Go to the tabular list for the E codes and check this code out, Start at the beginning of the code category.

√4th E849 Place of occurrence

Read down the column to review your choices for the required fourth digit.

E849.3 Industrial place and premises, warehouse

This completes the report. You are really becoming a great coder!

BRIDGE TO ICD-10-CM 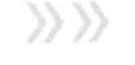

In ICD-10-CM's Table of Drugs and Chemicals, this column is titled *Adverse Effect* and will be found further to the right.

Therapeutic Use

The third column of the Table of Drugs and Chemicals to the right is titled Therapeutic use. As mentioned earlier in this chapter, codes for therapeutic use are reported when a properly prescribed drug was taken in the correct dose by the correct person but an unexpected reaction occurred (an adverse reaction).

LET'S CODE IT! SCENARIO

Whitney Shoal, a 27-year-old female, goes to Dr. Curtis because of chest congestion. He writes a prescription for penicillin, 250 mg, po, q8h and Whitney takes it to the pharmacy to be filled. She begins taking the pills that evening—as prescribed by Dr. Curtis. By the next day, her whole body is covered with a rash. She comes to see Dr. Curtis today for treatment of the rash.

Let's Code It!

Whitney had an *adverse reaction to penicillin,* the medication that Dr. Curtis prescribed to her. She was taking the medication for *therapeutic* (a remedy or to cure) reasons, and she suffered an unexpected response, breaking out in a rash. You need two codes: one to report the effect plus an E code. The effect that the penicillin had on Whitney was a rash. Turn to the alphabetic index, and look up *rash.* Review all the indented terms before deciding which one looks best.

Rash, drug (internal use) 693.0

It matches the situation perfectly. Let's turn to the tabular list and confirm the code's accuracy. Remember to look for notations and directions.

Start at

√4th 693 Dermatitis due to substances taken internally

Be certain to read the EXCLUDES note carefully. Did you notice the first one that states

EXCLUDES adverse effect NOS of drugs and medicines (995.20)

Whitney had an adverse effect of a drug, but this notation does not apply to her case because of the NOS included there. You should remember that NOS stands for Not Otherwise Specified. However, Dr. Curtis *did* specify the details of this event. If you are not certain, go ahead and look up the complete code description for 995.20.

995.20 Unspecified adverse effect of unspecified drug, medicinal, and biological substance

This confirms that code 995.20 is not accurate for this encounter between Whitney and Dr. Curtis because you know the specific adverse effect (the rash) and you know the specific drug (the penicillin). So, let's go back to code category 693 and keep reading down the column to review all of the choices for the required fourth digit.

693.0 Dermatitis due to drugs and medicines

Notice that this code also has an EXCLUDES note: EXCLUDES that due to drugs in contact with skin (692.3) Does this apply to Whitney? Go back to the documentation and check. What route of administration was used for this drug? Drugs in contact with skin would relate to a cream or ointment. The scenario does not state that she took the penicillin by mouth; however, it does state "pills" that informs us it was oral medication. So, this EXCLUDES note does not apply to this case.

Hey, did you also notice the directive? *Use additional E code to identify drug.*

But you remembered that already, didn't you? Let's go now to the Table of Drugs and Chemicals and look up penicillin:

Penicillin (any type) . . .

The first column shows the suggested poisoning code. Should you use this code? No. It was neither a poisoning nor a toxic effect; it was an adverse reaction to medication properly prescribed by a physician, used in the correct way by the intended person. So continue moving to the right. It was not an accident, so look at the code in the third column, *Therapeutic use.*

Penicillin (any type) E930.0

Let's check this in the tabular list and begin reading the notations under the heading:

Drugs, medicinal, and biological substances causing adverse effects in therapeutic use (E930-E949)

INCLUDES correct drug properly administered in therapeutic or prophylactic dosage, as the cause of any adverse effect, including allergic or hypersensitivity reactions

As always, check the EXCLUDES notation carefully, also. We are in the right place, so far, so move down the column to

√4th E930 Antibiotics

There's another EXCLUDES notation. Interesting, this time, ICD-9-CM is telling us that we need to know the original reason the antibiotic was prescribed. Read down the column and review the choices for the required fourth digit.

«« KEYS TO CODING

In addition to the term "pills," the terms "tablets," "capsules," or "caplets" would also relate a route of administration that was "by mouth." Or, you can look back in Whitney's chart and look for Dr. Curtis' notes when he first prescribed the penicillin. The route of administration would have certainly been specified then.

E930.0 Drugs, medicinal and biological substances causing adverse effects in therapeutic use, Antibiotics, Penicillins

Excellent. You now have the codes you need to properly report why Whitney was cared for: 693.0 and E930.0. Great job!

Suicide Attempt

BRIDGE TO ICD-10-CM »»

In ICD-10-CM's Table of Drugs and Chemicals, this column is titled *Poisoning Intentional self-harm.*

The fourth column in the Table of Drugs and Chemicals suggests E codes to explain that a poisoning or toxic effect was self-inflicted, also referred to as a *Suicide attempt.* These codes indicate that the overdose or toxic substance was taken with the full intent of causing one's own death.

YOU CODE IT! CASE STUDY

Rudy Gabriel, a 19-year-old male, was found, slumped over his desk, unconscious. Next to him was an empty bottle of secobarbital, recently filled. His roommate, Danny, called the ambulance, and they went to the emergency room. Danny stated that Rudy was very depressed after breaking up with his girlfriend and flunking his final exam in art history. After pumping Rudy's stomach, Dr. Hamilton documented that Rudy had fallen into a coma as a result of this attempt to commit suicide.

You Code It!

Read Dr. Hamilton's notes on his encounter with Rudy. Can you determine the best, most appropriate diagnosis code or codes for this encounter?

Step 1: Read the case completely.

Step 2: Abstract the notes: Which key words can you identify relating to the reason Dr. Hamilton cared for Rudy?

____

Step 3: Query the provider, if necessary.

Step 4: Code the diagnosis or diagnoses.

____

Step 5: Code the procedure(s): Emergency room visit.

Step 6: Link the procedure codes to at least one diagnosis code to confirm medical necessity.

Step 7: Back code to double-check your choices.

KEYS TO CODING »»

You might think you should also include a code that Rudy was unconscious. However, this is included in the coma code. Coma is a persistent state of unconsciousness, so there is no reason to duplicate the information with another code that states relatively the same thing.

Answer

Did you find the correct codes?

967.0 Poisoning by sedatives and hypnotics, barbiturates

780.01 Alteration of consciousness, coma

E950.1 Suicide and self-inflicted poisoning, barbiturates

Great!

Assault

The fifth column in the Table of Drugs and Chemicals suggests E codes to explain that a poisoning or toxic effect was done to intentionally cause harm to someone. The codes found in the *Assault* column specify that a person purposely poisoned the patient with the intention of inflicting illness, injury, or death. It implies attempted murder.

BRIDGE TO ICD-10-CM

In ICD-10-CM's Table of Drugs and Chemicals, this column is titled *Poisoning Assault.*

YOU CODE IT! CASE STUDY

Feeling nauseous and weak, Alma Masters came into Dr. Taylor's office. Alma's skin was unusually pale. After some tests it was determined that her lethargy and nausea were caused by arsenic poisoning. Alma told Dr. Taylor that her marriage was very bad and she suspected that her husband might be trying to kill her, and he had recently bought pesticide containing arsenic. Dr. Taylor documented this as a posioning by assault.

You Code It!

Which diagnosis code or codes will you use to properly report Alma's encounter with Dr. Taylor?

Step 1: Read the case completely.

Step 2: Abstract the notes: Which key words can you identify relating to the reason Dr. Taylor cared for Alma?

____

Step 3: Query the provider, if necessary.

Step 4: Code the diagnosis or diagnoses.

____

Step 5: Code the procedure(s): Office visit, lab tests.

Step 6: Link the procedure codes to at least one diagnosis code to confirm medical necessity.

Step 7: Back code to double-check your choices.

Answer

Did you find the correct codes?

985.1 Toxic effect of other metals, arsenic and its compounds

787.02 Nausea alone

780.79 Malaise and fatigue, other malaise and fatigue, lethargy

E962.1 Assault by poisoning, other solid and liquid substances

Terrific!

Undetermined

This is a bit different than "unspecified," which means the physician may know but didn't document the detail. The codes from the *Undetermined*

BRIDGE TO ICD-10-CM

In ICD-10-CM's Table of Drugs and Chemicals, this column is titled *Poisoning Undetermined.*

column are to be used only if the record does not state what caused the poisoning, most often because this information is just not yet known. The code might arise if, for example, the patient is unconscious and it cannot be determined how or why the poisoning happened. Remember, the detail missing here is the why—the intent—of the poisoning. You must be careful to never assume. It might appear that a child was abused (assault); however, it really could have been an accident. Sometimes, an investigation may need to occur before the intention can be determined.

YOU CODE IT! CASE STUDY

Benito Vanelli, an 86-year-old male, was brought into the emergency room by ambulance from his home. He was weak and disoriented, and his skin was pale and clammy. Dr. Jackson ran some blood tests and determined that Benito's symptoms were caused by dehydration. The dehydration was caused by an overdose of Lasix. However, because of Benito's altered mental state, no one can determine whether the overdose was an attempted suicide, an accident because he had forgotten that he had taken his regular dose, or if someone was trying to kill him.

You Code It!

Benito's situation is very sad. Which diagnosis codes will you use to report his encounter with Dr. Jackson?

Step 1: Read the case completely.

Step 2: Abstract the notes: Which key words can you identify relating to why Dr. Jackson cared for Benito?

Step 3: Query the provider, if necessary.

Step 4: Code the diagnosis or diagnoses.

Step 5: Code the procedure(s): ED visit, blood tests.

Step 6: Link the procedure codes to at least one diagnosis code to confirm medical necessity.

Step 7: Back code to double-check your choices.

BRIDGE TO ICD-10-CM

ICD-10-CM adds an additional category to this section of reporting, titled *Underdosing*. This is identified with the sixth character, and has its own column on the Table of Drugs and Chemicals.

ICD-10-CM EXAMPLE

A patient is told to take acetaminophen by his doctor.

The patient has an adverse effect (breaks out in a rash); this is reported with code T39.1×5.

The patient takes only half the dosage and still has pain; this is reported with code T39.1×6.

Answer

Did you find the correct codes?

974.4 Poisoning by other diuretics

276.51 Dehydration

E980.4 Poisoning by other specified drugs and medicinal substances, injury undetermined whether accidentally or purposely inflicted.

Good job!

SUBSTANCE INTERACTIONS

When the cause of the poisoning or toxic effect is the **interaction** between two substances (e.g., drugs and alcohol), then you will need to report both substances involved.

You will need one poisoning code for *each* substance causing the reaction, one or more codes to accurately report the effect of the interaction, and one E code to report the intent for *each* substance.

Interaction

The mixture of two or more substances that change the effect of any of the individual substances.

««« CODING TIP

Double up your codes to report a substance interaction: P.P.E.E.E.

LET'S CODE IT! SCENARIO

Meryl Brighton was prescribed Zyprexa (olanzapine), a psychotropic, by her psychiatrist Dr. Cauldwell, for treatment of her bipolar disorder. Meryl mentioned that her family doctor, Dr. Wall, had her on Norvasc (amlodipine), an antihypertensive, for her high blood pressure. Dr. Cauldwell told Meryl to stop taking the Norvasc while on the Zyprexa. Meryl forgot and took both medicines at the same time. Suffering a dangerous case of severe hypotension, she was rushed to the ED by ambulance.

Let's Code It!

Meryl was diagnosed with *severe hypotension* as a *result of taking both Zyprexa and Norvasc.* She was told *not* to take both medications, but she did anyway. It means that you need to code the incident as a poisoning because that was not the way the drug was prescribed by her physician.

First, you will need your poison codes—one for Zyprexa and one for Norvasc. Let's begin with the Zyprexa. You know three ways to look the medication up in the Table of Drugs and Chemicals:

1. By brand name: Zyprexa
2. By chemical name: olanzapine
3. By drug category: psychotropic

Neither Zyprexa nor olanzapine are shown in the table; however, you will find a listing for

Psychotropic agents
    Specified NEC

Use the codes on the line for *Specified psychotropic agents NEC,* because the physician did specify which drug Meryl took; it is just not elsewhere classified. The suggested code to report that Meryl was poisoned by Zyprexa is 969.8.

Turn to the tabular list, and check the complete code description: Begin with

√4th 969 Poisoning by psychotropic agents

Read the EXCLUDES note carefully. It doesn't apply to this case. Did you notice that this code does require a fourth digit? Keep reading down

««« KEYS TO CODING

Interactions can occur between two or more drugs, drugs and alcohol or other drinks, drugs and food, or many other combinations. For example, you might notice a warning "Don't take this drug with milk or other dairy products." This is a warning provided to prevent an interaction.

the column, carefully considering all the other codes to find the most accurate.

969.8 Poisoning by psychotropic agents, other specified psychotropic agents

Return to the Table of Drugs and Chemicals. On the same line, find the suggested E code for reporting that Meryl took it accidentally. Remember, she forgot the physician's instructions. Find and confirm it in the tabular list.

Start reading at

√4th E854 Accidental poisoning by other psychotropic agents

There are no notations or directives, so keep reading through all of the fourth digit choices including their descriptions. You will find that the most accurate code is

E854.8 Accidental poisoning by other psychotropic agents

Good work. Now, YOU CODE IT! and find the poisoning code and the E codes to report that Meryl was also poisoned by the Norvasc. Again, you know the three ways to look this up on the Table of Drugs and Chemicals:

1. By brand name: Norvasc
2. By chemical name: amlodipine
3. By drug category: antihypertensive

Look it up on the table, and confirm the codes in the tabular list. Did you find

972.6 Poisoning by agents primarily affecting the cardiovascular system, other antihypertensive agents

E858.3 Accidental poisoning by agents primarily affecting cardiovascular system

Excellent! Now, you need one more—the code for the effect, or reaction, that this drug interaction had on Meryl. What was the diagnosis for Meryl when she was taken to the ED? Severe hypotension. (Read carefully, since this is *hypo*tension, not *hyper*tension.)

Turn to the alphabetic index and find

Hypotension (arterial) (constitutional) 458.9

Go to the tabular list and begin reading at

√4th 458 Hypotension

You can see that this code includes hypopiesis and EXCLUDES several conditions that are not relevant to this case. Therefore, read down the column to determine the most accurate code description. Did you go right to the code suggested by the alphabetic index?

458.9 Hypotension, unspecified

Before you choose this, read the description for the code directly above 458.9.

458.8 Other specified hypotension

Code 458.8 is more accurate because the notes *do* indicate that Meryl's hypotension was caused by the poisoning—and that is a specific detail that cannot be described by any other code.

You now have five codes for this encounter. Let's put them in the correct order. Remember the tip: P. P. E. E. E. First, you will need to list the poisoning codes. The order does not matter.

969.8 Poisoning by psychotropic agents, other specified psychotropic agents

972.6 Poisoning by agents primarily affecting the cardiovascular system, other antihypertensive agents

Next, you will need to report the effect of the poisoning—hypotension.

458.8 Other specified hypotension

Now, report the two E codes to indicate the intent of the poisoning—accidental . . . one for each of the medications involved in the interaction.

E858.3 Accidental poisoning by agents primarily affecting cardiovascular system

E854.8 Accidental poisoning by other psychotropic agents

You remember that your last reported code will be the place of occurrence code. In this case,

E849.0 Place of occurrence, home

Great! You've coded a substance interaction.

««« **BRIDGE TO ICD-10-CM**

The guidelines for reporting drug or substance interactions remain the same for ICD-10-CM.

««« **BRIDGE TO ICD-10-CM**

Remember that it will be the seventh (7th) character of the code that will report a late effect, also known as sequela. "Late effects are reported using the seventh character extension "S" for sequela. These codes should be used with any report of a late effect or sequela resulting from a previous injury."

LATE EFFECTS OF POISONINGS

The late effects of an adverse effect, a poisoning, or a toxic effect can be troublesome for patients and require additional care. Remember to PaCE the late effects of an injury or poisoning being treated. Refer to Chap. 2 if you need a review on how to code such situations.

SEQUENCING OF CODES

For Poisonings

The coding tip "P.E.E. is for Poison" is also a memory tip to remember the sequence of the codes: First-listed: the Poisoning code, followed by the code or codes for the Effect the poison had on the patient. Last, the E code or codes to report the intent of the poisoning.

For Adverse Effects

Remember that there is no P (poisoning code) in adverse effect; therefore, your first-listed code or codes are those that report the Effect the medication had on the patient—the unexpected adverse reaction of the patient, followed by the E code to report the drug was being taken therapeutically.

«« **KEYS TO CODING**

PaCE the coding of the late effect of an injury or poisoning:

P stands for Problem being treated (scarring, mental retardation, paralysis, etc.)

C stands for Cause—the late effect code identifying the original injury or poisoning from the 905-909 range

E stands for the External cause—the E code—used to report the late effect of how the original poisoning occurred (specific E late effects codes). For example: E929.2 Late effect of accidental poisoning

«« **KEYS TO CODING**

E codes can *never, never, never* be listed first, or alone.

BRIDGE TO ICD-10-CM

The guidelines will tell you "A code from categories T36-T65 is sequenced first, followed by the code(s) that specify the nature of the adverse effect, poisoning, or toxic effect." (Note: This sequencing instruction does not apply to underdosing codes [fifth or sixth character "6" for example T36.0x6-].) Codes for underdosing should never be assigned as principal or first-listed codes. If a patient has a relapse or exacerbation of the medical condition for which the drug is prescribed because of the reduction in dose, then the medical condition itself should be coded.

CHAPTER SUMMARY

Individuals can come into contact with a substance that disagrees with their body chemistry for many reasons. An allergic reaction, accidentally taking too many pills, depression leading to a suicide attempt, environmental factors—any of these and more can cause a person to suffer a health-related incident.

Adverse effects, poisonings, and toxic effects can be very serious to the health of an individual. Complex chemical interactions in the human body equate to complex coding processes to accurately report what has happened. Remember the tips you learned: P.E.E. is for poison, and there is no P in adverse reaction! These cute sayings can help you ensure that all the important information is coded.

Chapter 6 Review
Coding Poisonings and Adverse Reactions

1. Thinking they are candy, Bobby eats a whole bottle of Grandma's blood pressure pills. This is an example of a(n)
   a. Poisoning.
   b. Adverse effect.
   c. Toxic effect.
   d. Late effect.

2. To properly code a poisoning, you need at least one code to report each of these except
   a. Quantity of the poison.
   b. E code to report intent.
   c. Poisoning code.
   d. Code to identify the effect of the poison.

3. Drugs and chemicals are listed on the table in all of these manners except
   a. The brand name.
   b. The chemical name.
   c. The drug category.
   d. The size of the dose.

4. The columns in the ICD-9-CM Table of Drugs and Chemicals include
   a. Suicide attempt.
   b. Malignant.
   c. Toxin.
   d. Adverse effect.

5. An adverse effect will use an E code from the ICD-9-CM Table of Drugs and Chemicals' column titled
   a. Unspecified.
   b. Poison.
   c. Accident.
   d. Therapeutic use.

6. A substance interaction will require at least ________________ codes.
   a. One
   b. Five
   c. Three
   d. Six

7. An example of a brand name of a drug is
   a. Antacid.
   b. Sedative.
   c. Tylenol.
   d. Barbiturate.

8. The Table of Drugs and Chemicals does not include a specific listing for
   a. Lettuce opium.
   b. Adhesives.
   c. Marsh gas.
   d. Vodka.

9. An example of a toxin is
   a. Asbestos.
   b. Penicillin.
   c. Wasp sting.
   d. Rolaids.

10. Raymond has shortness of breath and heart palpitations after accidentally taking his wife's heart medicine. The first-listed code will be
   a. The code for shortness of breath.
   b. The code for heart palpitations.
   c. The code for poisoning.
   d. The E code for accidental use.

YOU CODE IT! Practice

CHAPTER 6. Coding Poisonings and Adverse Reactions

1. Billy Selas, a 3-year-old male, was brought into the ED in a coma, a result of his accidentally ingesting his mother's oral contraceptives.

____

2. Karen Anne Washington, a 6-year-old female, was brought into her pediatrician's office because of having trouble swallowing. Dr. Lakemont determined she had stricture of the esophagus due to her father giving her lye to drink.

____

3. Maurice Goodwin, a 4-year-old male, was carried into the ED, listless. Blood tests show that he was poisoned by eating the lead paint off the windowsill in his parents' garage.

____

4. Roger Dennis, a 43-year-old male, was found unconscious in his car. The garage door was closed, and the motor was running. At the emergency room, Dr. Lexington determined that Roger was in a coma due to carbon monoxide poisoning. Paramedics found a suicide note next to Roger on the seat of the car.

____

5. Belle Delong, a 16-year-old female, was diagnosed with a vitamin deficiency due to an overdose of laxatives. She was trying to lose weight for the prom and didn't realize the potential hazards.

____

6. Edward Webber, a 63-year-old male, was at the medical center when he suffered a terrible attack of vertigo after being injected with dye for an intravenous pyelogram that his physician ordered.

____

7. Jeannette Lyman, a 33-year-old female, was having trouble with her stomach. Dr. Trevani diagnosed her with acute gastritis due to accidental overdose of Motrin.

____

8. Jay Royce, a 45-year-old male, went into cardiac arrest, caused by an accidental overdose of digoxin.

____

9. Dr. Lyles prescribed Tylenol with codeine for Jeannette Witsil. As a result, she suffered a localized edema.

____

10. Hector Rivera, a lawn care technician, was at work when he experienced respiratory distress after inhaling insecticide.

____

11. Paula Lewis misunderstood the instructions for her prescription of lisinopril. She took too many and went into cardiac arrest.

____

12. Jack Beasley had not slept in over a week. He accidentally overdosed on Sominex and came in suffering from nausea and vomiting.

____

13. Hailey Siegel, a 3-year-old female, was diagnosed with acute gastritis with hemorrhage, resulting from an accidental overdose of iron tablets.

____

14. Gray Norman fell into a coma as a result of an overdose of Sinequan.

____

15. Alana Lee is suffering from an electrolyte imbalance due to her intentional overdose of furosemide.

____

YOU CODE IT! Simulation

Chapter 6. Coding Poisonings and Adverse Reactions

On the following pages, you will see physicians' notes documenting encounters with patients at our textbook's health care facility, Taylor, Reader, & Associates. Carefully read through the notes, and find the best ICD-9-CM diagnosis codes for each case.

KEYS TO CODING »»

The fifth digit zero states "unspecified site" in its description. Use this VERY, VERY rarely. Think about it . . . how can a physician diagnose and treat a burn and not know exactly where it is?

2 foot

3 ankle

4 lower leg

5 knee

6 thigh (any part)

9 multiple sites of lower limb(s)

Example

Crystal Vasquez accidentally dropped a pot of boiling water on the floor, and the water splashed up and caused a second-degree burn on her foot.

945 Burn of lower limb

945.2 Burn of lower limb, blisters (second degree)

945.22 Burn of lower limb, blisters (second degree), foot

With one code, 945.22, you can tell the entire, specific story about Crystal's burn.

LET'S CODE IT! SCENARIO

Julian Ingles, a 15-year-old male, was working on a school project in the basement and accidentally released hot glue onto the palm of his hand. Dr. Tremont treated him for third-degree burns to the palm of his left hand.

Let's Code It!

Julian was diagnosed *with third-degree burns to his palm.* Let's turn to the alphabetic index and look up burns:

Burn

palm(s) 944.05

Turn to the tabular list, and read:

√4th 944 Burn of wrist(s) and hand(s)

There are no notations or directives, so read through your choices for the fourth digit.

√5th 944.3 Burn of wrist(s) and hand(s); full-thickness skin loss (third degree NOS)

That is much more specific and accurate. Now you have to review the fifth-digit choices for code 944. Did you notice that there is a digit to specify that the burn was on his palm? So the complete code to explain why Dr. Tremont treated Julian at this encounter is . . .

944.35 Burn of wrist(s) and hand(s); full-thickness skin loss (third degree NOS); palm

This code tells the complete story!

Multiple Burns

When you are coding one patient with multiple burns, you first must identify the anatomical site for each burn documented.

Determine the Category for Each Site

When reporting a patient with burns on multiple anatomical sites, you first need to identify the sites and determine which anatomical site groupings they fall into, as identified by ICD-9-CM code categories. Go through the documentation and align each reported site with a code category:

940 Eye and adnexa

941 Face, head, and neck

942 Trunk (including breast, chest wall, abdominal wall, back and buttock, and genitalia)

943 Upper limb (except wrist and hand)

944 Wrist and hand

945 Lower limb (including toes, foot, ankle, lower leg, knee, and thigh)

947 Internal organs (including mouth, pharynx, larynx, trachea, lung, esophagus, gastrointestinal track, vagina and uterus, and other)

Multiple Sites Fall Into Different Code Categories

When the various sites fall into different code categories, you will report one code for each burn. Sequence them with the most severe burn (determined by severity) listed first, following all other codes in decreasing order of severity.

Example

Madeline had a third-degree burn on the back of her right hand and a second-degree burn on her right forearm.

The burn on her hand is coded from the 944 code category, and the burn on her arm is coded from the 943 code category. Therefore, you will use both codes to completely report Madeline's injuries.

A third-degree burn is more severe than a second-degree burn, so you will report the two codes in this order:

944.36 Burn of hand, full-thickness skin loss (third-degree), back of hand

943.21 Burn of upper limb, blisters, epidermal loss (second-degree), forearm

Multiple Sites Fall Into the Same Code Category

When various sites fall into the same code category (the first three numbers of the code), you will report all of these sites with just one code.

If the burns are of different severity, use the fourth-digit that reports the *most severe* burn (determined by severity), the highest degree.

Then, identify that more than one specific site has been burned by using the fifth digit that reports "multiple sites."

«« KEYS TO CODING

Review the **ICD-9-CM Coding Guidelines, Section I. chapter 17. Injury and Poisoning (800-999),** subsection **c. Coding of burns, part 5 Assign separate codes for each burn site** and **part 1 Sequencing of burn and related condition codes** for more input on identifying what to code, what not to code, and in what order to put multiple codes. Use this to support your reading here, and as a reminder booster later on.

«« KEYS TO CODING

Review the **ICD-9-CM Coding Guidelines, Section I. chapter 17. Injury and Poisoning (800-999),** subsection **c. Coding of burns, part 2 Burns of the same local site** for more input on identifying what to code, what not to code, and in what order to put multiple codes. Use this to support your reading here, and as a reminder booster later on.

LET'S CODE IT! SCENARIO

Frank had a third-degree burn on his chin and second-degree burns on his nose and cheek.

Let's Code It!

KEYS TO CODING »»

The natural question you will ask now is, "Why not use a code from 946 Burns of multiple specified sites?"

I know this doesn't make sense, but here it is. The official guidelines, **Section I. chapter 17. Injury and Poisoning (800-999),** subsection **c. Coding of burns, 5. Assign separate codes for each burn site,** instruct you to use 946 "only when the location of the burns are not documented." The description of the category uses the word *specified,* and the instructions tell you to use this only when the sites are *not specified.* However, that is the guideline.

Let's begin by abstracting Frank's condition. He has:

3rd degree burn on his chin
2nd degree burn on his nose
2nd degree burn on his cheek

In the alphabetic index, turn to the term *burn.* You will notice that the long, long list of terms indented beneath this main term all identify anatomical sites, the location on the body that has been burned. Find the suggested codes for all three of Frank's burns:

Burn, chin, third-degree 941.34
Burn, nose, second-degree 941.25
Burn, cheek, second-degree 941.27

Notice that the code category 941 is the same for all three sites: chin, nose, and cheek. Therefore, you use only one code to report these burn sites. Turn to code 941 in the tabular list:

√4th 941 Burn of face, head, and neck

The only excluded diagnosis is a burn of the mouth. Frank's mouth has not been affected, so you need to read down the column to review all of the choices for the required fourth-digit. Now, you need to determine which 4th digit to use. The burn on his chin is a third-degree burn [4th digit = 3] but the burns on his nose and cheek are only second-degree burns [4th digit = 2]. Should you report both? The guidelines direct you to report only one code . . . with the fourth digit that reports the MOST SEVERE of all of these burns, so you need to use the fourth digit of 3.

√5th 941.3 Burn of face, head, and neck, full-thickness skin loss (third degree NOS)

Read up the column to the box below 941 to review your choices for the required fifth digit.

The fifth digit 4 reports his chin was burned.
The fifth digit 5 reports his nose was burned
The fifth digit 8 reports his neck was burned.

Again, the guidelines tell you that you must combine these all into one accurate code. Take a look at the fifth digit 9 that reports multiple sites of face, head, and neck. Perfect.

Put it all together and get the most accurate code that tells the whole story:

941.39 Burn of face, head, and neck, full-thickness skin loss (third-degree), multiple sites

(NOTE: You may remember from chapter 2 that you will need E codes to report how Frank became burned and where he was when he got burned. This exercise is designed to focus on the guidelines for reporting burns, so we are going to skip these codes, here. You can practice this on your own.)

Extent

The next code you have to report is the **extent**, or percentage, of the body involved.

The three-digit category for reporting the extent of a burn is 948. This code requires a total of five digits to be valid no matter what the extent of the burn. Turn to code 948 in the tabular list.

√4th 948 Burns classified according to extent of body surface involved

The required *fourth digit* will identify the percentage of the patient's *entire body* that is affected by any and all burns, of all degrees (severity). The code descriptions describe this as *percentage of body surface, also known as TBSA (total body surface area).*

The percentages may be specified by the physician in his or her notes. Statements like, "third-degree burns over 10% of the body" or "7% of the body burned" will give you the information you need to find the correct fourth digit for code 948. However, other times, the physician may not use a number, and you will have to calculate the percentage yourself. To do this you can use the rule of nines.

The **rule of nines** is used to estimate the total body surface area (TBSA) that has been affected by the burns. The body is divided into sections, each section representing 9% of the human body (see Fig. 7-2).

Head and neck 9%
Arm, right 9%
Arm, left 9%
Chest 9%
Abdomen 9%
Upper back 9%
Lower back 9%
Leg, right, anterior (front) 9%
Leg, right, posterior (back) 9%
Leg, left, anterior (front) 9%
Leg, right, posterior (back) 9%
Genitalia 1%

As you read through the physician's notes, be aware of the anatomical site, not only for your site code but so that you can use the information to calculate the extent of the body involved in the burns.

Example

Alice was burned on her lower back and the back of her left leg.

Lower back (9%) + left leg, back (9%) = total body surface (18%)

√5th 948.1 Burns extent of body surface, 10–19 percent of body surface

Extent

The percentage of the body that has been affected by the burn.

Rule of nines

A general division of the whole body portioned out to represent 9 percent used for estimating the extent of a burn.

«« KEYS TO CODING

Reporting a burn to a patient's eye, adnexa, or internal organ does not require an extent code (948) because the surface is already a limited area.

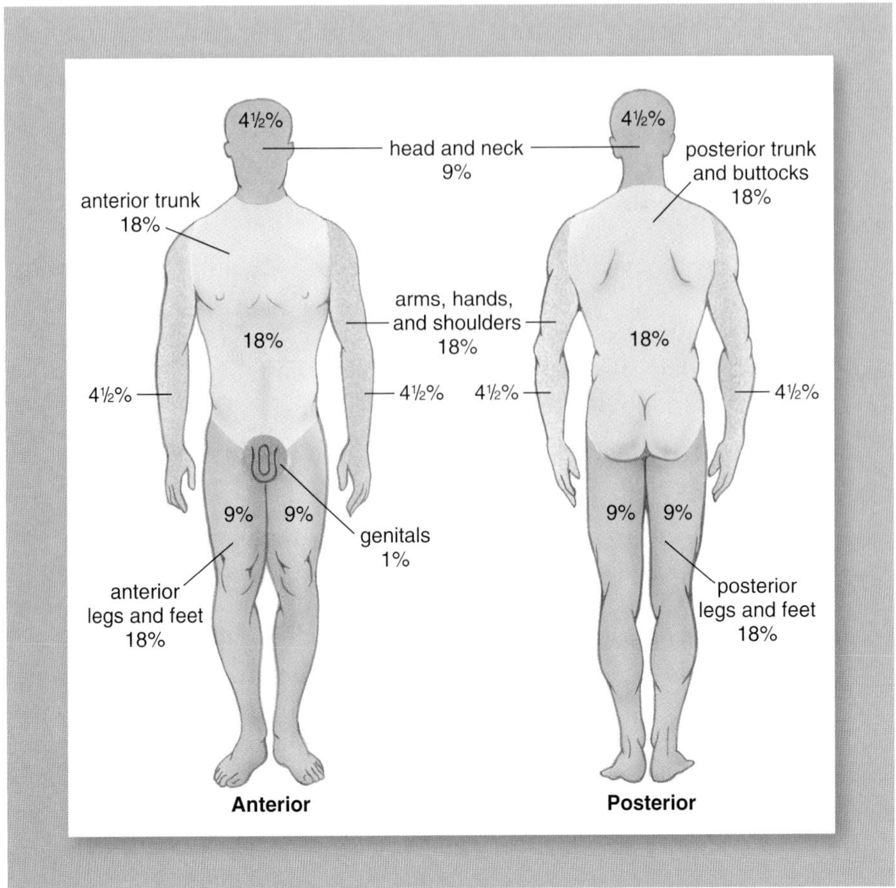

Figure 7-2 Using the Rule of Nines to Estimate the Extent of Burns.

Next, you must determine the most accurate fifth digit for this code. The *fifth digit* identifies the percentage of the patient's body that is *suffering with third-degree burns* only. You can also use the rule of nines to calculate the percentage of area affected by third-degree burns to find the best fifth digit.

KEYS TO CODING »»

For code category 948 make the following calculations:

4th digit = calculation of TBSA for ALL degrees of burns affecting the body

5th digit = calculation of TBSA for ONLY 3rd degree burns affecting the body

Example

Gregory had third-degree burns on his right arm and second-degree burns on the front of his right leg.

Right arm (9%) + right leg, front (9%) = total body surface (18%)

√5th 948.1 Burns extent of body surface, 10–19 percent of body surface

Third degree, right arm (9%) = total third-degree (9%)

948.10 Burns extent of body surface, 10–19 percent of body surface, less than 10 percent with third degree

Of course, these percentages are general—to be used for estimation purposes. As you look at the code descriptions for the fourth and the fifth digits, you will see that choices for code 948 all have descriptors that only require you to know the percentage of the body involved within a 10% range. Therefore, you don't have to worry too much about narrowing down the number.

When you are determining the fourth and fifth digits for code 948, you may have to add the percentages for several anatomical sites together. While everyone knows that the rule of nines is an estimation and not expected to be precise, it is a professional coder's job to be as specific as possible. Therefore, you want to adjust the percentage, as appropriate.

Example

The right arm is estimated at 9%. That is the entire arm.

If only a patient's upper arm is burned, you can estimate that to be 4.5%; from the elbow to the wrist would be estimated at 3% and the hand estimated at 1.5%. You can understand that if only both forearms were burned, it would not be accurate to report that 18% of the patient's body was burned; you would consider the burn to be 6%.

CODING TIP

If a patient does not have *any* third-degree burns, then the fifth digit is zero.

BRIDGE TO ICD-10-CM

In ICD-10-CM, code categories T31 and T32 report the extent of the body burned, just as code category 948 does. You will continue to use the rule of nines to calculate the TBSA.

LET'S CODE IT! SCENARIO

Arthur Bucholtz, a 28-year-old male, was trying to start a campfire when the flames flared and burned him on his right hand, right forearm, and right elbow. He was rushed to the emergency room, where Dr. Mathers determined that he had third-degree burns on his hand and forarm and second-degree burns on his elbow.

Let's Code It!

Dr. Mathers diagnosed Arthur with *third-degree burns* on his *hand and forearm* and *second-degree burns* on his *elbow.* Go to the alphabetic index, and look up *burn* and go down the indented list to find each site burned:

Burn, hand, third degree 944.30

Burn, forearm, third degree 943.31

Burn, elbow, second degree 943.22

Does the tabular list confirm the codes? Let's check each one:

√4th 944 Burn of wrist(s) and hand(s)

You can see that a fourth digit is required, so read down the column to

√5th 944.3 Burn of hand, full-thickness skin loss (third degree NOS)

The burns on Arthur's hand were documented as third-degree, so that is correct. Now, you need to determine the required fifth digit. Read up to the box containing all of the fifth-digit choices and review them all.

944.30 Burn of hand, full-thickness skin loss (third degree NOS), hand unspecified site

This code tells the whole story about the burn to Arthur's hand. Now, look at the other codes suggested by the alphabetic index.

Burn, forearm, third degree 943.31

Burn, elbow, second degree 943.22

8 Coding Musculoskeletal Conditions

KEY TERMS

- Aftercare
- Cartilage
- Closed fracture
- Dislocation
- Fracture
- Malunion
- Nonunion
- Open fracture
- Pathologic
- Sprain
- Subluxation

LEARNING OUTCOMES

8.1 Distinguish between a fracture and a dislocation.

8.2 Determine if a fracture is open or closed.

8.3 Identify the appropriate segment of anatomical site involved.

8.4 Differentiate between pathological, spontaneous, and stress fractures.

8.5 Apply the guidelines for coding late effects of fractures.

8.6 Discern between an open and closed dislocation.

The human body is made up of 206 bones and a network of muscles, ligaments, tendons, and connective tissues—the components of the musculoskeletal system.

Conditions that affect the musculoskeletal system, such as a **fracture** (of **cartilage** or bone) or **dislocation,** can dramatically affect an individual's quality of life. Activities and functions—walking, sitting, standing—are all accomplished by the use of one's bones, muscles, and ligaments. As a professional coding specialist, it is important to understand the coding guidelines and conventions relating to conditions of the musculoskeletal system in general, and orthopedics—the medical specialty that concentrates on treating deformities and disorders of bone structure and associated muscles and ligaments.

Fracture

Broken cartilage or bone.

Cartilage

Tough, connective, nonvascular tissue.

Dislocation

The displacement of a limb, bone, or organ from its customary position.

CONGENITAL MUSCULOSKELETAL CONDITIONS

As the human body develops during gestation, problems can occur with the formation of a baby's bones. Some of the most common conditions include

- Clubfoot
- Developmental dysplasia of the hip
- Muscular dystrophy

You will learn how to code congenital conditions in Chap. 10 of this textbook.

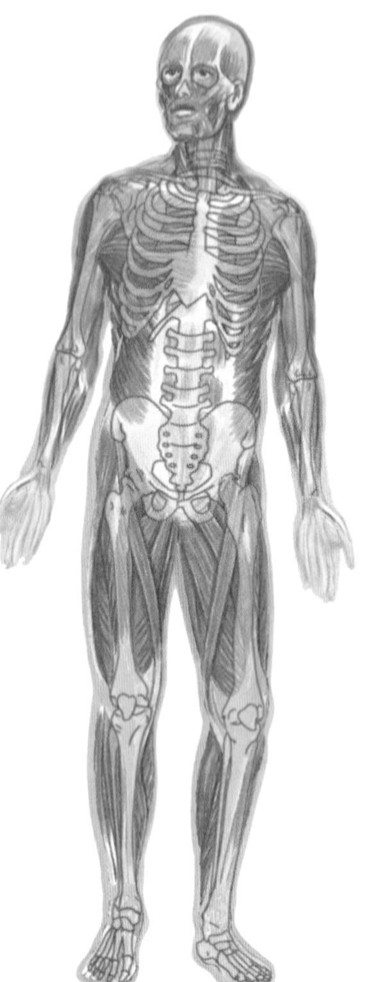

CODING TRAUMATIC FRACTURES

When a patient is diagnosed with a traumatic fracture, you need to know certain important elements in order to code the fracture properly. Think of *S.O/C.S. + E.* (pronounced *socks-ee*) for *s*ite, *o*pen/*c*losed, *s*egment, and *e* code. (See Fig. 8-1.)

S stands for Site—which anatomical site was fractured

O/C stands for Open or Closed . . . is the fracture diagnosed as an open fracture or a closed fracture

S stands for Segment—which segment of the specific bone was fractured.

\+

E stands for the E code—how did the patient become injured and where (at what location was the patient when he or she became injured).

This acronym can help you remember what details you will need to gather from the documentation to determine the correct code. When reporting traumatic fractures, each specific site is coded individually.

«« KEYS TO CODING

Review the **ICD-9-CM Coding Guidelines, Section I. chapter 17. Injury and Poisoning (800-999),** subsection **b. Coding of traumatic fractures** for more input on identifying what to code, what not to code, and in what order to put multiple codes. Use this to support your reading here, and as a reminder booster later on.

Site

First, you must know which bone has been fractured. The first three digits (the code category) of the diagnosis code identify the general anatomical site.

Fracture of skull, 800–804

Fracture of neck and trunk, 805–809

Fracture of upper limb, 810–819

Fracture of lower limb, 820–829

Open or Closed

Next, to choose the correct fourth digit of the code you will need to know whether it is an **open fracture** or a **closed fracture.** The physician's notes may use one of the following alternate terms for an open fracture:

- Compound
- Infected

Open fracture

A fracture in which the broken bone has protruded through the skin; fracture with a wound.

Closed fracture

A fracture in which the broken bone has not protruded through the skin.

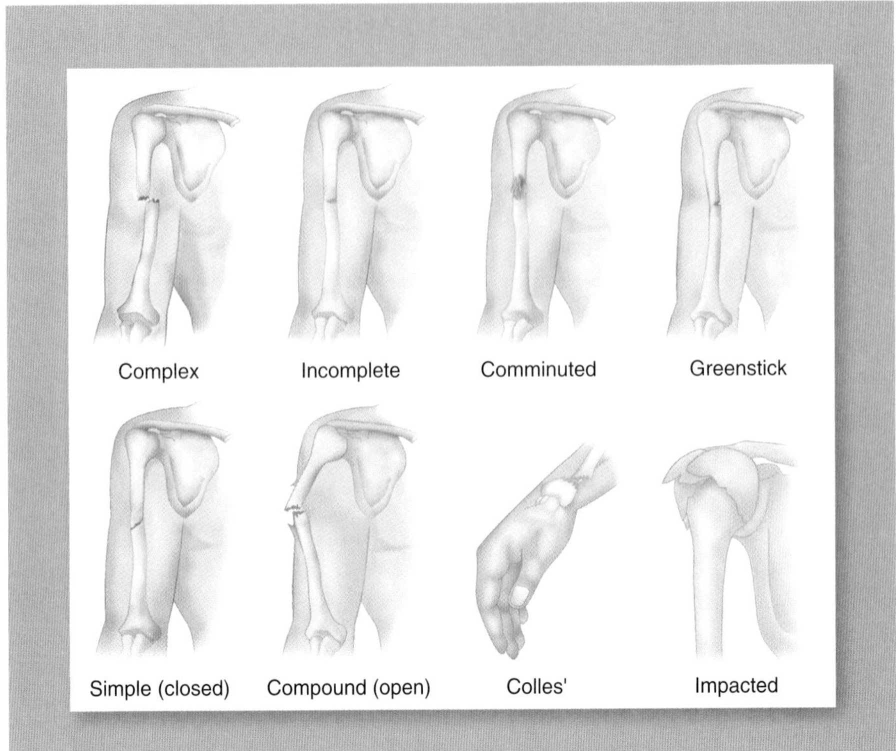

Figure 8-1 Different Types of Fractures.

CODING TIP »»

For fractures, if the documentation does not specify whether the fracture is open or closed, it should be coded as closed. This guideline remains the same in ICD-10-CM.

- Missile
- Puncture
- With foreign body

KEYS TO CODING »»

You don't have to memorize all of these alternate terms for open and closed fractures. Your ICD-9-CM book lists them, along with other coding guidelines, at the beginning of Chapter 17 Injury and Poisoning–right above code category 800.

Example

805.3 Fracture of vertebral column, dorsal [thoracic], open

814.04 Fracture of carpal bone, closed, pisiform

The physician may not always specifically state that the fracture is closed, and instead use one of these alternate terms for a *closed* fracture:

- Comminuted
- Depressed
- Elevated
- Fissured
- Fracture NOS
- Greenstick
- Impacted
- Linear
- Simple
- Slipped epiphysis
- Spiral

KEYS TO CODING »»

"Unspecified" should rarely be used. Check the report from the radiologist, and/or query the doctor first. Think about it . . . how can a physician diagnose and treat a fracture and not know where the fracture is located?

Segment

Depending upon the code category, the fourth or the fifth digit will be determined by the specific portion, or segment, of the bone that was fractured. The terms used to describe the bone segment may include

- Condyle, supracondylar, lateral condyle, medial condyle
- Coronoid process, olecranon process
- Ramus
- Symphysis
- Intracranial, subarachnoid, subdural, extradural
- Cervical, dorsal, lumbar, sacrum
- Acetabulum, pubis, ilium
- Upper end, shaft, surgical neck, anatomical neck
- Unspecified

Example

821.21 Fracture of femur, lower end, closed, condyle, femoral

812.31 Fracture of humerus, shaft, open, shaft of humerus

E Code

As you learned in Chap. 2, whenever a patient suffers an injury, you have to assign an E code to explain how and where the injury happened.

««« KEYS TO CODING

If you are not certain which term applies to the segment of the bone, begin with the code category (the three digit subsection), and then review all of the choices within. This will help you know what term to look for in the notes. For example, you know right away from the notes that the patient's humerus (bone between the shoulder and the elbow) was fractured, but what term would identify the "segment" of the bone?

812 Fracture of humerus

812.0 Upper end

812.1 Upper end

812.2 Shaft or unspecified part

812.3 Shaft or unspecified part

812.4 Lower end

812.5 Lower end

Now, you can go back to the documentation and look for the term "upper end," "shaft," or "lower end" to know which fourth digit to use.

LET'S CODE IT! SCENARIO

Calvin Clyde, a 16-year-old male, was tackled during a football game. His leg twisted when he fell to the ground, and he was brought to the emergency room (ER) by his father. Dr. Baker looked at the x-rays and determined that Calvin had a closed fracture of the fibular shaft. A thigh-to-toe cast was applied, and Calvin was sent home.

Let's Code It!

Dr. Baker diagnosed Calvin with *a closed fracture of the fibular shaft.* Let's use our acronym for coding fractures: S.O/C.S. + E. When you read Dr. Baker's notes, you can answer the questions:

Site = fibula
Open/Closed = closed
Segment = shaft
+
E = tackled in a football game

Turn to the alphabetic index and look up:

Fracture, Fibula, Shaft 823.21

BRIDGE TO ICD-10-CM

The guidelines for reporting a traumatic fracture in ICD-10-CM remain the same. However, the ICD-10-CM code will include a seventh character to report whether this is the initial encounter for treatment, a subsequent encounter, or an encounter for treatment of a sequela (late effect).

A initial encounter for closed fracture

B initial encounter for open fracture

D subsequent encounter for fracture with routine healing

G subsequent encounter for fracture with delayed healing

K subsequent encounter for fracture with nonunion

S sequela

Let's turn to the tabular list to confirm this code is the most accurate choice. Begin reading at

√4th 823 Fracture of tibia and fibula

The EXCLUDES notes do not include any diagnosis related to Calvin's diagnosis, so keep reading down the column to find the required fourth digit. To determine this, you need to know what segment of the bone was fractured. Go back to the notes. Dr. Baker wrote the fracture was to Calvin's *"fibular shaft"* so you need to find the fourth digit that reports this fact.

√5th 823.2 Fracture of tibia and fibula, shaft, closed

√5th 823.3 Fracture of tibia and fibula, shaft, open

Is Calvin's fracture open or closed? The notes state he has a *"closed fracture."* Great! Now, you need to read up the column to determine the correct fifth digit. Take a look in the box at your choices.

0 tibia alone

1 fibula alone

2 fibula with tibia

Did Dr. Baker mention any injury to Calvin's tibia in his notes? No. Therefore, the correct fifth digit is 1. Put this all together to get code:

823.21 Fracture of tibia and fibula, shaft, closed, fibula alone

Perfect. Now, you need an E code to explain how this happened. Turn to the E code alphabetic index in volume 2, section 3. According to the notes, Calvin was tackled during a football game. How will you look this up? *Play*—no. *Sports*—no. Try *tackle:*

Tackle in sport E886.0

Check this suggested code in the tabular list of the E codes:

√4th E886 Fall on same level from collision, pushing, or shoving, by or with other person

This code category *excludes* someone who was crushed or pushed by a crowd or human stampede. This does not apply to Calvin's circumstances, so keep reading down the column.

E886.0 In sports (tackles in sports)

There is an EXCLUDES note here directing you to different codes if the patient was "kicked, stepped on, struck by object, in sports." Is this what happened to Calvin? No, the notes state he was tackled and fell to the ground. Therefore, you have found the correct E code for this case.

E886.0 Fall on same level from collision, pushing, or shoving, by or with other person in sports.

Now, you have the codes that will correctly report why Dr. Baker cared for Calvin: 823.21 and E886.0. Good work!

MULTIPLE FRACTURES

In cases where a patient suffers more than one diagnosed fracture, the guidelines instruct you to code each fracture separately. Remember from the beginning of this chapter, "When reporting traumatic fractures, each specific site is coded individually." This is different from the guidelines for coding burns (Chap. 7) when you were directed to combine multiple burns under the same three-digit category into one code. With fractures, each will be represented by its own code, even if it is the same limb or same bone.

Example

Raymond broke his foot. He was diagnosed with a fractured calcaneus and a fractured astragalus.

825.0 Fracture of the calcaneus, closed

825.21 Fracture of the astragalus

«« KEYS TO CODING

Review the **ICD-9-CM Coding Guidelines, Section I. chapter 17. Injury and Poisoning (800-999),** subsection **b. Coding of traumatic fractures, 2. Multiple fractures of same limb and 3. Multiple unilateral or bilateral fractures of same bone** for more input on identifying what to code, what not to code, and in what order to put multiple codes. Use this to support your reading here, and as a reminder booster later on.

Multiple Fracture Combination Category

There are two combination fracture codes listed in the ICD-9-CM:

819 Multiple fractures involving both upper limbs and upper limb with rib(s) and sternum

INCLUDES Arm(s) with rib(s) or sternum

Both arms [any bones]

828 Multiple fractures involving both lower limbs, lower with upper limb, and lower limb(s) with rib(s) and sternum

INCLUDES Arm(s) with leg(s) [any bones]

Both legs [any bones]

Leg(s) with rib(s) or sternum

Note, however, that you are only to use the multiple fracture codes with the following reasons:

1. When the medical record (physician's notes)do not provide enough detail, or specific information, for you to accurately assign a fourth or fifth digit
2. When the reporting form (such as the CMS 1500 claim form) limits the number of codes that you can use to convey the data.

What does this mean? To provide greater clarity, let's use a scenario to illustrate the proper use of either of these codes: 819 and 828.

Dean was playing on the monkey bars and lost his grip, falling to the ground. Dr. Kennison, at the ER, determined that his left clavicle, his humerus, and his wrist were fractured, as well as three left ribs.

1. You don't have enough information in the documentation to specifically and accurately determine a fracture code. To code these fractures, you need more information, including what section of the clavicle, what segment of the humerus, and specifically which carpal bones. The only element of this diagnosis that you can code accurately from what you have in this scenario is the fractured

ribs [807.03 Fracture ribs, closed, three ribs]. This notation is telling you that you can use the one code, 819 Multiple fractures involving upper limb with ribs, rather than all the others because you don't have complete documentation. (Note: In reality, you are responsible for querying the physician to get the specifics to code all of the fractures separately and accurately. This is the more professional and proper way to report these injuries.)

2. There is not enough room on the claim form. The CMS-1500 claim form includes space for up to 4 diagnosis codes, and the UB-04 (CMS-1450) includes form locators to report up to 18 diagnosis or condition codes. You are permitted to use code 819 or 828 to save room. You can see this with our scenario for Dean: individual codes for his clavicle, arm, wrist, and ribs, plus the E codes for how and where he was injured totals six codes. The CMS-1500 claim form only has room for four codes. You can see where using 819 would help you complete this claim form and still tell the whole story.

In any event, if you ever have the occasion to use either code 819 or 828, it is advised that you append a letter of explanation along with the claim to provide the additional details.

KEYS TO CODING »»

Review the **ICD-9-CM Coding Guidelines, Section I. chapter 17. Injury and Poisoning (800-999),** subsection **b. Coding of traumatic fractures, 4. Multiple fracture categories 819 and 828** for more input on identifying what to code, what not to code, and in what order to put multiple codes. Use this to support your reading here, and as a reminder booster later on.

Example

Tasha was on the balcony of her second-floor apartment when she leaned against the railing, which gave way. She fell the two stories and landed on her right side. She suffered a fractured sternum, three fractured ribs, a fractured humerus, a fractured radius, and a fractured ulna. In this case, it would be permissible to use code 819.0 to report the encounter to her insurance carrier—along with E882 Fall from balcony, of course.

KEYS TO CODING »»

Review the **ICD-9-CM Coding Guidelines, Section I. chapter 17. Injury and Poisoning (800-999),** subsection **b. Coding of traumatic fractures, 5. Multiple fractures sequencing** for more input on identifying what to code, what not to code, and in what order to put multiple codes. Use this to support your reading here, and as a reminder booster later on.

Multiple Fracture Code Sequencing

When multiple fractures are treated, the codes should be listed indicating the most severe fracture first, with any other diagnosis codes following in order of decreasing seriousness. When the patient is diagnosed with multiple fractures of an equal severity, list the codes in anatomical order, beginning at the head and continuing in order toward the feet.

Example

Neil has a compound fracture of the neck of the scapula and a simple fracture of the nasal bones. A compound fracture is more severe.

811.13 Fracture of scapula, open, neck of scapula

802.0 Fracture of face bones, nasal bones, closed

Roseanne has a closed fracture of the coccyx and a closed fracture of the T7-T12 vertebrae. These fractures are of equal severity, and the thoracic vertebrae are closer to the head than the coccyx.

805.2 Fracture of vertebral column, without mention of spinal cord injury, dorsal [thoracic], closed

805.6 Fracture of vertebral column, without mention of spinal cord injury, coccyx, closed

KEYS TO CODING »»

Review the **ICD-9-CM Coding Guidelines, Section I. chapter 17. Injury and Poisoning (800-999),** subsection **f. 1. A. Complications of care** for more input on identifying what to code, what not to code, and in what order to put multiple codes. Use this to support your reading here, and as a reminder booster later on.

COMPLICATIONS OF FRACTURES

Most often, complications arising from a fracture are related to a surgical repair of the fracture. These should be reported with the appropriate codes as per the documentation along with a complications code. For example,

998.31 Disruption of internal operation (surgical) wound

OR

707.07 Plaster ulcer, heel

LATE EFFECTS OF FRACTURES

Malunion and **nonunion** are each considered to be a late effect of an earlier fracture. In such cases, you need to follow the appropriate guidelines for coding a late effect (see Chap. 2), even if the physician's notes do not specifically use the words "late effect." Use either code 733.81 Malunion of fracture or 733.82 Nonunion of fracture.

PATHOLOGIC AND SPONTANEOUS FRACTURES

When a fracture is the result of a disease that has weakened the bone structure, rather than caused by an external source (injury), you will *not* code from the Fracture subsection (800–829) but from the fifth-digit choices under 733.1 **Pathologic** fracture. You will choose the appropriate fifth digit based on the anatomical site of the fracture. In such cases, you will not need an E code because no external cause was involved.

STRESS FRACTURES

A stress fracture, also known as a fatigue fracture, is caused by continual weight-bearing actions such as long periods of walking, athletics, or ballet dancing. Physicians believe that a stress fracture occurs when a weakness in the supporting muscle fails to reduce the pressure on the bone. This type of fracture is most often associated with the bones in the leg or foot (codes 733.93, 733.94, and 733.95).

Example

Craig Dillion took up marathon running and developed a stress fracture of the fifth metatarsal of his right foot: code 733.94

AFTERCARE FOR FRACTURES

After the initial treatment for the fracture, whether traumatic, pathologic, or stress-induced, the physician will normally see the patient during the healing process and recovery. This is known as **aftercare.** Typically, the follow-up encounters will involve an adjustment to medication, the change or removal of a cast, or the adjustment or removal of a fixation device.

Malunion

A fractured bone that did not heal correctly; healing of bone that was not in proper position or alignment.

Nonunion

A fractured bone that did not heal back together; no mending or joining together of the broken segments.

«« BRIDGE TO ICD-10-CM

Patients with late effects of a fracture will have their fracture codes include a seventh character:

G subsequent encounter for fracture with delayed healing

K subsequent encounter for fracture with nonunion

S sequela

Pathologic

Related to, or caused by, disease.

«« KEYS TO CODING

Review the **ICD-9-CM Coding Guidelines, Section I. chapter 13. Diseases of Musculoskeletal and Connective Tissue (710-739),** subsection **a. Coding of pathologic fractures** for more input on identifying what to code, what not to code, and in what order to put multiple codes. Use this to support your reading here, and as a reminder booster later on.

«« CODING TIP

Even though there is no "*code underlying disease*" notation with fracture codes, you might want to add a code for the disease or condition to complete the report. Remember, your job is to tell the ***whole story.***

Aftercare

Follow-up monitoring of the patient's condition after the primary treatment has been completed.

KEYS TO CODING »»

When reporting a visit for aftercare of a traumatic fracture, match the documentation to the appropriate code description for the fourth and fifth digits with regard to the reason for the aftercare and which anatomical site was fractured.

All codes within the V54 code category require both fourth and fifth digits, with the sole exception of V54.9 Unspecified orthopedic aftercare.

Review the **ICD-9-CM Coding Guidelines, Section I. chapter 17. Injury and Poisoning (800-999),** subsection **b. Coding of traumatic fractures, 1. Acute fractures vs. aftercare** for more input on identifying what to code, what not to code, and in what order to put multiple codes. Use this to support your reading here, and as a reminder booster later on.

Subluxation

A partial dislocation.

BRIDGE TO ICD-10-CM »»

The guidelines for reporting a patient's pathologic fracture remains the same. However, the code will include a seventh character to provide additional information:

A initial encounter for fracture

D subsequent encounter for fracture with routine healing

G subsequent encounter for fracture with delayed healing

K subsequent encounter for fracture with nonunion

P subsequent encounter for fracture with malunion

S sequela of fracture

Aftercare codes are reported for those encounters between the provider and the patient that take place after the initial treatment for the fracture—the treatment that involved the diagnosis, possible manipulation of the fracture, and placement of the cast or other device. Codes from this V code category reports the routine care during the recovery and healing process. The code will be determined by specifics of the patient's condition and treatment:

V54.0 Aftercare involving internal fixation device

V54.1 Aftercare for healing traumatic fracture

V54.2 Aftercare for healing pathological fracture

V54.8 Other orthopedic aftercare

V54.9 Unspecified orthopedic aftercare

Example

Lamar Dresden broke his right ulna after a fall from the jungle gym. He is here to see Dr. Bowen to get his cast removed. Code V54.12.

DISLOCATIONS

The process of coding a dislocation or **subluxation** is similar to the process for coding a fracture.

The first piece of information you need from the physician's notes is the anatomical *site* of the dislocation. It will bring you to the three-digit category for the diagnosis code.

Example

√4th 831 Dislocation of shoulder

√4th 837 Dislocation of ankle

The next thing you need to know is whether or not the dislocation is *open* or *closed*, just as in the case of a fracture. There are alternate terms used for these descriptors.

An open dislocation may also be termed:

- Compound
- Infected
- With foreign body

A closed dislocation may also be termed:

- Complete
- Dislocation NOS
- Partial
- Simple
- Uncomplicated

The last clinical element that you will need to know is the specific location of the dislocation within the anatomical site area.

Example

Anterior, posterior, inferior

Medial, lateral, obturator

When you put all the components together, you will be able to determine the accurate four- or five-digit code for the diagnosis.

Example

Johanna hurt her wrist. She was diagnosed with a dislocated carpometacarpal.

833	Dislocation of wrist
833.0	Dislocation of wrist, closed
833.04	Dislocation of wrist, closed, carpometacarpal (joint)

PATHOLOGIC DISLOCATION

A dislocation described as pathologic, or spontaneous, indicates that the cause of the dislocation was not an injury but a disease or other biological cause. In such cases, the diagnosis will be coded from the subcategory √5th 718.2 Pathological dislocation and not from any of the codes in the dislocation subsection (830–839). Specification of anatomical site is reported with the fifth digit.

BRIDGE TO ICD-10-CM

As mentioned previously, aftercare will be reported with a seventh character of the fracture code.

The section of ICD-10-CM titled Aftercare Z codes are not permitted to be used for aftercare of an injury.

CODING TIP

If the physician does not specify whether the dislocation is open or closed, you should code the condition as closed.

LET'S CODE IT! SCENARIO

Annette Pringle, a 27-year-old female, was learning to rock climb at her gym. As she was scaling the wall, her foot slipped, and Annette grabbed on with her right hand, pulling something in her shoulder. The severe pain caused her to stop by her physician's office on her way home. Dr. Vega took x-rays and determined that she had an inferior dislocation of the humerus, right side. Dr. Vega put Annette's right arm into a sling and gave her a prescription for a pain reliever.

CODING TIP

In addition to pathologic dislocations, recurrent dislocations and congenital dislocations are coded from three-digit categories different than those reporting an injury.

Let's Code It!

Dr. Vega diagnosed Annette with an *inferior dislocation of the humerus*, right side. Turn to the alphabetic index and look up *dislocation, humerus.* Read down and see:

Dislocation, humerus, proximal, inferior (closed) 831.03

Even though Dr. Vega's notes didn't specify proximal, that was necessary to get to inferior—anatomically. Now, turn to the tabular list and confirm the code.

Start reading at

√4th 831 Dislocation of shoulder

The EXCLUDES note mentions the sternoclavicular joint and the sternum. However, Annette dislocated her humerus, so you can keep reading down the column to find that required fourth digit.

Bacterial Inflammatory Conditions

- *Septic arthritis:* Bacterial invasion of a joint causing inflammation
- *Osteomyelitis:* Bone infection

Metabolic Conditions

- *Gout:* Identifiable urate deposits in the joints
- *Osteoporosis:* Loss of bone mass
- *Osteitis deformans (Paget's disease):* Painful deformities of both external and internal bone structures

Degenerative Diseases

- *Neurogenic arthropathy:* Loss of sensation in the joints that results in progressive deterioration

Chronic Diseases

- *Arthritis:* Swelling and stiffness of joints
- *Osteoarthritis:* Deterioration of the joint cartilage

Skeletal Deviations

- *Hallux valgus:* Bursa and callus formation at the bony prominence
- *Kyphosis (adult):* Degeneration of intervertebral disks (See Fig. 8-2.)
- *Herniated disk (slipped disk, ruptured disk):* Extruded vertebral disk
- *Scoliosis:* Lateral curvature of the spine (See Fig. 8-2.)

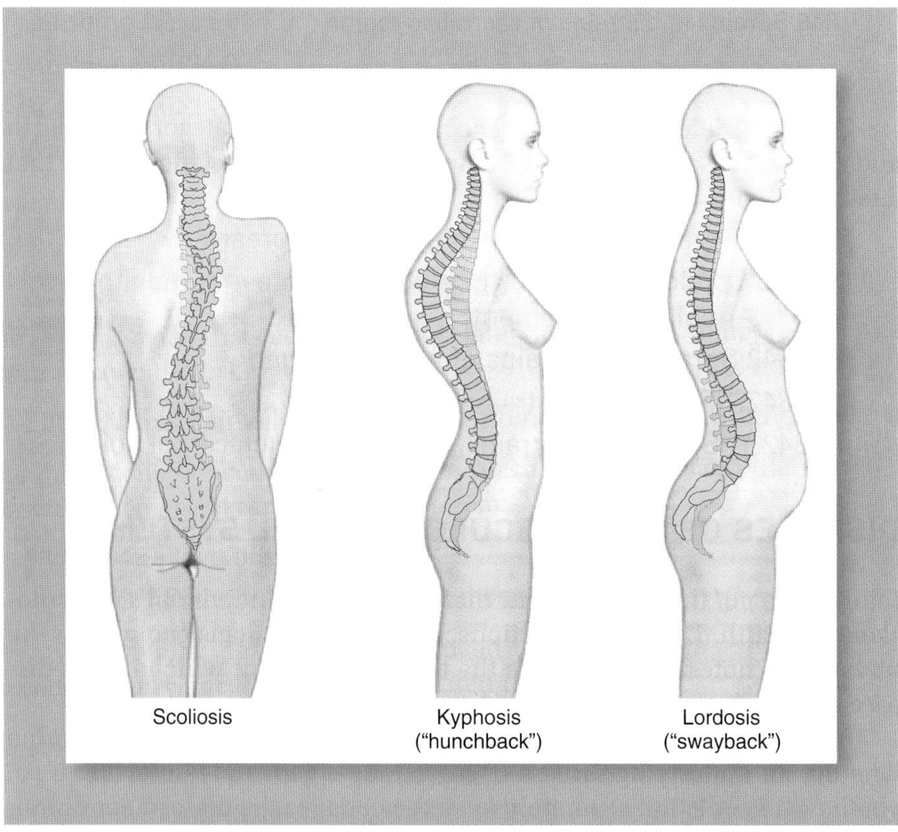

Figure 8-2 The Three Types of Spinal Curvatures.

LET'S CODE IT! SCENARIO

Everett Rotarine, a 43-year-old male, was having pain that his orthopedist, Dr. Nixon, identified as excessive bone resorption, the osteoclastic phase of Paget's disease. X-rays and a urinalysis showing elevated levels of hydroxyproline confirmed the osteoclastic hyperactivity. He comes in today to discuss the test findings and treatment options.

Let's Code It!

Dr. Nixon diagnosed Everett with Paget's disease. You may remember that this is an eponym and will be shown in the ICD-9-CM alphabetic index, so let's turn to find the suggested codes.

Paget's disease (osteitis deformans) 731.0

Notice the long list of additional descriptors of this condition indented beneath this listing. Look at the scenario again. There is no mention of any of these terms in the documentation, so let's go to the tabular list to check this code out. Find

√4th 731 Osteitis deformans and osteopathies associated with other disorders classified elsewhere

You know that "osteitis deformans" is correct because the alphabetic index included this as a nonessential modifier. However, this code category states "AND osteopathies associated with other disorders classified elsewhere" and that is not in our documentation at all. Are you in the wrong place?

Remember, you learned in Chap. 3 that the word "and" in ICD-9-CM really means "and/or." So, let's keep reading.

731.0 Osteitis deformans without mention of bone tumor

Paget's disease of bone

731.1 Osteitis deformans in diseases classified elsewhere

Code first underlying disease as:

Malignant neoplasm of bone (170.0–170.9)

Both code descriptions include osteitis deformans, but the rest of the description changes. Did the physician mention anything about a bone tumor or a malignancy in the notes? Go back and read them again. There is no mention of a bone tumor or any malignancy. Therefore, the most accurate code is

731.0 Osteitis deformans without mention of bone tumor

«« KEYS TO CODING

Read carefully! Paget-Schroetter syndrome may begin with the same name, but it is a different condition than Paget's disease.

YOU CODE IT! CASE STUDY

After completing a full course of radiation treatments for a malignant tumor, Tarlissa Montgomery started having trouble with her back. Dr. Panocchi diagnosed her with scoliosis as a result of the radiation.

You Code It!

Go through the steps of coding, and determine the diagnosis code(s) that should be reported for this encounter between Dr. Panocchi and Tarlissa.

Step 1: Read the case completely.

Step 2: Abstract the notes: Which key words can you identify relating to why Dr. Panocchi cared for Tarlissa?

Step 3: Query the provider, if necessary.

Step 4: Code the diagnosis or diagnoses.

Step 5: Code the procedure(s): Office visit

Step 6: Link the procedure codes to at least one diagnosis code to confirm medical necessity.

Step 7: Back code to double-check your choices.

Answer

Did you find the correct code?

737.33 Scoliosis due to radiation

Review the other code choices to be certain.

Idiopathic means "with no known cause." But the notes DO state a cause of her scoliosis—the radiation. So 737.30 cannot be correct.

Is there an associated condition documented by the physician? There is none, so 737.43 cannot be correct.

Tarlissa was not born with scoliosis; it developed as a result of her having radiation treatments so 754.2 cannot be correct.

KEYS TO CODING »»

How do you know if you need additional codes when the ICD-9-CM book doesn't tell you? Remember that your job is to tell the *whole story*. Look at our example of Sidney Brody. He was diagnosed with "acute staphylococcal osteomyelitis of the pelvic region." Code 730.05 reports acute osteomyelitis of the pelvic region but NOT the staphylococcal infection. There is more to the story than the one code 730.05 can tell, so you now know you need another code, to tell the rest of the details–041.10 Staphylococcus, unspecified

Now . . . with both codes and only both codes you have the *whole story*.

Muscular/Connective Tissue Conditions

- *Tendinitis:* Painful inflammation of the tendons
- *Bursitis:* Painful inflammation of the bursae
- *Epicondylitis (tennis elbow):* Inflammation of the extensor tendons of the forearm
- *Achilles tendon contracture:* Shortening of the tendocalcaneus
- *Carpal tunnel syndrome:* Compression of the nerve at the wrist
- *Torticollis:* Neck deformity involving spastic sternocleidomastoid neck muscles

Example

Sidney Brody is diagnosed with acute staphylococcal osteomyelitis of the pelvic region.

730.05 Acute osteomyelitis, pelvic region

041.10 Staphylococcus, unspecified

If a traumatic injury caused, or was involved, in the development of the condition, be certain to include the appropriate E code or codes.

Example

Lilly Allendale was diagnosed with ankylosis of the shoulder after her last parachute jump.

> 718.51 Ankylosis of joint, shoulder region
>
> E844.7 Other specified air transport accident, parachutist

YOU CODE IT! CASE STUDY

Jerome Hermann, a 9-year-old male, has been having a persistent pain in his right thigh that has been getting worse over the last few weeks. It is also very difficult for him to rotate his right hip. His mother brings Jerome to see Dr. Allen, an orthopedist. Dr. Allen diagnoses Jerome with Legg-Calvé-Perthes disease at the head of his femur.

You Code It!

Go through the steps of coding, and determine the diagnosis code(s) that should be reported for this encounter between Dr. Allen and Jerome Hermann.

Step 1: Read the case completely.

Step 2: Abstract the notes: Which key words can you identify relating to why Dr. Allen cared for Jerome?

____

Step 3: Query the provider, if necessary.

Step 4: Code the diagnosis or diagnoses.

____

Step 5: Code the procedure(s): Office visit, physical exam, x-ray.

Step 6: Link the procedure codes to at least one diagnosis code to confirm medical necessity.

Step 7: Back code to double-check your choices.

Answer

Did you find the correct code?

> 732.1 Juvenile osteochondrosis of hip (Legg-Calvé-Perthes)

Good job!

CHAPTER SUMMARY

Bones, muscles, tendons, and ligaments throughout the human body play an important part in the quality of life of every individual. The musculoskeletal system can sustain injury in many different ways: fractures, dislocations, sprains, and strains. The injuries can be the result of an external cause (of course, requiring the addition of an E code), stress, or disease.

It is a professional coding specialist's responsibility to accurately report the complete nature of the patient's musculoskeletal concern.

BRIDGE TO ICD-10-CM

The Musculoskeletal section (codes M00–M99) includes all conditions in one place:

M00–M02	Infectious arthropathies
M05–M14	Inflammatory polyarthropathies
M15–M19	Osteoarthritis
M20–M25	Other joint disorders
M26–M27	Dentofacial anomalies [including malocclusion] and other disorders of jaw
M30–M36	Systemic connective tissue disorders
M40–M43	Deforming dorsopathies
M45–M49	Spondylopathies
M50–M54	Other dorsopathies
M60–M63	Disorders of muscles
M65–M67	Disorders of synovium and tendon
M70–M79	Other soft tissue disorders
M80–M85	Disorders of bone density and structure
M86–M90	Other osteopathies
M91–M94	Chondropathies
M95	Other disorders of the musculoskeletal system and connective tissue
M96	Intraoperative and postprocedural complications and disorders of musculoskeletal system, not elsewhere classified
M99	Biomechanical lesions, not elsewhere classified

CHAPTER 8 Review

Coding Musculoskeletal Conditions

1. The three-digit category for a fracture code is determined by the fracture's
   a. Severity.
   b. Anatomical site.
   c. The type of fracture.
   d. The external cause.

2. The terms *greenstick* and *spiral* refer to
   a. Open fractures.
   b. Open dislocations.
   c. Closed fractures.
   d. Closed dislocations.

3. If the physician's notes do not specify open or closed, you must code it as
   a. Closed.
   b. Open.
   c. Unspecified.
   d. Not otherwise specified.

4. When coding a fracture, the fourth and/or fifth digit will be determined by
   a. The bone that was fractured.
   b. The status of the fracture.
   c. The type of treatment performed.
   d. The portion or segment of the bone that was fractured.

5. The terms *acetabulum, symphysis,* and *condyle* refer to
   a. Segments of a bone.
   b. Types of fractures.
   c. Diseases of the bone.
   d. Late effects of fractures.

6. When coding multiple fractures, the first code should identify
   a. The lowest portion of the body affected.
   b. The most severe fracture.
   c. The right side before the left side.
   d. The least severe fracture.

7. A pathologic fracture is coded
   a. The same way a closed fracture is coded.
   b. The same way an open fracture is coded.
   c. The same way a dislocation is coded.
   d. From a different three-digit category.

8. An infected dislocation is coded as
   a. A dislocation NOS.
   b. An open dislocation.
   c. A closed dislocation.
   d. A fracture.

9. Pathologic dislocations are also called
   a. Stress dislocations.
   b. Complicated dislocations.
   c. Spontaneous dislocations.
   d. Subluxations.

10. Cartilage is
    a. Tissue.
    b. Bone.
    c. Joint.
    d. Organ.

YOU CODE IT! Practice

Chapter 8. Coding Musculoskeletal Conditions

1. Norman Wilhelm, an 86-year-old male, was stepping off the train when the car jerked forward. He fell and injured his leg. He was diagnosed with a torus fracture of the tibia and fibula.

   ___

2. Olivia Campbell, a 13-year-old female, stepped off a curb the wrong way and hurt her ankle. X-rays confirmed Dr. Conner's diagnosis of a trimalleolar fracture.

   ___

3. Ivan Scotto, a 19-year-old male, dove into a lake, while swimming with his friends, and hit the bottom. Dr. Polarris diagnosed him with a C1–C4 fracture with spinal cord injury.

   ___

4. Sylvia York, a 43-year-old female, was driving down Main Street, was involved in a car accident, and suffered an open fracture of the shaft of her left humerus.

   ___

5. Clayton Harrison, a 25-year-old male, was in a hang glider when he lost control and fell into the river. He was diagnosed with a fractured acetabulum.

   ___

6. Walter Baumann has been a Shriner for many years. He was given the privilege to ride the elephant in its annual circus parade. Halfway around, he fell off the animal and suffered four fractured ribs.

   ___

7. Francine Baumann was trying to help her husband, Walter, after he fell from the elephant. The elephant stepped on her left foot and caused a fracture of the metatarsal bones.

   ___

8. Lee Rogers, a 39-year-old male, was in astronaut training when he hit his head in the weightlessness simulator. He was unconscious for 15 minutes. Dr. Sousman determined that Lee had a fractured parietal bone.

   ___

9. Colleen O'Donnell, a 33-year-old female, slipped and fell in her bathtub, which resulted in a fractured left radius with ulna, lower end, and a posterior dislocation of the left elbow.

____

10. Robert Emory, a 15-year-old male, was on his skateboard when he dislocated the medial meniscus of his left knee.

____

11. Elaine Gregory, a 79-year-old female, was diagnosed with a pathologic fracture of the humerus due to postmenopausal osteoporosis.

____

12. Bennett Bernardo, a 47-year-old male, has been morbidly obese for over a decade. Dr. Jaffe diagnoses him with a stress fracture of the metatarsals.

____

13. Everett Callman, a 33-year-old male, was diagnosed with a pathologic fracture of the vertebrae due to a metastatic carcinoma of the bone from the lung, upper lobe.

____

14. Janine Samuels was struck, by her opponent, on the side of the head while boxing. Janine suffered a dislocated jaw.

____

15. Isis Graham, a 5-year-old female, fell from the monkey bars at the playground and fractured the shaft of her clavicle.

____

YOU CODE IT! Simulation

Chapter 8. Coding Musculoskeletal Conditions

On the following pages, you will see physicians' notes documenting encounters with patients at our textbook's health care facility, Taylor, Reader, & Associates. Carefully read through the notes, and find the best ICD-9-CM code or codes for each case.

TAYLOR, READER, & ASSOCIATES
A Complete Health Care Facility
975 CENTRAL AVENUE • SOMEWHERE, FL 32811 • 407-555-4321

PATIENT: FRACMANN, GERALD
ACCOUNT/EHR #: FRACGE001
Date: 04/25/11

Attending Physician: Willard B. Reader, MD

S: Patient is a 29-year-old male who states that his car was struck from behind by another car. He was driving on the highway near his office. Patient is complaining of severe neck pain and difficulty turning his head.

O: PE reveals tightness upon palpitation of ligaments in neck and shoulders, most pronounced C3 to C5. X-rays are taken of head and neck including the cervical vertebrae. Radiological review denies any fracture.

A: Dislocation of fourth cervical vertebra

P:
1. Cervical collar to be worn during all waking hours
2. Rx Vicodin (hydrocodone) 500 mg po prn
3. 1,000 mg aspirin qid
4. Pt to return in 2 weeks for follow-up

Willard B. Reader, MD

WBR/pw D: 04/25/11 09:50:16 T: 04/30/11 12:55:01

Find the best, most accurate ICD-9-CM code(s).

___

___

___

TAYLOR, READER, & ASSOCIATES
A Complete Health Care Facility
975 CENTRAL AVENUE • SOMEWHERE, FL 32811 • 407-555-4321

PATIENT: WHITMAN, ELOISE
ACCOUNT/EHR #: WHITEL01
Date: 09/16/11

Attending Physician: Suzanne Taylor, MD

S: This new Pt is a 31-year-old female who was involved in an accident when the motorcycle she was riding was struck by a car. She is complaining about some neck pain. She has tingling into her hand and her feet. She states that her arm hurts when she tries to pull it overhead. A friend apparently told her that she should likely need to see a spine doctor, but somehow she came to see me first. PMH is remarkable for kidney trouble. Past bronchoscopy, laparoscopy, and kidney stone surgery, otherwise noncontributory as per the medical history form completed by the patient and reviewed at this visit.

O: Ht 5′5″ Wt. 179 lb. R 16. Pt presented in a sling. She was told to use it by the same friend. She states if she does not use it, her arm does not feel any different, so I had her remove it. On exam, the left shoulder demonstrates full passive motion. She has normal strength testing. She has no deformity. She has some tenderness over the trapezial area. The reflexes are brisk and symmetric. X-rays of her chest 2 views and C spine AP/LAT are relatively benign, as are complete x-rays of the shoulder.

A: Linear fracture of the second cervical vertebra, and an anterior dislocation of the humerus

P: 1. Rx Naprosyn.
2. Referral to PT
3. Referral to orthopedist

Suzanne Taylor, MD

ST/mg D: 9/16/11 09:50:16 T: 9/18/11 12:55:01

Find the best, most accurate ICD-9-CM code(s).

TAYLOR, READER, & ASSOCIATES
A Complete Health Care Facility
975 CENTRAL AVENUE • SOMEWHERE, FL 32811 • 407-555-4321

PATIENT: BRADLEY, MICHAEL
ACCOUNT/EHR #: BRADMI001
Date: 09/20/11

Attending Physician: Willard Reader, MD

S: Pt is a 37-year-old male who was involved in a fist fight at a local bar the previous evening. He complained of an ache in the area of his right eye as well as severe pain around his left ear.

O: Ht 5′10.5″ Wt. 209 lb. R 19. Surface hematoma evident in the area surrounding the left eye socket reaching to the upper cheek. Head x-ray of the right side confirmed a closed fracture of the right mandible.

A: Black eye; fracture of the right mandible, angle (closed)

P: 1. Wire right jaw
2. NPO except liquids for 3 weeks
3. Cold wet compresses on eye prn4. Return for follow-up in 3 weeks

---

Willard Reader, MD

WR/mg D: 09/20/11 09:50:16 T: 09/22/11 12:55:01

Find the best, most accurate ICD-9-CM code(s).

____

____

____

TAYLOR, READER, & ASSOCIATES
A Complete Health Care Facility
975 CENTRAL AVENUE • SOMEWHERE, FL 32811 • 407-555-4321

PATIENT: ALLISON, JOANNA
ACCOUNT/EHR #: ALLIJO01
Date: 09/16/11

Attending Physician: Suzanne R. Taylor, MD

S: Pt is a 23-year-old female who fell from the porch in front of her house and hurt her back. She states that the pain is mostly in her lower back. She denies any personal history of back problems. She states she had trouble sitting up and finds slight relief when lying flat. She claims she cannot bend over at all because the pain is too severe.

O: Ht 5′7″ Wt. 129 lb. R 16. X-rays of back, l1–l5 A/P/ and lateral. Films confirm a nondisplaced compression fracture of L1 and L2 vertebral bodies.Patient is placed into a back brace and told to get bed rest.

A: Nondisplaced compression fracture L1–L2

P: 1. Rx Tylenol with codeine for pain, as directed
2. Referral to PT
3. Referral to orthopedist

Suzanne R. Taylor, MD

SRT/pw D: 9/16/11 09:50:16 T: 9/18/11 12:55:01

Find the best, most accurate ICD-9-CM code(s).

TAYLOR, READER, & ASSOCIATES
A Complete Health Care Facility
975 CENTRAL AVENUE • SOMEWHERE, FL 32811 • 407-555-4321

PATIENT:	CONTINALE, THEODORE
ACCOUNT/EHR #:	CONTTH001
Date:	08/11/11
Attending Physician:	Willard B. Reader, MD

S: Pt is a 50-year-old male who fell down the icy front steps of his house. He hit his head on the concrete step and sustained a head injury, but did not lose consciousness. He also noted that his right ankle swelled up and was so painful he could not put his weight on it.

O: Ht 5′11″ Wt. 187 lb. R 20. T 98.6. BP 130/95 Patient sent to radiology for x-rays of right ankle—A/P/L views as well as the skull. Physical examination HEENT: Pt denies any problems with vision, PERLA. X-rays indicate a closed trimalleolar fracture of the medial and lateral malleolus with anterior lip of tibia involvement. No fracture of skull revealed.

A: Fracture of trimalleolar with involvement of the medial and lateral malleolus and anterior lip of tibia; mild brain concussion.

P: 1. Pt to return 3 weeks
2. Rx Tylenol with codeine for pain
3. Patient sent to casting room for short leg cast. Triped cane provided for walking

---

Willard B. Reader, MD

WBR/pw D: 08/11/11 09:50:16 T: 08/13/11 12:55:01

Find the best, most accurate ICD-9-CM code(s).

9 Coding Obstetrics and Gynecology

KEY TERMS

Abortion
Antepartum
Gestation
Gravida
Gynecologist
Obstetrician
Para
Postpartum
Prenatal
Puerperium

LEARNING OUTCOMES

9.1 Apply guidelines for coding all aspects of pregnancy.
9.2 Determine the correct codes for reporting complications of pregnancy.
9.3 Correctly report labor and delivery encounters.
9.4 Distinguish between antepartum and postpartum conditions.
9.5 Report the late effects of obstetric complications accurately.
9.6 Explain the different types of abortive occurrences.

Gynecologist
A physician specializing in the care of the female reproductive organs.

Obstetrics
A health care specialty focusing on the care of women during pregnancy and the puerperium.

Puerperium
The time period from the end of labor until the uterus returns to normal size, typically 3 to 6 weeks.

Gravida
An alphanumeric (G1, G2, G3, etc.) that indicates how many times a woman has been pregnant in her life.

Para
An alphanumeric that identifies the number of times a woman has given birth, designated on the chart as P1, P2, etc.; had a fetus reach viability.

Females of all ages may go to the **gynecologist** (GYN) for specialized health care. An **obstetrician (OB)** is a physician who focuses on care during pregnancy and the **puerperium.** An OB-GYN includes both types of services in his or her practice.

As she matures, the fact that a woman has or has not been pregnant should be reported as a relevant part of the patient's history. You may see notations identifying the woman's **gravida** and **para,** often written as G# P#. The number following the letter reports how many times this woman has been pregnant (gravida [G]) or given birth (para [P]).

G1 P1 tells you that this woman has been pregnant once and given birth once.

G1 P2 tells you that this woman has been pregnant once and given birth twice—twins!!

G2 P1 tells you that this woman has been pregnant twice and given birth once—if she is pregnant now, this is her second pregnancy; if she is not pregnant now, she may have had a miscarriage in the past.

Example

Joellen is pregnant for the second time. The first time she was pregnant, she suffered a miscarriage in her tenth week. Her chart will indicate G2 P0—it is her second pregnancy, but, as yet, she has not given birth.

PRENATAL VISITS

Normal Pregnancy

Routine outpatient **prenatal** checkups are very important to the health and well-being of both the mother and the baby. For a healthy pregnant woman, the visits are typically scheduled at specific points throughout the pregnancy, as determined by the number of weeks of **gestation.**

When coding routine visits, with the patient having no complications, you will choose from the available V codes. Remember that you will use a V code when the patient is not encountering the health care provider because of any current illness or injury. A healthy, pregnant woman is neither.

V22.0 Supervision of normal first pregnancy

V22.1 Supervision of other normal pregnancy

You will know which code to use based on the physician's notes as to the woman's gravida status.

Example

Alana, a 23-year-old female, G1 P0, is 10 weeks pregnant and is seen by Dr. Carter for a routine checkup. No problems. Everything is fine.

V22.0 Supervision of normal first pregnancy

Sharon, a 27-year-old female, G3 P2, is 10 weeks pregnant and is seen for a routine checkup. No problems. Everything is fine.

V22.1 Supervision of other normal pregnancy

Sharon has been pregnant before. The term "other" in the code description means "other than first" pregnancy.

High-Risk Pregnancy

In cases where the pregnancy is considered to be medically high risk, you will use a code from code category V23 Supervision of high-risk pregnancy for the routine visit instead of V22.0 or V22.1.

You will determine the fourth digit, and possibly fifth digit, for the V23 code by the reason stated in the physician's notes that the pregnancy is considered high-risk. The reason might be a history of infertility (V23.0), a very young mother (V23.83), an older mother (V23.81), or another issue.

Examples

V23.7 Supervision of high-risk pregnancy, insufficient prenatal care

V23.81 Supervision of high-risk pregnancy, elderly primigravida

Prenatal

Prior to birth; also antenatal.

Gestation

The length of time for the complete development of a baby from conception to birth; on average 40 weeks.

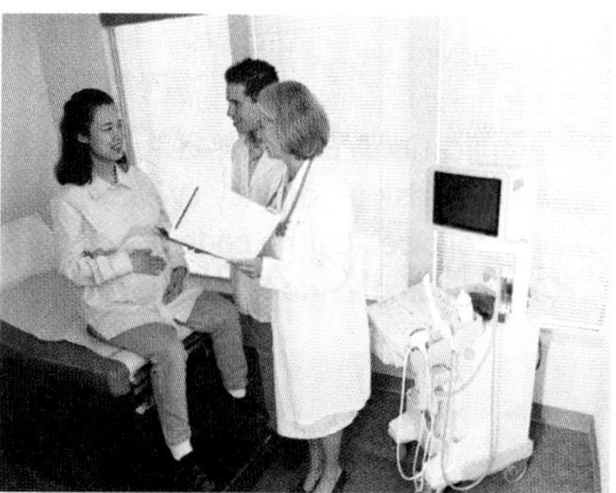

«« KEYS TO CODING

The physician may not necessarily state "high-risk" in the notes, so you will need to read all information carefully—as you always do—to make certain you catch the details. For example, the notes may simply state, "*This 37-year-old female is 19 weeks pregnant with her first child . . .* ". This tells you that the most accurate code for this routine visit is V23.81 Supervision of high-risk pregnancy, elderly primigravida.

The definition of "elderly primigravida" is a woman who will be 35 years of age or older at the projected date of delivery for her first pregnancy.

«« BRIDGE TO ICD-10-CM

Routine prenatal visits with no complications will be reported from code category

Z34 Encounter for supervision of normal pregnancy or O09 Supervision of high-risk pregnancy.

TAYLOR, READER, & ASSOCIATES
A Complete Health Care Facility
975 CENTRAL AVENUE • SOMEWHERE, FL 32811 • 407-555-4321

PATIENT NAME: CABOT, OLIVIA
MRN: CABOOL01

Operative Report

Date: 5 September 2011
Preoperative DX: 1. First trimester missed abortion; 2. Undesired fertility
Postoperative DX: same
Operation: 1. Dilation and curettage with suction; 2. Laparoscopic bilateral tubal ligation using Kleppinger bipolar cautery.
Surgeon: Rodney L. Cohen, MD
Assistant: None
Anesthesia: General endotracheal anesthesia
Findings: Pt had products of conception at the time of dilatation and curettage. She also had normal-appearing uterus, ovaries, fallopian tubes, and liver edge.
Specimens: Products of conception to pathology
Disposition: To PACU in stable condition.

Procedure: The patient was taken to the operating room, and she was placed in the dorsal supine position. General endotracheal anesthesia was administered without difficulty. The patient was placed in dorsal lithotomy position. She was prepped and draped in the normal sterile fashion. A red rubber tip catheter was placed gently to drain the patient's bladder. A weighted speculum was placed in the posterior vagina and Deaver retractor anteriorly. A single-tooth tenaculum was placed in the anterior cervix for retraction. The uterus sounded to 9 cm. The cervix was dilated with Hanks dilators to 25 French. This sufficiently passed a #7 suction curet. The suction curet was inserted without incident, and the products of conception were gently suctioned out. Good uterine cry was noted with a serrated curet. No further products were noted on suctioning. At this point, a Hulka tenaculum was placed in the cervix for retraction. The other instruments were removed.

Attention was then turned to the patient's abdomen. A small vertical intraumbilical incision was made with the knife. A Veress needle was placed through that incision. Confirmation of placement into the abdominal cavity was made with instillation of normal saline without return and a positive handing drop test. The abdomen was then insufflated with sufficient carbon dioxide gas to cause abdominal tympany. The Veress needle was removed and a 5-mm trocar was placed in the same incision. Confirmation of placement into the abdominal cavity was made with placement of the laparoscopic camera. Another trocar site was placed two fingerbreadths above the pubic symphysis in the midline under direct visualization. The above noted intrapelvic and intraabdominal findings were seen. The patient was placed in steep Trendelenburg. The fallopian tubes were identified and followed out to the fimbriated ends. They were then cauterized four times on either side. At this point, all instruments were removed from the patient's abdomen. This was done under direct visualization during the insufflation. The skin incisions were reapproximated with 4-0 Vicryl suture. The Hulka tenaculum was removed without incident.

The patient was placed back in the dorsal supine position. Anesthesia was withdrawn without difficulty. The patient was taken to the PACU in stable condition. All sponge, instrument, and needle counts were correct in the operating room.

Rodney L. Cohen, MD 09/05/11 10:40:36

Find the best, most appropriate ICD-9-CM code(s).

TAYLOR, READER, & ASSOCIATES
A Complete Health Care Facility
975 CENTRAL AVENUE • SOMEWHERE, FL 32811 • 407-555-4321

PATIENT NAME: ALEXANDER, JORY
MRN: ALEXJO01

Operative Report

Date: 4 September 2011

Preoperative DX: 1. Chronic pelvic pain; 2. History of endometriosis; 3. Right adnexal mass, probable endometrioma

Postoperative DX: same

Operation: Total abdominal hysterectomy with bilateral salpingo-oophorectomy and lysis of pelvic adhesions with procedure of unusual difficulty secondary to endometriosis.

Surgeon: Rodney L. Cohen, MD

Assistant: None

Anesthesia: General endotracheal intubation by Dr. Kastorman

Findings: See body of dictation

Procedure: The patient was taken to the operating room, and she was placed supine on the table. Underwent general anesthesia with endotracheal intubation without complication. The patient had Foley catheter inserted. Was prepped and draped in a sterile fashion for abdominal procedure. Scalpel was used to make a vertical midline incision in elliptical fashion removing the previously noted dense abdominal scar, taken down through subcutaneous tissue to the level of the anterior rectus sheath, nicked in its midline and extended the length of the incision. Blunt dissection through the midline rectus muscles exposing the peritoneum, sharply entered the midline, extended the length of the incision down to the bladder. Balfour self-retaining retractor was put into place, elevated with blue towels with care taken to avoid posterior nervous injury. Initial attempts to pack the bowel off the field were difficult as there were significant adhesions between the colon and the previous area of the left adnexectomy and the endometrioma that was on the right side. Through an extensive and lengthy dissection, the bowel was carefully dissected from the pelvis with both blunt and sharp dissection with care to avoid bowel injury. The right adnexa was then carefully dissected by both blunt and sharp dissection off the sidewall to avoid ureteral injury. After freeing up all tissue, the packing was removed from the abdomen, and the bowel was again repacked away from the operative site, and then the hysterectomy was proceeded with in the usual fashion. Bilaterally, the utero-ovarian ligaments were cross-clamped with Kelly clamp for traction. The uterus was elevated. Bilaterally, the round ligaments were identified, cross-clamped with Heaney clamps, severed with pelvic scissors and ligated with 0-Vicryl suture in a Heaney-ligature-type fashion. The bladder was sharply dissected of the lower uterine segment. Bilaterally, the uterine arteries were skeletonized, cross-clamped with Heaney clamps, severed with pelvic scissors, and then ligated with 0-Vicryl suture. The remaining portion of the cardinal ligaments were then cross-clamped with Heaney clamp, severed with pelvic scissors, and ligated with 0-Vicryl suture in Heaney ligature type fashion. At the uppermost portion of the vagina, the angles were cross-clamped with Heaney clamp and severed with pelvic scissors, and the uterus, cervix, and remaining right adnexa were then removed from the vaginal cuff.

Bilaterally, the angles were ligated with 0-Vicryl suture in Heaney-ligature-type fashion, and the central portion of the vaginal cuff was closed with a 0-Vicryl suture in a running interlocking fashion.

Continued

The pelvis was copiously irrigated and inspected, noted to be clean and dry with the exception of some small bleeding sites overlying the region of the right ureter in the region of the extensive dissection. These were cauterized and clipped with care taken to avoid a ureteral injury. There was a small tissue ooze due to the extensive dissection, and Gelfoam was placed in the site.

Prior to this, a look at all operative sites revealed good homeostasis. All pedicles revealed good homeostasis. All instrumentation was removed. The fascia and peritoneum were closed in a bulk fashion using 0-PDS suture in a running mixed simple interlocking fashion starting from the superior margin of the incision and running to the midline, starting from the inferior margin of the incision and running to the midline.

Subcutaneous tissue was irrigated and inspected and noted to be clean and dry. It was drawn together in the midline with 3-0 plain suture in a running simple fashion, and then the skin was reapproximated with a 4-0 Vicryl suture in subcuticular fashion. Steri-Strips and overlying pressure dressing were applied. The patient was awakened on her own, breathing on her own in good condition, and transferred to the recovery room.

Rodney L. Cohen, MD. 09/04/11 12:43:45

Find the best, most appropriate ICD-9-CM code(s).

____

____

____

TAYLOR, READER, & ASSOCIATES
A Complete Health Care Facility
975 CENTRAL AVENUE • SOMEWHERE, FL 32811 • 407-555-4321

PATIENT NAME: MC DOUGAN, ZENA
MRN: MCDOZE01
Date: 7 September 2011

OB Ultrasound

FINDINGS: A single fetus is seen in the breech presentation with limb motion and heart motion visualized. No organ abnormalities are seen. The placenta lies posteriorly and is grade 1. The amount of amniotic fluid is within normal limits.

The estimated menstrual age based on:

BPD of 6.4 cm = 25.5 weeks FL of 5.1 cm = 27.0 weeks
AC of 21.9 cm = 26.0 weeks HC of 25.1 cm = 26.5 weeks

Average = 26.3 weeks

The ratios of:	Normal Ratios
FL to BPD = 79%	(79% +/− 8)
FL to AC = 23%	(22% +/− 2)
HC to AC = 1.15%	(1.13 +/− 0.9)

Estimate fetal weight is 1,000 grams
The cephalic index = 70% (70–80)

IMPRESSION/INTERPRETATION: Normal appearing intrauterine pregnancy estimated to be 26.3 weeks menstrual age. No fetal abnormalities are identified. The fetus is currently in the breech presentation.

Diane Colon, MD. 09/07/11 11:47:39

Find the best, most appropriate ICD-9-CM code(s).

___

___

___

TAYLOR, READER, & ASSOCIATES
A Complete Health Care Facility
975 CENTRAL AVENUE • SOMEWHERE, FL 32811 • 407-555-4321

PATIENT NAME: CANSECCA, APRIL
MRN: CANSAP01

Operative Report

Date: 10 September 2011

Preoperative DX: 1. Menometrorrhagia refractory to medical treatment; 2. Endometrial mass; 3. Adnexal masses with normal CA-125

Postoperative DX: same

Operation: Supracervical hysterectomy, bilateral salpingo-oophorectomy

Surgeon: Rodney L. Cohen, MD

Assistant: None

Anesthesia: General endotracheal

Procedure: The patient was taken to the OR, was placed in the supine position, and was prepped and draped in the usual sterile manner. A Foley catheter was inserted into the bladder to drain the urine. A Pfannenstiel skin incision was made with a knife and carried down to the fascia. The fascia was nicked in the midline and extended bilaterally. Kochers were used to grasp the superior portion of the fascia that was separated sharply and bluntly in the midline. Kochers were then used to grasp the inferior portion of the fascia, which was separated sharply and bluntly. The rectus muscles were separated. Hemostats were used to grasp the peritoneum and extend superiorly under direct visualization and inferiorly under translumination. The bladder flap was developed and pushed well of the low uterine segment. The Balfour self-retaining retractor was placed and the bowel packed with warm moist laps. Two curved Kelly clamps were placed across the corneal area of the uterus on each side. The right round ligament was placed on stretch. A 0-Vicryl was used to suture ligate this ligament. The anterior and posterior leaves off the broad ligament were then opened. The same procedure was done to the left. The infundibulopelvic ligament on the right was then identified. The ureter was found to be well out of the way, and a curved Heaney clamp × 2 was placed across the infundibulopelvic ligament and this ligament excised. A 0-Vicryl free tie, as well as a 0-Vicryl suture ligation was performed with good homeostasis. Next, the same procedure was done on the left, obtaining the left round ligament and infundibulopelvic ligament in the same manner. Next, the bladder flap was dissected off the low uterine segment and cervix. Once this was done appropriately, the uterine artery on the left side was skeletonized and curved. Heaney clamps were used to obtain these. Suture ligation was performed with 0-Vicryl. The uterine artery was then obtained on the right. Straight Heaney used in succession to obtain the cardinal ligaments. The patient was noted to have endometriosis on her ovaries, as well as a lot of oozing with aberrant blood vessels at this time, and it was decided to go ahead with a supracervical hysterectomy due to the nature of the patient's tissue and difficulty of going any deeper into the pelvis. A Bovie was used to cauterize and remove the fundal portion of the uterus and lower uterine segment, and a portion of the cervix as well. The remaining cervical stump was cauterized en mill, and 0-Chromic was first used to reapproximate the inside edges of the cervix; then 0-Vicryl was used on the outside through the cervix in a running locking manner for homeostasis. Once this was done, all areas were inspected for any further bleeding. Bovie cautery or figure-of-eight sutures were placed as necessary. The bladder flap was placed over the cervical stump in the midportion. A 2-0 Chromic was used to anchor this. The right ureter was identified and found to be peristalsing normally. The left ureter could not be seen but was palpated low in the pelvis. Irrigation was performed.

Continued

No further bleeding was noted, so all the instruments were removed, counts are correct, the rectus muscles were reapproximated with 0-Chromic in an interrupted manner. The fascia was closed with 0-Viscryl in the running manner. The subcutaneous tissue was thoroughly irrigated, and the skin was closed with staples. This ended the procedure. The patient tolerated it well and went to recovery room in good condition.

Rodney L. Cohen, MD. 09/10/11 09:24:26

Find the best, most appropriate ICD-9-CM code(s).

10 Coding Congenital and Pediatric Conditions

KEY TERMS

- Anomaly
- Apgar
- Clinically significant
- Congenital
- Low birth weight (LBW)
- Morbidity
- Mortality
- Neonate
- Perinatal
- Prematurity

LEARNING OUTCOMES

10.1 Differentiate between the mother's chart and the baby's chart.
10.2 Correctly code the infant's birth.
10.3 Distinguish between neonatal and perinatal.
10.4 Code clinically significant conditions accurately.
10.5 Distinguish between congenital and childhood conditions.
10.6 Apply guidelines for coding observation and evaluation for an infant.

Most of the time, the arrival of a baby is a joyous occasion. It is always a wondrous event. A **neonate** is the focal point of so much attention. Every year more than 4 million babies are born—about seven babies every minute— in the United States.

Neonate

An infant from birth to 1 month of age.

An assessment of the baby's health begins almost immediately after delivery. Gestational assessment determines the baby's physical maturity, the neuromuscular maturity is established, and an **Apgar** test is usually performed.

Apgar

Assessment of a neonate's condition based on five areas: muscle tone, heart rate, reflex response, skin color, and breathing.

The Apgar test, devised by Virginia Apgar in 1952, provides the doctor and health care team with a quick health assessment of the infant. The test is performed at one minute and then again at five minutes after the baby is born. If the score is low, the physician may decide to do the test again at 10 minutes. Table 10-1 shows you what an Apgar score indicates about a neonate.

KEYS TO CODING »»

No codes from ch. 15 Newborn (Perinatal) Guidelines (760-779) are permitted to be reported on the maternal–the mother's chart or record.

Once the baby is born, he or she gets his or her own chart. From that point forward, anything having to do with the baby is coded for the baby and stays off the mother's chart.

TABLE 10-1 Apgar Scoring for Newborns

Score	Interpretation
0–3	Baby needs immediate lifesaving procedures.
4–6	Baby needs some assistance; requires careful monitoring.
7–10	Normal.

CODING TIP

APGAR is derived from the following:

Activity (muscle tone)
Pulse rate (heart rate)
Grimace (reflex response)
Appearance (skin color)
Respiration (breathing)

CODING THE BIRTH

You may remember from Chap. 9 that the very last code directly relating to the baby that is placed on the mother's chart is an outcome of delivery code from category V27. The *very first code on the baby's chart* will be from the range V30–V39 Liveborn infants according to type of birth. This V code is used to report a newborn baby that is being treated by a health care professional and is always the principal (first-listed) code. A code from this category can only be used once, at the time of birth.

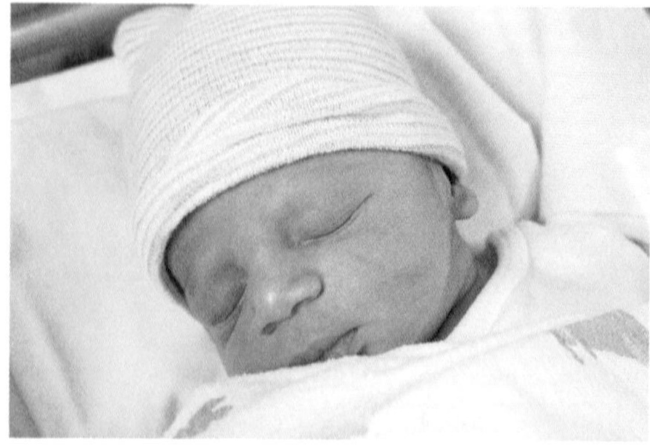

Example

Luci-Anne was just born in the delivery room of Barton Hospital: code V30.00

Joshua was born in the taxi on the way to the hospital and was just admitted for a newborn checkup: code V30.1

Hashem, and his twin brother, Yahya, were born by cesarean at Barton Hospital: code V31.01

KEYS TO CODING

Review the **ICD-9-CM Coding Guidelines, Section I. chapter 15. Newborn (Perinatal) Guidelines (760-779),** subsection **b. Use of codes V30-V39** for more input on identifying what to code, what not to code, and in what order to put multiple codes. Use this to support your reading here, and as a reminder booster later on.

LET'S CODE IT! SCENARIO

Richard Harold was born via vaginal delivery in the Carrolton Birthing Center at 10:58 A.M. on September 1. He weighed 8 lb 5 oz and was 21 inches long, with Apgar scores of 9 and 9. Dr. Smith, a pediatrician, performed a comprehensive examination immediately following Richard's birth. Baby Ricky was sent home at 6:30 P.M. in the care of his mother, Katherine.

BRIDGE TO ICD-10-CM

You will follow these same exact steps when ICD-10-CM is implemented. This process will not change. Only the way the codes look will change.

Let's Code It!

Ricky was just born, and this is his first health care chart. As you learned, his very first code must be from the V30–V39 range.

As with all other cases, begin in the alphabetic index. What should you look up? Birth would be a logical choice. However, when you turn to this term in the ICD-9-CM alphabetic index, you are going to see a long list of adjectives . . . none of which apply to Ricky, or any other

CODING TIP

You know that the V30-V39 code *must* be first-listed because the baby has to be born before anything else can be documented on his or her chart.

baby, being born without a problem. As you look down the list, you may notice this item:

Birth
  Infant—see Newborn

OK, you have nothing to lose. Let's go look up the term Newborn.

Newborn (infant)(liveborn)

And another long list of additional terms. Look through them all and notice the complete reference to

Newborn
  Single
    Born in hospital (without mention of cesarean delivery or section) V30.00
    With cesarean delivery or section V30.01
    Born outside hospital
      Hospitalized V30.1
      Not hospitalized V30.2

CODING TIP »»

Be careful! Only the fourth digit of zero for code V30 requires a fifth digit.

KEYS TO CODING »»

Code V39 Unspecified should be used very, very rarely. Think about it . . . how could you possibly be reporting a baby being born without the physician knowing how many babies were born at this delivery? If single, twin, etc. is not documented, you must query the physician.

You will see a similar listing for Newborn, twin, and Newborn, multiple NEC. Check Dr. Smith's notes. It is documented that Ricky was a "*single, liveborn* baby." Also, he was born in the *Carrolton* Birthing Center which is *not a part of a hospital.* In addition, Dr. Smith's notes state that this was a "vaginal delivery," meaning it was not cesarean delivery. The last piece of information you need to know is this: was Ricky hospitalized or not? The notes state *"Baby Ricky was sent home"* so the answer is no.

Therefore, the code suggested by the alphabetic index is V30.2

Let's go to the tabular list and look at our choices.

Begin with

√4th V30 Single liveborn

You can clearly see the symbol telling you that a fourth digit is required. The fourth-digit choices are

√5th 0 Born in hospital
1 Born before admission to hospital
2 Born outside hospital and not hospitalized

The documentation clearly indicates that Ricky was born outside of a hospital and he was not hospitalized (he was sent home with his mother). Therefore, the correct code is

V30.2 Single liveborn, born outside hospital and not hospitalized

You got it!

CONGENITAL ANOMALIES

Every now and then, during the course of gestation, something goes wrong, and the baby develops a **congenital** defect, or **anomaly.** The defects may affect the baby's entire system or one organ or portion of the body. Some anomalies are cosmetic, affecting only the appearance of the child, whereas others can impede or prevent function.

Anomalies that have been documented in the United States over the last several years include:

- Central nervous system anomalies, including hydrocephalus and spina bifida
- Circulatory and respiratory defects, including heart malformations
- Gastrointestinal anomalies, including rectal stenosis and esophageal atresia
- Urogenital anomalies, including malformed genitalia and renal agenesis
- Musculoskeletal and integumentary anomalies, such as club foot, cleft lip, and diaphragmatic hernia
- Chromosomal anomalies, such as Down syndrome

Some states require the reporting of congenital anomalies on the baby's birth certificate. In any case, all health concerns documented must be reported for statistical tracking, as well as reimbursement.

When the baby is born and a congenital condition is identified and documented, the condition is to be reported with a code from the 740–759 range and placed after (secondary to) the birth code (V30–V39).

Congenital anomalies can be identified the next day or any time later. When appropriate, the congenital defect code may be used as a principal, or first-listed, code whenever the condition is addressed by a physician or other health care professional. Even though the issue is developed during gestation, a congenital anomaly can be treated at any point in one's lifetime. These codes are not used exclusively for babies.

Sadly, it is possible that one baby may be affected by more than one defect. When this is the case, list the code for each condition in order of severity, reporting the worst or most life threatening first, followed by the rest of the codes listing them in decreasing severity down to least. If the severity of two or more conditions is considered to be equal, or unknown, list them in order starting with the top of the body, reporting them from head to toe.

Example

Marshall was born today at Barton Hospital. Dr. Meneudo did a thorough examination and diagnosed a left-sided, incomplete cleft lip and palate: V30.00 and 749.22

Nikita Baranski is 7 months old and is admitted to the hospital for treatment of her congenital cortical and zonular cataract of her left eye: 743.32

Congenital

A condition existing at the time of birth.

Anomaly

Abnormal, or unexpected, condition.

«« KEYS TO CODING

Review the **ICD-9-CM Coding Guidelines, Section I. chapter 14 Congenital Anomalies (740-759)** and **chapter 15 Newborn (Perinatal) Guidelines (760-779),** subsection **part g. Congenital anomalies in newborns** for more input on identifying what to code, what not to code, and in what order to put multiple codes. Use this to support your reading here, and as a reminder booster later on.

«« CODING TIP

A congenital defect code (740-759) should be used *whenever* the condition is treated, regardless of the age of the patient–whether it be 9 months, 9 years, or 90 years.

«« BRIDGE TO ICD-10-CM

Congenital anomalies are reported with codes from a different chapter than other neonatal conditions: ICD-10-CM chapter 17 Congenital malformations, deformations, and chromosomal abnormalities (Q00-Q99).

LET'S CODE IT! SCENARIO

Marianna Vermicelli was born 2 weeks ago with polydactyly of the right foot, with a total of five normal toes and two extra digits that do not contain bony structures. She is brought to the Barton Ambulatory Surgical Center by her mother so Dr. Tempano can tie off and remove the extra digits.

Let's Code It!

Dr. Tempano is treating Marianna's *polydactyly* condition of her *toes* today. Let's turn to the alphabetic index and look this up:

Polydactylism, polydactyly 755.00
  Fingers 755.01
  Toes 755.02

You can see clearly that Marianna's condition has affected her toes, not her fingers, so let's go to the tabular list and confirm this code:

√4th 755 Other congenital anomalies of limbs

Notice the EXCLUDES note that specifically states "excludes those deformities classifiable to 754.0–754.8."

What does that mean? It means that you need to check code category 754 to confirm that this diagnosis is not better reported with a code from:

√4th 754 Certain congenital musculoskeletal deformities

INCLUDES nonteratogenic deformities which are considered to be due to intrauterine malposition and pressure

Polydactyly is a condition of the musculoskeletal system so you need to read through the fourth digit choices.

754.0 Of skull, face, and jaw
754.1 Of sternocleidomastoid muscle
754.2 Of spine
√5th 754.3 Congenital dislocation of hip
√5th 754.4 Congenital genu recurvatum and bowing of long bones of leg
√5th 754.5 Varus deformities of feet
√5th 754.6 Valgus deformities of feet
√5th 754.7 Other deformities of feet
√5th 754.8 Other specified nonteratogenic anomalies

Do any of these codes accurately describe Marianna's diagnosis? No. Now, you can return to code category 755 and read through those four digit choices.

√5th 755.0 Polydactyly

This is great! This matches what Dr. Tempano wrote. This code requires a fifth-digit, so keep reading down the column to find the most accurate fifth-digit.

755.02 Polydactyly, of toes

Now, you have the correct code for Marianna's report. Because she was born 2 weeks ago, you will *not* use a code from any of the V30–V39 categories. Therefore, your diagnosis coding is done for this encounter with Dr. Tempano. Good job!

««« CODING TIP

If the admission for a suspected condition without signs or symptoms occurs on the date of birth, report a code from category V29 after (second to) the V30-V39 code. If the admission occurs after the first day through the 28th day of life, you are permitted to use a code from the V29 category as a principal diagnosis.

PERINATAL CONDITIONS

After the baby is born, any condition that develops during his or her first 28 days will be coded from the range 760–779 Certain conditions originating in the **perinatal** period.

At times, a newborn (during the perinatal period) is suspected of having an abnormal condition, and the physician feels it wise to admit the baby to the hospital for observation and evaluation. The baby, however, has no signs or symptoms of the condition. You cannot code this until a determination, or result, is made by the physician. This determination will direct you how to code this situation.

1. If the condition is found to exist, code the condition, signs, or symptoms as stated in the diagnostic statement in the physician's notes.
2. If the condition is found *not* to exist, choose the appropriate code from the V29 category.

If the physician has ordered the admission of the baby for observation and evaluation based on specifically stated signs and/or symptoms, do not use a code from the V29 category. Instead, code those specific signs and/or symptoms.

Perinatal

The time period from before birth to the 28th day after birth.

«« KEYS TO CODING

Review the **ICD-9-CM Coding Guidelines, Section I. chapter 15. Newborn (Perinatal) Guidelines (740-779),** sections **a. General perinatal rules** and **d. Use of category V29** for more input on identifying what to code, what not to code, and in what order to put multiple codes. Use this to support your reading here, and as a reminder booster later on.

Example

Dr. Jenkins decides to admit Harris, 3 days old, for observation. It was discovered that his mother drank alcohol heavily during her first trimester, and Dr. Jenkins is concerned about possible neurologic defects. Happily, all the tests are negative, and Harris is diagnosed as a healthy baby boy: V29.1 Observation for suspected neurologic condition.

««« BRIDGE TO ICD-10-CM

Code categories P00-P04 will be used to report those cases in which a healthy neonate is admitted for evaluation for a suspected condition that is found to be nonexistent. The guidelines for these code categories are the same as they are for ICD-9-CM's V29 code category.

CLINICALLY SIGNIFICANT CONDITIONS

The guidelines state that you must code all clinically significant conditions noted on the baby's chart during the standard newborn examination. The problem may be your concern as to how you, as a coder, can be sure to determine what is **clinically significant** and what is not. Good news! It is not your decision to make. It can only be determined by the

Clinically significant

Signs, symptoms, and/or conditions present at birth that may impact the child's future health status.

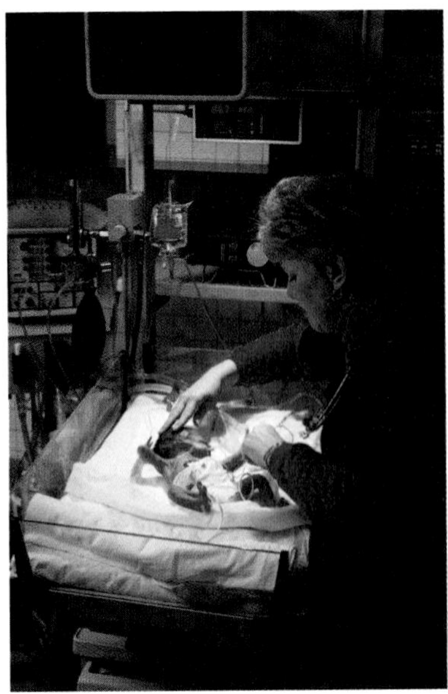

physician. However, you must ensure that the documentation gives you the diagnostic conditions that support any of the following:

- Therapeutic treatments performed. For example, the baby is placed on a respirator.
- Diagnostic procedures done. For example, additional and specific blood tests are performed on the baby.
- Keeping the baby in the hospital longer than usual. For example, the physician is concerned about an issue so he or she does not discharge the baby yet.
- Increased monitoring or nursing care. For example, the physician orders 24-hour private duty nursing care for continuous monitoring.
- Any implication that the child will need health care services in the future as a result of a condition, sign, or symptom that can be identified now. For example, there is evidence that there may be brain damage as a result of the birth process; however, this cannot be confirmed until the child is about 2 years old.

There are times when a physician is very specific about the perinatal condition; however, the ICD-9-CM book does not provide a newborn (perinatal) code with enough detail to report the situation accurately. In such cases, you are to use code 779.89 for other specified conditions originating in the perinatal period and follow it with an additional code for the specific condition.

When a congenital or perinatal condition has been resolved and no longer has an impact on the child's health and well-being, you have to assign a code from the range V10–V15 Personal history of.

KEYS TO CODING »»

Review the **ICD-9-CM Coding Guidelines, Section I. chapter 15. Newborn (Perinatal) Guidelines (740-779),** subsection **a. 4. Code all clinically significant conditions** for more input on identifying what to code, what not to code, and in what order to put multiple codes. Use this to support your reading here, and as a reminder booster later on.

PREMATURITY AND FETAL GROWTH CONDITIONS

The documented age (weeks of gestation completed at birth) and weight of the neonate very often influence his or her health quality. When a baby is born prematurely, it often means that organs, bones, muscles, and other elements have not had enough time to finish developing. Commonly, such babies do not grow to the necessary size and are born with a **low birth weight (LBW).** It may result in the baby not being strong enough to completely grow, fight off disease, or even stay alive.

You will find the codes needed to report an infant's prematurity and LBW, as documented in the physician's notes, with code categories:

√4th 764 Slow fetal growth and fetal malnutrition

√4th 765 Disorders relating to short gestation and low birth weight

Remember: You cannot determine whether a condition or concern with the baby has been caused by either **prematurity** or LBW. You will use codes from those categories only when the physician's notes identify the cause-and-effect of a diagnosis. When the documentation leads you to a code from the 764 Slow fetal growth and fetal malnutrition category, code 765.0 Extreme immaturity (with the appropriate fifth digit), or 765.1

Low birth weight (LBW)

A baby born weighing less than 5 lb 8 oz, or 2,500 grams.

Prematurity

Birth occurring prior to the completion of 37 weeks gestation.

CODING TIP »»

Usually, the physician will write the baby's birth weight in grams. However, you should learn how to convert from pounds and ounces to grams:

1 ounce = 28.375 grams

1 pound = 16 ounces = 454 grams

1 gram = 0.0022 pound

Other preterm infants (with the appropriate fifth digit), you will be able to determine the correct fifth digit from the birth weight noted in the baby's chart.

Also, you can see that both 765.0*x* Extreme immaturity and 765.1*x* Other preterm infants code choices include a notation beneath the code description that tells you this code *implies* a birth weight of either under 1,000 grams or between 1,000 and 2,499 grams.

One more thing these codes have in common . . . they both include the notation "Use additional code for weeks of gestation (765.20–765.29)."

Although the notation does not appear, the guidelines state that the same rule applies when using a code from the 764 category—that you must use a code from 765.20–765.29 to report the number of weeks gestation completed. Again, this detail should be included in the physician's notes so that you can determine the correct code.

««« KEYS TO CODING

Review the **ICD-9-CM Coding Guidelines, Section I. chapter 15. Newborn (Perinatal) Guidelines (740–779),** subsection **i. Prematurity and fetal growth retardation** for more input on identifying what to code, what not to code, and in what order to put multiple codes. Use this to support your reading here, and as a reminder booster later on.

YOU CODE IT! CASE STUDY

Michael Young was born today at 27 weeks gestation by cesarean section at Barton Hospital. He weighed 945 grams at birth, and his lungs are immature. Dr. Forsyth admits Michael into the neonatal intensive care unit (NICU) with a diagnosis of extreme immaturity delivered by cesarean section.

You Code It!

Read through Dr. Forsyth's notes on Michael Young, and find the correct diagnosis code or codes.

Step 1: Read the case completely.

Step 2: Abstract the notes: Which key words can you identify relating to why Dr. Forsyth cared for Michael?

____

Step 3: Query the provider, if necessary.

Step 4: Code the diagnosis or diagnoses.

____

Step 5: Code the procedure(s): Birth.

Step 6: Link the procedure codes to at least one diagnosis code to confirm medical necessity.

Step 7: Back code to double-check your choices.

Answer

Did you find the correct codes?

V30.01 Single liveborn, born in hospital, delivered by Cesarean delivery

765.03 Extreme immaturity, 750–999 grams

765.24 Weeks of gestation, 27–28 completed weeks of gestation

««« CODING TIP

Only a physician can diagnose an infant as premature or LBW. You cannot code this simply from documentation stating the statistics. The physician must document the actual diagnosis.

««« CODING TIP

In the case of Michael Young, the reason you will not code the lung immaturity is because it is a sign or symptom for his extreme immaturity diagnosis. It is not coded separately.

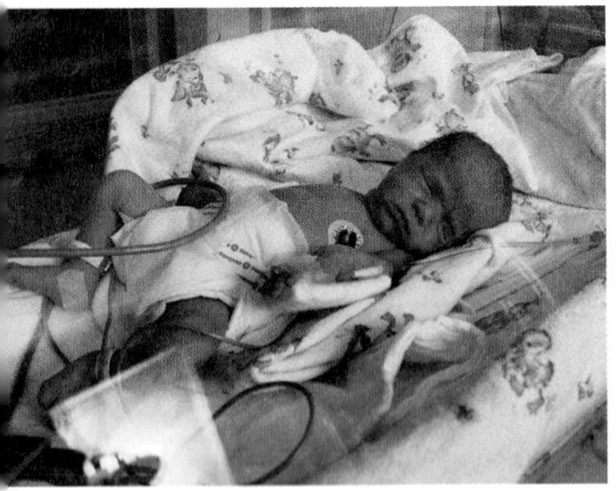

«« CODING TIP

Neither code 038 Septicemia nor code 995.9x Systemic inflammatory response syndrome is used on newborn charts.

PERINATAL SEPTICEMIA (SEPSIS)

Many things are dealt with differently when they exist in a newborn rather than an adult. A diagnosis of septicemia is one such instance. Let's say that Dr. Frances diagnoses Judy, a 15-day old newborn, with septicemia. When you look *septicemia* up in the alphabetic index, read carefully. You will see

> Septicemia, septicemic (generalized) (suppurative) 038.9

There is a long list of descriptors indented beneath this. It seems that you don't have any additional information, so let's turn to the tabular list to check:

> √4th 038 Septicemia

This certainly matches, doesn't it? Professional coding specialists need to be very careful, so let's read the EXCLUDES note, as you always do, to be certain. You will see

> EXCLUDES septicemia (sepsis) of newborn (771.81)

This is exactly why these EXCLUDES notes are there. To help you if you land in the wrong place. So, turn to 771 in the tabular list to double-check.

> √4th 771 Infections specific to the perinatal period

Read the INCLUDES and EXCLUDES notes carefully. OK, it seems you are in the correct location this time. You need a fourth digit, so read down the column. The best choice is:

> √5th 771.8 Other infection specific to the perinatal period

There is a notation that directs you to

> Use additional code to identify organism or specific infection

Isn't it great when the book actually TELLS you what additional codes you will need? Absolutely. Be certain to follow that direction, and if this detail is not included in the notes, you will need to either consult the lab report in the chart or query the physician. Read down the column to find the most accurate fifth digit:

> 771.81 Septicemia (sepsis) of newborn

There is another notation below that directs you to

> Use additional codes to identify severe sepsis (995.92) and any associated acute organ dysfunction, if applicable.

Unlike the previous notation, this "Use additional code" includes the phrase "if applicable." This directs you to check the notes to confirm whether or not this additional condition is diagnosed. If it is, you need to include these additional codes. If not, don't worry about it.

KEYS TO CODING »»

Review the **ICD-9-CM Coding Guidelines, Section I. chapter 15. Newborn (Perinatal) Guidelines (740-779),** subsection **j. Newborn sepsis** for more input on identifying what to code, what not to code, and in what order to put multiple codes. Use this to support your reading here, and as a reminder booster later on.

MATERNAL CONDITIONS AFFECTING THE INFANT

When the physician's notes specify that a mother's illness, injury, or condition had a direct impact on the baby's health, you will include a code on the baby's chart from the range of 760–763 Maternal causes of perinatal **morbidity** and **mortality.**

Morbidity

The status of being diseased.

Mortality

Cause of death.

Conditions in the mother, such as high blood pressure, the presence of certain infections, or an abnormal uterus or cervix, can increase the possibilities that the baby might be born prematurely and with a LBW. A mother's heart, kidney, and/or lung problems might also affect the baby's health.

While the reasons are not completely understood by physicians, a woman may experience spontaneous *p*remature *r*upture *o*f the *m*embranes (PROM), which results in spontaneous preterm labor. There is virtually nothing that can be done to prevent the situation that so often leads to the birth of a premature, LBW baby.

Premature, LBW babies are more likely to be at risk for developing certain conditions now and later in life. This is why it is so important that the documentation and the coding accurately report the baby's situation from the beginning. Some of the most common conditions include:

- Breathing problems, including respiratory distress syndrome (RDS)
- Periventricular and/or intraventricular hemorrhage (bleeding in the brain)
- Patent ductus arteriosus (PDA), a dangerous heart problem
- Necrotizing enterocolitis (NEC), an intestinal problem that leads to difficulties in feeding
- Retinopathy of prematurity (ROP)
- Low body temperature (caused by a lack of body fat used by newborns to maintain normal body temperature), which promotes slow growth, breathing problems, and other complications
- Apnea, an interruption in breathing
- Jaundice, a result of incomplete liver development
- Anemia
- Bronchopulmonary dysplasia, also known as chronic lung disease
- Infections, due to the inability of immature immune systems to fight off bacteria and viruses

«« KEYS TO CODING

Review the **ICD-9-CM Coding Guidelines, Section I. chapter 15. Newborn (Perinatal) Guidelines (740-779),** subsection **f. Maternal causes of perinatal morbidity** for more input on identifying what to code, what not to code, and in what order to put multiple codes. Use this to support your reading here, and as a reminder booster later on.

YOU CODE IT! CASE STUDY

Suzette Collier was born, full term, at Barton Hospital vaginally. Her mother has been an alcoholic for many years and would not stop drinking during the pregnancy. Suzette was diagnosed at birth with fetal alcohol syndrome and admitted into the NICU.

You Code It!

Read the notes on Suzette, and find the most accurate diagnosis code(s).

Step 1: Read the case completely.

Step 2: Abstract the notes: Which key words can you identify relating to why Suzette was cared for?

____

Step 3: Query the provider, if necessary.

Step 4: Code the diagnosis or diagnoses.

Step 5: Code the procedure(s): Birth.

Step 6: Link the procedure codes to at least one diagnosis code to confirm medical necessity.

Step 7: Back code to double-check your choices.

Answer

Did you find the correct codes?

V30.00 Single liveborn, born in hospital, with no mention of cesarean delivery

760.71 Noxious influences affecting fetus or newborn via placenta or breast milk, alcohol (fetal alcohol syndrome)

Terrific!

ROUTINE WELL-BABY CHECKUPS

Once released from the hospital, all children should have regularly scheduled checkups with their pediatrician or family physician. The encounters, just like adult physicals and other checkups, are coded from V code categories, including:

√4th V20 Health supervision of infant or child

You will need to identify the patient's age to determine which code to use:

V20.2 Routine infant or child health check—health check for child over 28 days old

√5th V20.3 Newborn health supervision for child under 29 days old

V20.31 Health supervision for newborn under 8 days old

V20.32 Health supervision for newborn 8 to 28 days old

√4th V21 Constitutional states in development

BRIDGE TO ICD-10-CM

Routine well-baby and child checkups will be reported with the same process. Just the codes will look differently.

You will notice that V21 includes additional digits to identify which particular concern is an issue, addressed by the physician during this encounter.

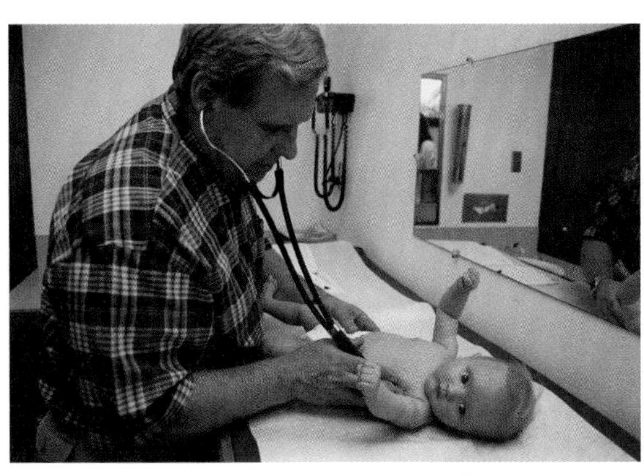

V21.0 Period of rapid growth in childhood

V21.1 Puberty

V21.2 Other adolescence

√5th V21.3 Low birth weight status

V21.8 Other specified constitutional states in development

V21.9 Unspecified constitutional state in development

For the most part, V21.3- is the only code in the category that refers to services for LBW newborns. That is because, as you learned earlier in this chapter, a baby born with LBW is at risk for developing additional health concerns—many of which will need continued monitoring and/or treatment.

TAYLOR, READER, & ASSOCIATES
A Complete Health Care Facility
975 CENTRAL AVENUE • SOMEWHERE, FL 32811 • 407-555-4321

PATIENT: TOBIAS, TRISTA
MRN: TOBITRI01
Procedure Performed: Newborn Reevaluation
Date: 07/10/11

Attending Physician: Pravdah H. Jeppard, MD

This is an 18-month-old female who is brought into the Emergency Department by her mother in a carriage. Upon arrival, child is sleeping. Skin is hot to touch. She is irritable initially upon awakening but then lethargic. Occasional wimper. Mother reports loose yellow stool. Also reports child has been coughing and vomiting over the past 6 days. Child was seen in clinic for an ear infection and has been on Amoxicillin 125mg/5ml for 3 days.

Allergies: NKA

Growth/Development: WNL

W 30lbs. T104.3 AR 158 R 60 BP 103/58 Pulse Ox 99% Abdomen is distended. Tachypenic. Lungs clear. Eyes clear, pupils reactive. No eye contact is made. CBC, CMET, BCx1, CXR ordered.

Admit to hospital pediatrics unit.

Admitting Diagnoses: Hypokalemia, fever, anemia

Pravdah H. Jeppard, MD

PHJ/mg D: 07/10/11 09:50:16 T: 07/15/11 12:55:01

Find the best, most accurate ICD-9-CM code(s).

TAYLOR, READER, & ASSOCIATES
A Complete Health Care Facility
975 CENTRAL AVENUE • SOMEWHERE, FL 32811 • 407-555-4321

PATIENT: BELGUM, ALLEN
ACCOUNT/EHR #: BELGAL001
Date: 05/15/11

Attending Physician: Pravdah H. Jeppard, MD

Consultant: Vivian Pixar, MD

REASON FOR CONSULTATION: Rule out retinopathy of prematurity

FINDINGS & RECOMMENDATIONS OF CONSULTANT: The patient was born on 04/13/11, with a birth weight of 2,620 grams, gestational age of 36 weeks, highest recorded PO2 of 310.

PHYSICAL EXAMINATION: Exam this date shows normal external exam, well-dilated pupils. Indirect exam shows clear media, normal optic nerves and retinae both eyes with normal retinal vessel extension to the periphery without evidence of retinopathy.

IMPRESSION: Normal retinal exam

RECOMMENDATIONS: See patient again in 3 months

Vivian Pixar, MD

VP/mg D: 05/15/11 09:50:16 T: 05/20/11 12:55:01

Find the best, most accurate ICD-9-CM code(s).

TAYLOR, READER, & ASSOCIATES
A Complete Health Care Facility
975 CENTRAL AVENUE • SOMEWHERE, FL 32811 • 407-555-4321

PATIENT: EDWARDS, MANUEL
ACCOUNT/EHR #: EDWAMA001
Date: 10/10/11

PREOP DIAGNOSIS: Anoxic encephalopathy, neuromuscular incoordination
POSTOP DIAGNOSIS: Same
OPERATION: Gastrostomy
SURGEON: Robert R. Singer, MD
ANESTHESIOLOGIST: John Katzman, MD

INDICATIONS FOR OPERATION: This is a neonatal patient who weights approximately 2,200 grams. The child has severe anoxic encephalopathy, cannot be fed without an NG tube. The child had an upper GI which shows minimal reflux. The child was brought to the operation room at this time for a gastrostomy.

PROCEDURE; The patient was placed in the supine position under general endotracheal anesthesia and the abdomen was prepped and draped in the usual sterile manner. A midline upper abdominal incision was made. The abdomen was entered. The stomach was grasped with a Babcock clamp and brought up to the wound. Two concentric purse strings of 3-0 silk were placed. A 12 Malecot catheter was placed in the stomach through a stab wound in the center of the purse string. The two purse strings were tied consecutively and the stomach was packed to the GE tube. The Malecot catheter was brought out through a separate stab wound in the left upper quadrant. The stomach was sutured to the abdominal wall using 3-0 chromic. A suture was placed on the outside to secure the gastrostomy tube and prevent it from being dislodged. The midline incision was closed with interrupted 3-0 silk. The skin was closed with 5-0 plain subcuticular stitches. A Steri-strip dressing and Telfa were placed at the GE tube site. The patient tolerated the procedure well and was taken back to the neonatal unit in fair condition.

Robert R. Singer, MD

RRS/mg D: 10/10/11 09:50:16 T: 10/13/11 12:55:01

Find the best, most accurate ICD-9-CM code(s).

____

____

____

11 Coding Infectious Diseases

KEY TERMS

- Asymptomatic
- Bacteremia
- Human immunodeficiency virus (HIV)
- Infectious
- Pathogen
- Septic shock
- Sepsis
- Septicemia
- Severe sepsis
- Systemic inflammatory response syndrome (SIRS)
- Tuberculosis

LEARNING OUTCOMES

11.1 Apply the guidelines for coding diagnoses with HIV.

11.2 Correctly code testing and test results for infectious diseases.

11.3 Distinguish between septicemia and SIRS.

11.4 Identify the differences between sepsis and severe sepsis.

11.5 Place the codes for severe sepsis in the correct sequence.

11.6 Determine the correct guidelines for coding tuberculosis.

Many conditions and illnesses can be disseminated from one individual to another. **Infectious** diseases are spread by personal contact, such as a hand shake or the exchange of bodily fluids; other diseases can be spread by the touch of a doorknob that has been handled by someone else.

You have heard about some of these conditions, such as meningitis, hepatitis, **tuberculosis,** and **human immunodeficiency virus (HIV).**

As a coding specialist, your vulnerability to infectious diseases and conditions while on the job is limited. However, you should realize that protecting your health is the basis for certain safety protocols, such as wearing gloves and using special waste receptacles. As long as you follow important safety policies, there is no reason to be afraid.

Infectious

A condition that can be transmitted from one person to another.

Tuberculosis

An infectious condition that causes small rounded swellings on mucous membranes throughout the body.

Human immunodeficiency virus (HIV)

A condition affecting the immune system.

Sepsis and Septic Shock Relating to Pregnancy or Newborns

As you read in Chap. 9, a woman who has had an ectopic pregnancy, a molar pregnancy, or an abortion AND has been diagnosed with sepsis or septic shock, will not be reported with a code from category 038 like other septic patients. Instead, you will use a code from the range 630–639, as appropriate by the notes, for example

639.0 Genital tract and pelvic infection (sepsis NOS, Septicemia NOS) following conditions classifiable to 630–638

639.5 Shock (postoperative) (septic) following conditions classifiable to 630–638

As reviewed in Chap. 10, a newborn baby diagnosed with sepsis or septicemia will be reported with

√5th 771.8 Other infection specific to the Perinatal period

+ A code to identify the organism or specific infection

As the guidelines direct (1C15j. Newborn Sepsis), it is not necessary to use a code from 995.91 Systemic inflammatory response syndrome (SIRS), sepsis on a newborn's record because code 771.8x already reports the presence of sepsis. However, when the documentation supports a diagnosis for severe sepsis, you are instructed to report, in addition to the above codes,

995.92 Systemic inflammatory response syndrome (SIRS), severe sepsis

+ a code for documented acute organ dysfunction

Let's say you forgot. Go to septicemia in the ICD-9-CM alphabetic index:

Septicemia, septicemic [generalized (suppurative)] 038.9

Then, go to the tabular list to confirm, and of course, you start reading

√4th 038 Septicemia

The first thing you see is the note "Use additional code for systemic inflammatory response syndrome (SIRS)(995.91–995.92)." Keep reading

EXCLUDES . . . .

During labor (659.3)

Following ectopic or molar pregnancy (639.0)

Postpartum, puerperal (670)

Septicemia (sepsis) of newborn (771.81)

That complicating abortion (634–638 with .0, 639.0)

You can see that the ICD-9-CM book is reminding you when a diagnosis of septicemia from code category 038 is not correct.

Septic Condition Resulting from Surgery

Should a patient develop sepsis from an infection as a complication of a surgical procedure, you will list a code for that situation first. In the alphabetic index, find

Septicemia, septicemic, postoperative 998.59

«« KEYS TO CODING

Review the **ICD-9-CM Coding Guidelines, Section I. chapter 1. Infectious and Parasitic Diseases (001-139),** subsection **b7. Sepsis and septic shock complicating abortion and pregnancy** and **b9. Newborn sepsis** for more input on identifying what to code, what not to code, and in what order to put multiple codes. Use this to support your reading here, and as a reminder booster later on.

In the tabular list, find

√4th 998 Other complications of procedures, not elsewhere classified

Read down the column to review your choices for the required fourth digit:

√5th 998.5 Postoperative infection

Read the EXCLUDES notes. You will see that there is one specific item that would be easy to code incorrectly from this subcategory:

Postoperative obstetrical wound infection (674.3)

While there are other diagnoses also included, an obstetrical surgical wound, such as an abdominal wound from a C-section performed, is the only EXCLUDES condition also described as a "postoperative infection." This is a great example of why it is so important to read carefully.

998.59 Other postoperative infection, septicemia, postoperative

Don't forget the notation below this code:

"Use additional code to identify infection"

Then, continue with the usual coding sequence for sepsis, as reviewed earlier in this chapter.

KEYS TO CODING »»

Review the **ICD-9-CM Coding Guidelines, Section I. chapter 1. Infectious and Parasitic Diseases (001-139),** subsection **b. 10. Sepsis due to a post-procedural infection** for more input on identifying what to code, what not to code, and in what order to put multiple codes. Use this to support your reading here, and as a reminder booster later on.

YOU CODE IT! CASE STUDY

Gregory Parrale, a 31-year-old male, had his appendix taken out last week. He comes to Dr. Gorman's office for his postsurgical follow-up visit, and Dr. Gorman finds the surgical wound is erythematous, swollen, and painful to the touch. He takes a swab of the fluid oozing from the site. The lab confirms a postoperative staph infection.

You Code It!

Go through the steps of coding, and determine the diagnosis code(s) to be reported for this encounter between Dr. Gorman and Gregory Parrale.

Step 1: Read the case completely.

Step 2: Abstract the notes: Which key words can you identify relating to why Dr. Gorman cared for Gregory?

Step 3: Query the provider, if necessary.

Step 4: Code the diagnosis or diagnoses.

Step 5: Code the procedure(s): Office visit, blood tests.

Step 6: Link the procedure codes to at least one diagnosis code to confirm medical necessity.

Step 7: Back code to double-check your choices.

Answer

Did you find the correct codes?

998.59 Other postoperative infection

041.10 Staphylococcus, unspecified

Good job!

SYSTEMIC INFLAMMATORY RESPONSE SYNDROME WITHOUT INFECTION

Systemic inflammatory response syndrome (SIRS) can develop in patients who have not developed an infection. Instead the reaction may occur due to the presence of a burn or other trauma, a malignant neoplasm, or the presence of pancreatitis. In such cases, coding the condition will change slightly. You will code the following sequence:

1. The code for the underlying condition (e.g., 943.31 Third-degree burn of forearm)
2. The code for SIRS from the subcategory √4th 995.9 Systemic inflammatory response syndrome
3. The code for the acute organ dysfunction, when applicable

If the documentation indicates that the patient later developed an infection, you will code the diagnosis of SIRS as shown earlier in the chapter, along with the additional code for the underlying trauma or condition.

METHICILLIN-RESISTANT *STAPHYLOCOCCUS AUREUS*

Methicillin-resistant *Staphylococcus aureus* (MRSA) is a bacterial (staph) infection that is essentially unaffected by certain antibiotics. MRSA is spread from one person to another by direct contact with the infection, such as touching a skin bump or infection that is draining pus. MRSA can be spread directly, for example, by touching an infected person's rash, or it can be spread indirectly, such as by touching a used bandage contaminated with MRSA or by sharing a towel or razor that has come in contact with infected skin. One of the most frequent anatomic sites of MRSA colonization is the nose; bacteria can be found in nasal secretions.

Methicillin-Resistant *Staphylococcus Aureus* Colonization

When the patient is documented as having a MRSA screening or nasal swab test that is positive, yet there is no current illness, this is called colonization. Colonization indicates that the patient is a carrier. When this is the case, report either

V02.53 Carrier or suspected carrier, Methicillin susceptible Staphylococcus aureus (MSSA)

or

V02.54 Carrier or suspected carrier, Methicillin resistant Staphylococcus aureus (MRSA)

The ICD-9-CM coding guidelines state that it is possible for one patient to be a MRSA carrier AND have a current MRSA infection at the same encounter. When this is the case, you are permitted to report code V02.54 and a code for the MRSA infection.

KEYS TO CODING »»

Review the **ICD-9-CM Coding Guidelines, Section I. chapter 1. Infectious and Parasitic Diseases (001-139),** subsection **c. Methicillin Resistant Staphylococcus aureus (MRSA) Conditions** for more input on identifying what to code, what not to code, and in what order to put multiple codes. Use this to support your reading here, and as a reminder booster later on.

Methicillin-Resistant *Staphylococcus Aureus* Infection

There are some infections commonly known to be caused by the patient's current MRSA status. In these cases, ICD-9-CM provides a combination code that can be used—the one code instead of two different codes. Two examples of these combination codes are

038.12 Methicillin resistant Staphylococcus aureus septicemia

482.42 Methicillin resistant pneumonia due to Staphylococcus aureus

Notice that the code descriptions include both the MRSA plus_another infection: septicemia in the first code and pneumonia in the second.

BRIDGE TO ICD-10-CM 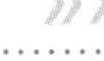

MRSA will be reported with

Z16 Infection with drug resistant microorganisms

"This category is intended for use as an additional code for infectious conditions classified elsewhere to indicate the presence of drug-resistance of the infectious organism." As you can see, ICD-10-CM has broadened the scope of the MRSA code.

Not all infections occurring at the same time a patient has a MRSA infection will have a combination code available. To properly report these diagnoses, code the current infection due to MRSA and the MRSA infection separately with code

041.12 Methicillin resistant Staphylococcus aureus

Example

Taneshia Novack was diagnosed with acute cystitis due to MRSA.

595.0 Acute cystitis

041.12 Methicillin resistant Staphylococcus aureus

TUBERCULOSIS

Tuberculosis (TB) is a threat to the community because it is highly contagious. You may have been required to take a TB skin test as a part of your entry into the health care field. *Mycobacterium tuberculosis*, the causative agent of TB, is a bacterial infection that is transmitted through the air. It means that someone can become infected by being coughed on by someone who has TB. One version of TB is called *latent tuberculosis infection (LTBI),* because it is dormant and may not show symptoms right away. That is why individuals must take a TB test, because not everyone that has been infected is symptomatic. Most types of TB and LTBI are successfully treated with medication.

There is a specific cultural group of people who will get a positive result to the skin test but not actually have the disease. A simple chest x-ray confirms that situation. Should you have a patient in such a circumstance, you will use code

795.5 Nonspecific reaction to tuberculin skin test without active tuberculosis

In cases where a patient tests positive for TB and actually does have the disease, you will choose the best, most appropriate code from the range 010–018 Tuberculosis. As you look through the section, you will notice that TB is a disseminated disease. While most people think of TB as a pulmonary infection, infiltrating only the lungs, it can actually leach throughout the body and be identified in many different anatomical sites. You have to know which anatomical site is infected with the TB bacterium so that you can find the most accurate code.

YOU CODE IT! CASE STUDY

Henry Kensington was brought into the emergency department (ED) by ambulance because he was having pain in his abdomen. Dr. Stanton diagnosed Henry with renal tuberculosis, confirmed histologically, with pyelonephritis.

You Code It!

Go through the steps of coding, and determine the diagnosis code or codes that should be reported for this encounter between Dr. Stanton and Henry Kensington.

Step 1: Read the case completely.

Step 2: Abstract the notes: Which key words can you identify relating to why Dr. Stanton cared for Henry?

___

Step 3: Query the provider, if necessary.

Step 4: Code the diagnosis or diagnoses.

___

Step 5: Code the procedure(s): Admission to hospital.

Step 6: Link the procedure codes to at least one diagnosis code to confirm medical necessity.

Step 7: Back code to double-check your choices.

Answer

Did you find the correct codes?

016.05 Tuberculosis of kidney, tubercle bacilli not found by bacteriological examination but tuberculosis confirmed histologically

590.81 Pyelitis or pyelonephritis in disease classified elsewhere

Terrific!

BACTERIAL INFECTIONS

Some bacterial infections that you will encounter in a typical health care facility are those that are foodborne, commonly called food poisoning. According to Centers for Disease Control (CDC), approximately 76 million cases of foodborne illness and 5,000 associated deaths occur in the United States annually. Do not let this fool you: These diagnoses are not poisonings (as far as coding goes); they are infections. Therefore, the diagnosis codes will not include E codes. Some of the most frequently seen bacterial infections, and their sources, are as follows:

- *Campylobacter:* From foods including raw poultry; raw meat; untreated milk*:* code 008.43
- *Listeria:* Untreated milk; dairy products; raw salads and vegetables: code 027.0
- *Salmonella:* Raw poultry; eggs; raw meat; untreated milk and dairy products: codes 003.x
- *Shigella:* Untreated water; milk and dairy products; raw vegetables and salads; shellfish; turkey; apple cider: codes 004.x
- *Vibrio:* Raw and lightly cooked fish and shellfish: code 005.81
- *Clostridium perfringens:* Animal and human excreta; soil; dust; insects; raw meat: code 005.2
- *Escherichia coli (E. coli 0157):* Human and animal gut; sewage; water; raw meat: codes 008.0x

Almost all the above infections induce symptoms of diarrhea, abdominal pain, nausea, fever, and vomiting. Other serious effects include dehydration, headache, and kidney damage or failure. Therefore, you must be careful not to report unnecessary codes for signs and symptoms that are actually included in a definitive diagnosis that has been made.

LET'S CODE IT! SCENARIO

Robyn Julianni, a 23-year-old female, came to see Dr. Chou due to severe abdominal pain. She had a fever and stated that she has had bloody diarrhea for the past 2 days. Dr. Chou's examination revealed that she was dehydrated as well. Robyn stated she ate at a new restaurant at the beach where she had a salad and a vegetable plate. After taking some tests, he diagnosed Robyn with Shigella dysenteriae *(bacillary dysentery).*

Let's Code It!

Dr. Chou found Robyn to be suffering from *Shigella.* Turn to the alphabetic index and find

Shigella (dysentery) (see also Dysentery, bacillary) 004.9

Turn to the tabular list, and check the code's complete description:

√4th 004 Shigellosis

There are no notations or directives, so read down the column to review all of the choices for the required fourth digit. The code suggested by the alphabetic index:

004.9 Shigellosis, unspecified

Is this the most accurate code? You will note that the other fourth-digit code choices for 004 want specifics on which group (A, B, C, or D) of the *Shigella* infection is present. Do you know? Dr. Chou did specify in the notes—*Shigella dysenteriae,* which matches the description for

004.0 Shigella dysenteriae

Therefore, 004.0 is the most accurate code available. Excellent!

OTHER INFECTIONS

There are a large number of infectious diseases that you may have to code, depending upon the type of facility that employs you, combined with geographic and other factors. Let's review some of the most common infections, their descriptions, and their code ranges.

Viral Hepatitis

Hepatitis (hepat = liver; -itis = inflammation) actually refers to several different viral infections. According to the Centers for Disease Control (CDC) viral hepatitis is the most prevalent cause of malignant neoplasms of the liver. Millions of people are living with one of these conditions in the United States. As you know, prevention is a much better path than treatment. For those coming to your facility to get a hepatitis vaccine, you will report one of these codes:

V01.79 Contact with or exposure to other viral diseases

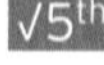
V02.6 Viral hepatitis carrier or suspected carrier

V05.3 Need for prophylactic vaccination and inoculation against single disease, viral hepatitis.

Viral Hepatitis, Type A

The CDC estimates that an additional 25,000 people each year become infected with viral hepatitis, type A, a viral infection of the liver caused by the hepatitis A virus (HAV). The virus can travel from person to person by personal contact, as with other infections. However, in addition, one can become infected by being exposed to contaminated water or ice. Shellfish harvested from sewage-contaminated water, as well as fruits, vegetables, and other foods that have been contaminated and eaten uncooked, may also carry the hepatitis A virus. Viral hepatitis A is reported with either

070.0 Viral hepatitis A with hepatic coma

or

070.1 Viral hepatitis A without mention of hepatic coma

Viral Hepatitis, Type B

Caused by the hepatitis B virus (HBV), viral hepatitis, type B, is transmitted through contact with infected bodily fluids, such as blood or semen. The infection can also be spread by the use of equipment that has been contaminated with the virus, which is why when getting a tattoo, body piercing, or even fingernail application, one must be careful that the needles and files have been sterilized properly. The CDC estimates 43,000 new cases of Hepatitis B are diagnosed each year. Viral hepatitis B is reported with either

√5th 070.2 Viral hepatitis B with hepatic coma

or

√5th 070.3. Viral hepatitis B without mention of hepatic coma

To choose the most accurate code, you have to know if the patient has a hepatic coma, whether or not the condition is identified as acute or chronic, and whether or not hepatitis D (delta) is involved.

Viral Hepatitis, Type C

The hepatitis C virus (HCV) infection is estimated by the Centers for Disease Control (CDC) to chronically affect 3.2 million people in the United States. It is considered to be the most widespread chronic bloodborne infection. Those individuals at the highest risk for infection are those using injected drugs. Each year, it is believed that an additional 17,000 individuals become hepatitis C positive. Report this diagnosis with one code from

070.41 Acute hepatitis C with hepatic coma

070.44 Chronic hepatitis C with hepatic coma

070.51 Acute hepatitis C without mention of hepatic coma

070.54 Chronic hepatitis without mention of hepatic coma

√5th 070.7 Unspecified viral hepatitis C

Viral Hepatitis, Type D

Also known as Hepatitis delta, this is a serious liver disease that requires the HBV (hepatitis B virus) to replicate itself. This condition is not seen often in the United States. Hepatitis D is transmitted through direct contact with infected blood, similar to how Hepatitis B is passed from one person to another. Currently, there is no vaccine for Hepatitis D. Hepatitis D is referred to as hepatitis delta in the ICD-9-CM code descriptions, and reported with codes

070.42 Hepatitis delta without mention of active hepatitis B disease with hepatic coma

070.52 Hepatitis delta without mention of active hepatitis B disease or hepatic coma

This may also be reported with the fifth digit 1 or 3 for Hepatitis B codes 070.2 and 070.3:

Fifth digit choices:

1 acute or unspecified, with hepatitis delta

3 chronic, with hepatitis delta

Viral Hepatitis, Type E

Occurrences of Hepatitis E in the United States are rare; it is known to be common in countries with poor sanitation and contaminated water supplies. This liver disease, caused by the Hepatitis E virus (HEV) does not lead to chronic infection. There is no vaccine currently approved by the FDA for Hepatitis E. Report this diagnosis with either

070.43 Hepatitis E with hepatic coma

070.53 Hepatitis E without mention of hepatic coma

Meningitis

Meningitis is the inflammation of the meningeal membranes of the brain and/or the spinal cord. Meningitis can be bacterial; however, it is more often the result of a viral infection. When meningitis is caught early, the prognosis is good and the complications are rare.

In order to code a diagnosis of meningitis, you have to know which virus or bacteria is at the core of the inflammation.

Example

Meningococcal meningitis 036.0

In some cases, ICD-9-CM will identify the requirement of a second code.

Example

Meningitis due to whooping cough 033.9 *[320.7]*

Tetanus (Lockjaw)

You are probably more familiar with the tetanus vaccine than you are with the disease. Tetanus is an infection of the nervous system and is caused by the entry of bacteria into the body through a break in the skin. It causes death in about 11% of all cases. The illness can be prevented by the administration of the tetanus toxoid, included in the DTaP, DT, and Td vaccines.

When the patient has come for inoculation with the tetanus toxoid only, you will use V03.7. However, read the notes carefully. If the DTP or DTaP was administered, use code V06.1. If the development of tetanus is a complication arising from the vaccination, use code 999.*x*. If it is a result of an incident, such as stepping on a rusty nail, report it with code 037 (plus an E code). Should this disease occur with or following an abortion or ectopic pregnancy, then you will report it as a complication of pregnancy, using 633.*x* or 639.*x*. And in cases where the tetanus is affecting a neonate, it will be reported with code 771.3.

Influenza

There is a reason why so much commotion is made annually about individuals getting their flu shots. A seemingly ordinary infection, influenza (commonly called the flu) can be deadly. It is caused by the influenza A

Step 5: Code the procedure(s): Office visit.

Step 6: Link the procedure codes to at least one diagnosis code to confirm medical necessity.

Step 7: Back code to double-check your choices.

Answer

Did you find the correct codes?

276.51 Dehydration

250.03 Diabetes mellitus, without mention of complications, type 1, uncontrolled

V15.81 Noncompliance with medical treatment

Good job!

Overdose of Insulin

KEYS TO CODING »»

When a patient suffers complications due to an overdose or an underdose of any drug, including insulin, an E code may also be needed to be reported, as per the guidelines for reporting adverse reactions and poisonings. See Chap. 6 to review the rules for coding these events.

KEYS TO CODING »»

Review the **ICD-9-CM Coding Guidelines, Section I. chapter 3. Endocrine, Nutritional, and Metabolic Disease and Immunity Disorders (240–279),** subsection **a. 6. Insulin Pump Malfunction** for more input on identifying what to code, what not to code, and in what order to put multiple codes. Use this to support your reading here, and as a reminder later on.

Patients with an insulin pump that malfunctions can dose themselves with a higher quantity of insulin than that prescribed by the attending physician. For such a case, you will use the following code (which is the same as an underdose):

996.57 Mechanical complication of other specified prosthetic device, implant, and graft, due to insulin pump

Follow that code with a poisoning code:

962.3 Poisoning by insulins and antidiabetic agents

And follow that code with the appropriate 250 Diabetes mellitus code and any other appropriate codes, including those codes identifying the reaction or conditions caused by the overdose.

If the patient delivers a dose of insulin manually and suffers an overdose, you will code it the same way you do any other poisoning, including the determination of the cause of the overdose (such as accident, attempted suicide, assault, etc.). Unless the health concern with the patient is an adverse reaction to the insulin and not related to the actual dosage, you will not use the code reporting therapeutic usage.

SECONDARY DIABETES MELLITUS

In a previous section of this chapter, you learned about reporting a diagnosis of DM (primary). That means that the condition was caused by a malfunction of the patient's pancreas. However, there are circumstances where diabetes is actually caused by medication or another condition or disease. When this is the case, the patient is diagnosed with secondary diabetes mellitus. This may be indicated in the physician's notes as *secondary* diabetes or as diabetes mellitus *due to* cystic fibrosis, *due to* pancreatic malignancy, *due to* a reaction to a specific drug, etc. Code category 249 Secondary diabetes mellitus contains the codes for reporting this specific condition, as well as any related manifestations, just as you did with primary diabetes mellitus.

√5th 249.0 Secondary diabetes mellitus without mention of complication

Secondary diabetes mellitus, caused by a drug, chemical, or other condition, may be diagnosed without any other manifestations.

√5th 249.1 Secondary diabetes mellitus with Ketoacidosis

Diabetic ketoacidosis (DKA), sometimes a life-threatening condition, develops when the individual's hyperglycemia doesn't receive proper treatment. Patients with secondary diabetes are at risk of developing DKA.

√5th 249.2 Secondary diabetes mellitus with hyperosmolarity

A patient with too high of a concentration of glucose in their body has diabetes with hyperosmolarity. Hyperosmolarity can cause the patient to fall into a nonketotic coma.

√5th 249.3 Secondary diabetes mellitus with other coma

Several aspects of the diabetic condition can cause an individual to slip into a coma. In any of these cases, other than a hyperosmolarity coma, you will use this fourth digit.

√5th 249.4 Secondary diabetes mellitus with Renal Manifestations

Renal manifestations affect those patients with secondary diabetes mellitus, as they do those with primary diabetes. Chronic kidney disease, diabetic nephrosis, and Kimmelstiel-Wilson syndrome are a few of the conditions seen in these patients. As with the other manifestations, you will need to report additional code(s) to provide the specific details.

√5th 249.5 Secondary diabetes mellitus with Ophthalmic Manifestations

Just as primary diabetes mellitus, secondary diabetes mellitus can cause problems with the patient's eyes and eye sight. Diabetic blindness, diabetic glaucoma, and diabetic retinal edema are a few of the conditions that may develop. You have to identify the specific ophthalmic complication with additional code(s).

√5th 249.6 Secondary diabetes mellitus with Neurological Manifestations

The nervous system can be affected by the presence of secondary DM in the body. Manifestations such as diabetic gastroparalysis and diabetic polyneuropathy can develop. You will need an additional code to specifically report the neurologic complication.

√5th 249.7 Secondary diabetes mellitus with Peripheral Circulatory Disorders

Diabetic gangrene is a condition that can cause tissue to become necrotic (die as a result of lack of blood). When gangrene is not caught early enough, the resulting treatment to stop the spread of necrosis is often amputation. Another manifestation reported with this subcategory is diabetic peripheral angiopathy, a disease involving the blood vessels of the extremities. An additional code will be required to specify the peripheral circulatory manifestations.

BRIDGE TO ICD-10-CM

Similarly to the way primary diabetes mellitus is handled, secondary diabetes mellitus is also separated into multiple code categories.

√4th E08 Diabetes mellitus due to underlying condition

√4th E09 Drug or chemical induced diabetes mellitus

E89.1 Post-procedural hypoinsulinemia (post-pancreatectomy hyperglycemia)

KEYS TO CODING »»

Review the **ICD-9-CM Coding Guidelines, Section I. chapter 3. Endocrine, Nutritional, and Metabolic Disease and Immunity Disorders (240-279),** subsection **a. 7. Secondary Diabetes Mellitus** for more input on identifying what to code, what not to code, and in what order to put multiple codes. Use this to support your reading here, and as a reminder booster later on.

√5th 249.8 Secondary diabetes mellitus with Other Specified Manifestations

Code 249.8*x* is your catchall fourth digit to report any of the numerous other complications of secondary diabetes. People with secondary diabetes mellitus are more likely to develop:

- hypoglycemia or hypoglycemic shock
- diabetic bone changes
- associated ulcerations

You will need an additional code to identify the specific complication.

√5th 249.9 Secondary diabetes mellitus with Unspecified Complication

You will remember that this code choice is an absolutely last resort, when the attending physician or the record provides no opportunity to obtain additional details.

Fifth Digit Choices

The fifth-digit choices for code category 249 Secondary diabetes mellitus are much simpler than those for 250. You only have two choices:

0 not stated as uncontrolled, or unspecified

1 uncontrolled

Essentially, if the notes specifically state the patient's secondary diabetes mellitus is currently uncontrolled, report the 249 code with a fifth digit of 1 (one). If not, report the 249 code with a fifth digit of 0 (zero).

DIABETES INSIPIDUS

Another type of diabetes that few people have heard of is *diabetes insipidus (DI).* DI is a disorder of water metabolism that is the result of an antidiuretic hormone (ADH) deficiency. Intracranial neoplastic or metastatic lesions, hypophysectomy or other neurosurgery, a skull fracture, or other head trauma that damages the neurohypophyseal structures can all incite DI. The condition can also result from infection. Diabetes insipidus is also known as *pituitary diabetes insipidus* and is coded using 253.5—from the subsection for disorders of the pituitary gland.

Nephrogenic diabetes insipidus, another form of DI, is a very rare congenital disturbance of water metabolism resulting from a renal tubular resistance to vasopressin. Interestingly, it is not coded from the congenital anomalies, but is reported using code 588.1—disorders resulting from impaired renal function.

YOU CODE IT! CASE STUDY

Chet McKeen, a 19-year-old male, comes to see Dr. Turner with complaints of extreme thirst and muscle weakness. During examination, Dr. Turner identifies that he had poor tissue turgor, dry mucous membranes, and hypotension. UA results show urine of low osmolality at 75 mOsm/kg. Dr. Turner diagnoses Chet with diabetes insipidus and prescribes Vasopressin IM qid.

You Code It!

Go through the steps of coding, and determine the diagnosis code(s) to be reported for this encounter between Dr. Turner and Chet McKeen.

Step 1: Read the case completely.

Step 2: Abstract the notes: Which key words can you identify relating to why Dr. Turner cared for Chet?

Step 3: Query the provider, if necessary.

Step 4: Code the diagnosis or diagnoses.

Step 5: Code the procedure(s): Office visit, urinalysis.

Step 6: Link the procedure codes to at least one diagnosis code to confirm medical necessity.

Step 7: Back code to double-check your choices.

Answer

Did you find the correct code?

253.5 Diabetes insipidus

Good job!

WEIGHT FACTORS

Obesity

The definitions of overweight, obese, and morbidly obese can get lost in societal norms and self-perception. Of course, the health care industry has its own official determinations of these conditions, further specified by reporting the patient's body mass index (BMI).

Overweight merely means weighing too much. This can be a reference to the individual's muscles, bones, fat, or fluid retention when calculated along with the person's height. This condition is calculated as a BMI of 25–29.9.

Obesity is a condition calculated as a body mass index (BMI) of 30–38.9. Typically, a person becomes obese when more calories are consumed than expended. Whereas some critics believe this is only caused by eating too much and not exercising enough, the facts are that one's genetics and current medications (including herbal supplements) can also influence this condition. Being diagnosed as obese is a true health condition that not only can result in self-esteem problems and social anxiety but also may increase the risk of developing diabetes, heart disease, arthritis, stroke, and even certain malignancies.

Morbid obesity is a patient's current overweight status to the extent that it actually interferes with normal, daily activities. This condition is calculated as a BMI over 39.

KEYS TO CODING »»

Several different types of health care professionals, such as a dietician or a nutritionist, may be involved in the care of a patient determined to be overweight, obese, or morbidly obese. However, the first time this diagnosis code is reported may only be coded from physician documentation.

Example

√4th 278 Overweight, obesity, and other hyperalimentation

√5th 278.0 Overweight and obesity

Use additional code to identify Body Mass Index (BMI) if known (V85.0–V85.54)

As you can see, ICD-9-CM reminds you to use an additional code to specify the patient's BMI.

BRIDGE TO ICD-10-CM »»

Overweight and obesity codes have more specificity:

√5th E66 Obesity due to excess calories

E66.1 Drug-induced obesity

E66.2 Morbid (severe) obesity with alveolar hypoventilation

E66.3 Overweight

E66.8 Other obesity

Body Mass Index

It is important for health care to determine specifically what is a healthy amount of body fat and what falls or rises to an unhealthy level. Body mass index (BMI) is a calculation using an individual's actual weight and current height to determine a workable measure of body fat. However, some people, such as athletes, may have a BMI that indicates that they are overweight even though there is no excess body fat. This can occur because BMI does not actually measure body fat but instead determines a ratio to work with. BMI is just one indicator of potential health risks related to an individual being outside of the normal weight range.

BMI ranges are listed differently for adults than they are for children and teens. The pediatric ranges, used for individuals aged 2–20, use the Centers for Disease Control's growth charts and take into account those normal differences in body fat for various ages as well as differences between males and females.

BRIDGE TO ICD-10-CM »»

The code category in ICD-10-CM is similar to V85 in ICD-9-CM

√4th Z68 Body mass index (BMI)

√4th V85 Body Mass Index

V85.0–V85.4 Adult BMI codes range

√5th V85.5 Body Mass Index, pediatric

Underweight

With all the discussion regarding how many people in the United States are overweight or clinically obese, the opposite—being underweight—can also cause health concerns. Unlike being overweight, abnormal weight loss or being underweight is reported with codes from the Symptoms, Signs, and Ill-Defined Conditions section of ICD-9-CM. In certain cases, the BMI will also need to be reported.

Example

√5th 783.2 Abnormal loss of weight and underweight

Use additional code to identify Body Mass Index (BMI) if known (V85.0-V85.54)

When a patient is diagnosed with an eating disorder, you may need more information from the physician before determining the correct code.

307.1 Anorexia nervosa

307.51 Bulimia nervosa

307.59 Loss of appetite of non-organic origin

When the cause of the anorexia has not been determined as organic (physiological) or nonorganic (psychological), you would report

783.0 Anorexia (loss of appetite)

«« KEYS TO CODING

While you may see issues of overweight status accompanying diagnoses such as DM or hypertension, in cases of underweight patients, be alert to initial or additional diagnoses of malnutrition.

OTHER METABOLIC DISORDERS

When you eat, it is your metabolism that processes that nutrition into energy. The chemicals in the digestive system portion out glucoses and acids from the carbohydrates, fats, and proteins in the food. This process is known as metabolization. The energy created by this can be used right away, such as when someone eats before taking a test or running a race. If the body doesn't need the energy at this time, the tissues in the liver, the muscular system, as well as the adipose (body fat) can store it for future use.

Dysfunction of the metabolic processes can interfere with the various systems of the body getting what they need to work properly. This may be a case of too little of a chemical needed, such as when the pancreas cannot create enough insulin (a condition known as diabetes mellitus). You have already learned about what havoc can be caused in the other organs and systems when this disorder continues. Metabolic disorders can also result in too much of a chemical being present in the body. For example, hyperchloremia is an excessive level of chloride anion in the blood and can cause tachycardia (rapid heart beat), hypertension, dyspnea (shortness of breath), and agitation.

The long list of metabolic diagnoses include:

- Acid lipase disease
- Amyloidosis
- Barth syndrome
- Central pontine myelinolysis
- Metabolic diseases of muscle
- Farber's disease
- G6PD deficiency
- Gangliosidoses
- Hunter syndrome
- Trimethylaminuria
- Lesch-Nyhan syndrome
- Lipid storage diseases
- Metabolic myopathies
- Mitochondrial myopathies
- Mucopolysaccharidoses (MPS)
- Mucolipidoses

- Type I glycogen storage disease
- Pompe disease
- Urea cycle disorder
- Hyperoxaluria
- Oxalosis

YOU CODE IT! CASE STUDY

Marilyn brought her 4-year old son, Elian, to his pediatrician, Dr. Willows. She was very distressed because he had eruptions on his arms, legs, and face that appeared after he had spent the day at the beach. She also noticed that his urine appeared to be reddish in color. Dr. Willows examined Elian, discovering that he had splenomegaly (enlargement of the spleen). The blood test came back positive for hemolytic anemia. Both of these conditions are signs of erythropoietic porphyria, also known as Gunther's disease. Dr. Willows diagnosed Elian with this condition.

You Code It!

Go through the steps of coding, and determine the diagnosis code(s) that should be reported for this encounter between Dr. Willows and Elian.

Step 1: Read the case completely.

Step 2: Abstract the notes: Which key words can you identify relating to why Dr. Willows cared for Elian?

____

Step 3: Query the provider, if necessary.

Step 4: Code the diagnosis or diagnoses.

____

Step 5: Code the procedure(s): Office visit, blood work.

Step 6: Link the procedure codes to at least one diagnosis code to confirm medical necessity.

Step 7: Back code to double-check your choices.

Answer

Did you find the correct code?

277.1 Disorders of porphyrin metabolism (porphyria)

Good job!

Thyroid Disorders

Above your collarbone, in your neck, is the thyroid gland. This gland secretes hormones as a part of the metabolic system of the body.

Hypothyroidism is a condition in which the thyroid converts energy more slowly than normal resulting in otherwise unexplained weight gain and fatigue. In addition, individuals with hypothyroidism may often feel cold or have greater sensitivity to cold temperatures.

Hyperthyroidism, also known as an overactive thyroid, secretes too many hormones, more than the body needs to function properly. Signs and symptoms include unexplained weight loss, rapid heart rate, and a sensitivity to heat.

Additional disorders of the thyroid include:

- Goiter
- Graves' Disease
- Hashimoto's Disease
- Thyroid Nodules
- Thyroiditis
- Myxedema

Conditions and diseases that are related or involve the thyroid and its function include:

- Celiac disease
- Iodine deficiency
- Thyroid eye disease: protruding, irritated eyes
- Thyrotoxic myopathy

YOU CODE IT! CASE STUDY

Gretel Hanson, a 63-day-old female, was having dyspnea and her cry sounded hoarse. In addition, Dr. Grissom noticed her skin color was jaundiced. Her mother stated that she is a good baby and sleeps all the time. After running a TSH blood test and performing a thyroid scan, he diagnosed her with infantile cretinism, also known as congenital hypothyroidism. Dr. Grissom also noted mild cognitive impairment, which is associated with the cretinism. He explained to Gretel's mother that the mental impairment is likely to be progressive.

You Code It!

Go through the steps of coding, and determine the diagnosis code(s) that should be reported for this encounter between Dr. Grissom and Gretel.

Step 1: Read the case completely.

Step 2: Abstract the notes: Which key words can you identify relating to why Dr. Grissom cared for Gretel?

____

Step 3: Query the provider, if necessary.

Step 4: Code the diagnosis or diagnoses.

____

Step 5: Code the procedure(s): Office visit, blood work.

Step 6: Link the procedure codes to at least one diagnosis code to confirm medical necessity.

Step 7: Back code to double-check your choices.

Answer

Did you find the correct code?

243 Congenital hypothyroidism

331.83 Mild cognitive impairment, so stated

Did you see the directive under code 243 to "Use additional code to identify associated mental retardation"? Good for you!!

CHAPTER SUMMARY

Diabetes mellitus is probably the most common of the conditions and diseases affecting the endocrine system. From the hypothalamus of the brain to the genitals, every part of this system, like all of the others that make up the human body, can malfunction or become diseased.

Coding Respiratory Conditions

13

KEY TERMS

Chronic obstructive pulmonary disease (COPD)
Exacerbation
Expiration
Influenza
Inspiration
Pneumonia
Pneumothorax
Respiration
Respiratory disorder
Status asthmaticus

LEARNING OUTCOMES

13.1 Differentiate between the different types of respiratory conditions.
13.2 Apply the guidelines for coding asthma accurately.
13.3 Accurately code chronic obstructive pulmonary disease (COPD) diagnoses and manifestations.
13.4 Determine the details needed to code pneumonia correctly.
13.5 Code infectious respiratory diseases accurately.
13.6 Determine the appropriate use of E codes when applicable to respiratory conditions.

As you know, breathing is a crucial part of life; the average person breathes approximately 25,000 times each day. The human body accomplishes this function via the respiratory system that is designed to process oxygen (O_2) and carbon dioxide (CO_2). The respiratory system includes many anatomical sites beginning with the nose and continuing down the windpipe to the lungs and the bronchi. The central nervous system controls respiration from the lateral medulla oblongata of the brain stem.

Respiration is the term used for what is commonly known as breathing and consists of two parts: **inspiration** (bringing oxygen into the body and delivering it into the circulatory system that then distributes the oxygen to the cells throughout the body), and **expiration** (getting rid of carbon dioxide).

Respiration
The physical process of acquiring oxygen and releasing carbon dioxide.

Inspiration
The physical process of acquiring oxygen.

Expiration
The physical process of expulsing carbon dioxide.

Specifically, the respiratory system includes the following parts:

The Upper Respiratory System

- Nose, nasal cavity, and nasal conchae
- Frontal and sphenoidal sinuses
- Internal nares
- Nasopharynx
- Hyoid bone
- Pharynx

The Lower Respiratory System

- Larynx (voice box)
- Trachea (windpipe)
- Bronchus
- Lungs (right and left)
- Bronchioles
- Diaphragm

RESPIRATORY DISORDERS

Respiratory disorder

A malfunction of the organ system relating to respiration.

A **respiratory disorder** can threaten a patient's quality of life and possibly his or her life itself. These individuals have difficulty breathing, thereby reducing the amount of oxygen taken in during inspiration. As a coding specialist, it is important for you to understand the factors involved in the patient's diagnosis, so you will know which additional codes are required. Respiratory disorders can arise from any of the following conditions:

Congenital: A problem started during the formation of the fetus in the womb

Example

Respiratory distress syndrome

Genetic: Inherited from family members

Example

Cystic fibrosis (CF), also know as *mucoviscidosis*

Infection: Caught from exposure to someone with the condition, or a carrier of the condition, a virus or bacteria

Example

Epiglottitis; influenza

Environmental: Caused by the air surrounding an individual

Example

Coal worker's pneumoconiosis; Legionnaires' disease; asbestosis

Trauma: Outside elements causing damage to any portion of the respiratory system

Pneumothorax

A condition by which air or gas is present within the chest cavity but outside the lungs.

Example

Respiratory acidosis caused by medullary injury; **pneumothorax**

Other organ failure, impaired heart function, and/or lung lymphatic drainage

Example

Pulmonary edema

Other condition in the body that affects respiratory function

Example

Pulmonary embolism

Manifestation of another disease

Example

Pleurisy

Lifestyle behaviors, caused by the voluntary inhalation of pollutants

Example

Cigarette smoke

Other conditions and issues

LET'S CODE IT! SCENARIO

Gayle Permanente, a 19-year-old female, was feeling very congested in her chest and was having trouble breathing. She went to see Dr. Matlock at the school clinic. After a complete physical examination (PE) and blood tests, he diagnosed her with an acute upper respiratory infection.

Let's Code It!

Dr. Matlock diagnosed Gayle with *acute upper respiratory infection.* Turn to the alphabetic index to *infection, respiratory, upper,* and find

Infection
  Respiratory
    Upper (acute) (infectious) NEC 465.9

Turn to code 465 in the tabular list, and check the description:

√4th 465 Acute upper respiratory infections of multiple or unspecified sites

Read the EXCLUDES note. Does it relate to Gayle's diagnosis? No, so keep reading down the column. Which fourth digit best reports Gayle's condition?

465.9 Acute upper respiratory infections of unspecified site

Good job!

«« KEYS TO CODING

Why is this unspecified code description acceptable? In this code description, "unspecified site" means that there is no confirmation of exactly where in the upper respiratory system the infection is located. Take a look again at the list of anatomical sites included in the upper respiratory system and you can see that this is reasonable.

PLEURAL DISORDERS

The pleura is made up of two membranes: the visceral pleura—a thin membrane that coats the outside of the lung; and the parietal pleura—a membrane that lines the inside of the thoracic (chest) cavity. Pleurisy, also known as pleuritis, identifies the presence of inflammation on one or both of the pleural membranes. This condition can cause pain to the patient with each breath. A virus is most often the cause. To report pleurisy, the alphabetic index provides a long list of possibilities that lead to a surprisingly short number of codes:

- √5th 010.1 Tuberculous pleurisy in primary progressive tuberculosis
- √5th 012.0 Tuberculous pleurisy
- 487.1 Influenza with other respiratory manifestations
- 511.0 Pleurisy without mention of effusion or current tuber culosis
- 511.1 Pleurisy with effusion, with mention of a bacterial cause other than tuberculosis
- 862.29 Injury to the pleura, without mention of open wound into the cavity
- 862.39 Injury to the pleura, with mention of open wound into the cavity

(Note: Of course, you remember that with either code 862.29 or 862.39 an E code should be reported to identify how the injury happened, as well as the place of occurrence.)

The very narrow space between these two membranes is referred to as the pleural space or pleural cavity. Normally, this space contains a tiny amount of fluid, just enough to enable the visceral pleura and the parietal pleura to move and function without irritation. If excess air or fluid gets into this space, it can cause pressure on the lung and prevent the patient from inhaling because the lung does not have the room required to expand as the oxygen is brought in. Plural space disorders include:

Pleural effusion:

The presence of excess fluid in the pleural cavity, frequently a manifestation of congestive heart failure

- √5th 511.8 Other specified forms of pleural effusion, except tuberculous
  - 511.81 Malignant pleural effusion
  - 511.9 Unspecified pleural effusion

Pneumothorax:

When excess air or gasses become present in the pleural space typically caused by respiratory disease such as chronic obstructive pulmonary disorder (COPD) or tuberculosis (TB)

- √5th 011.7 Tuberculous pneumothorax
- √4th 510 Empyema [an infection within the pleural space]

ICD-9-CM directs you to use an additional code to report the specific infectious organism:

√4th 512 Pneumothorax

512.0 Spontaneous tension pneumothorax

512.1 Iatrogenic pneumothorax (post-operative pneumothorax)

512.8 Other spontaneous pneumothorax

Hemothorax:

This condition identifies an accumulation of blood in the pleural cavity, most often caused by an injury to the thoracic cavity (the chest).

511.89 Other specified forms of pleural effusion, except tuberculous (hemothorax)

««« KEYS TO CODING

You may remember seeing this in a movie or television show: a doctor declares that the patient can't breathe because of a pneumothorax, then sticks a large needle into a patient's chest to let the air out; this, almost immediately, brings relief to the patient and his or her ability to breathe.

««« KEYS TO CODING

Why is a hemothorax coded as a type of pleural effusion? Remember that a pleural effusion is the accumulation of excessive fluid in the pleural space. Blood is a type of fluid.

PULMONARY EMBOLISM

As you probably remember, an embolus is the medical term for a blood clot (thrombosis) or other tiny piece of bone marrow fat (most often created by high cholesterol) that travels within the bloodstream. During its passage through the body, this embolus can get stuck in an artery and block the flow of blood through that area. When this occurs in the lungs, it is called a pulmonary embolism.

The presence of a pulmonary embolism can create serious problems for the patient, including dyspnea (shortness of breath), pain, and/or hemoptysis (coughing up blood). Over the course of time, a pulmonary embolism can result in permanent damage to the lung as well as damage to the organs being denied oxygen because of the blockage. A pulmonary embolism can also cause an infarction (necrotic tissue) due to the lack of oxygen to the cells. A large clot, or cluster of several clots, can result in the patient's death.

√4th 415 Acute pulmonary heart disease

√5th 415.1 Pulmonary embolism and infarction

415.11 Iatrogenic pulmonary embolism and infarction

415.12 Septic pulmonary embolism

415.19 Other pulmonary embolism and infarction

416.2 Chronic pulmonary embolism

««« BRIDGE TO ICD-10-CM

The guidelines for reporting these respiratory conditions remain the same in the transition to ICD-10-CM.

INFECTIOUS RESPIRATORY DISEASES

When an infectious organism causes a patient to be diagnosed with a respiratory disorder, you often have to report a separate code to identify which infectious organism is involved. In the tabular list, you will find the instruction directly under the following heading:

Diseases of the Respiratory System (460–519)

Use additional code to identify infectious organism.

As you can see, the instructional note is valid for all codes from and including 460–519. You may find the identified organism in the physician's notes, or you may need to refer to the pathology report.

LET'S CODE IT! SCENARIO

Mason Dominey, a 15-year-old male, came to see Dr. Siplin with a complaint of a sore throat, fever, cough, chills, and malaise. Dr. Siplin examined Mason, took a chest x-ray, and did a WBC count. After reviewing the results of the exam and tests, Dr. Siplin diagnosed Mason with adenovirus pneumonia.

Let's Code It!

BRIDGE TO ICD-10-CM

ICD-10-CM will provide more specific code categories, such as

√4th J12 Viral Pneumonia

√4th J13 Pneumonia due to Streptococcus pneumoniae

√4th J14 Pneumonia due to Hemophilus influenzae

√4th J15 Bacterial Pneumonia

Dr. Siplin identified Mason's health concern as *adenovirus pneumonia.* The alphabetic index will direct you to

Pneumonia
    Adenoviral 480.0

Will the tabular list confirm that it is the correct code? Turn to

√4th 480 Viral pneumonia

There are no notations or directions so keep reading to review all of the choices for the required fourth digit.

480.0 Pneumonia due to adenovirus

You will remember that when there is an infectious organism involved, you must code it. Dr. Siplin's notes identify it as the adenovirus. Should you use an additional code (079.0) or not? At the beginning of this subsection in the tabular list, directly under the heading

Diseases of the Respiratory System (460–519)

ICD-9-CM directs you to "Use additional code to identify infectious organism." Code 480.0 is within this range. However, the official guidelines, Section I. B. 11. Combination Code state, "Assign only the combination code when that code fully identifies the diagnostic conditions involved or when the alphabetic index so directs."

480.0 Pneumonia due to adenovirus

Professional coding specialists are responsible for relating the entire story with all specific details applicable to the diagnosis. This one code tells both the condition AND the infectious organism. There is no reason to provide a second code to repeat the same information. Therefore, the code on Mason's claim form will be 480.0 alone.

CHRONIC OBSTRUCTIVE PULMONARY DISEASE

Chronic obstructive pulmonary disease (COPD)
An ongoing obstruction of the airway.

One of the most common respiratory disorders that you may code is **chronic obstructive pulmonary disease (COPD).** It is estimated that as much as 10% of the world population over age 40 has a lung disorder that is parallel with COPD. COPD is distinguished by restricted airflow.

It is not fully reversible and, therefore, is a leading cause of disability and death. Clinically, there are three types of COPD:

- Chronic bronchitis
- Emphysema
- Asthma

While all three of these conditions are considered COPD, when coding the patient's diagnosis, ICD-9-CM does differentiate between them. As always, you will code what the attending physician documents. Therefore, determined by what the physician wrote, you may code:

√5th 491.2 Obstructive chronic bronchitis

√4th 492 Emphysema

√4th 493 Asthma

496 Chronic airway obstruction, not elsewhere classified

The diagnoses in the COPD section can be particularly complex. You will need to be very diligent as you read the terms in the physician's notes and those included in the code descriptions. It is, as always, crucial that you refer to the index and then verify the code in the tabular list.

«« CODING TIP

Code 496 is to be used with caution–*only* when the documentation does not provide additional specific details AND, for some reason, you are not able to query the physician for more details.

«« CODING TIP

Never, never, never, never code out of the alphabetic index. *Always* confirm the code by reading the complete description in the tabular list.

LET'S CODE IT! SCENARIO

Peggy Newman, a 63-year-old female, quit smoking last month after a two-pack-a-day habit that lasted 40 years. She came to see Dr. Michaels with an insidious onset of dyspnea, tachypnea, and malaise. PE showed use of her accessory muscles for respiration. Dr. Michaels took a chest x-ray, ECG, RBC count, and a pulmonary function test. The results directed a diagnosis of emphysema with chronic bronchitis.

Let's Code It!

Dr. Michaels diagnosed Peggy with *emphysema with chronic bronchitis.* The alphabetic index shows:

Emphysema
    With bronchitis
        Chronic 491.20

Go to the tabular list to confirm this code:

√4th 491 Chronic bronchitis

The EXCLUDES note shows only one diagnosis. Does it relate to Peggy's condition? No, so keep reading and review all of the choices for the required fourth digit.

√5th 491.2 Obstructive chronic bronchitis

Read carefully, there is another EXCLUDES note. But it does not apply to Peggy's diagnosis, so keep reading to find the correct fifth digit.

491.20 Obstructive chronic bronchitis without exacerbation, emphysema with chronic bronchitis

This one code reports the entire diagnosis.

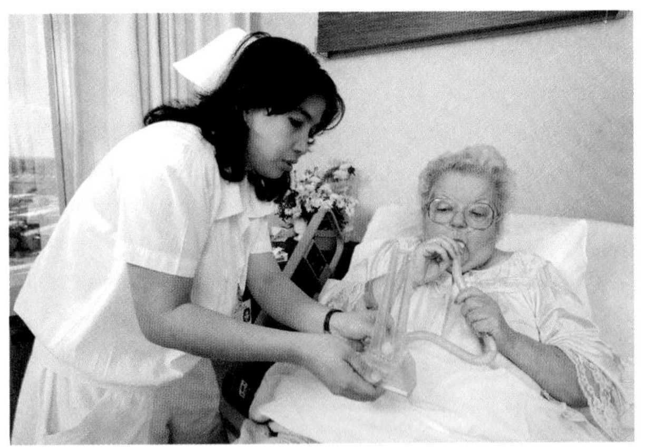

COPD with Asthma

You may notice that some of the codes in this section have the designation for acute **exacerbation** of asthma, COPD, or other related condition. It is a clinical term and can be assigned only by the attending physician.

Acute exacerbation of asthma indicates an increase in the severe nature of a patient's asthmatic condition. The patient may be suffering from wheezing or shortness of breath, commonly called an asthma attack. **Status asthmaticus,** however, is a life-threatening condition and is a diagnosis indicating that the patient is not responding to therapeutic procedures. If a patient is diagnosed with status asthmaticus *and* COPD or acute bronchitis, the status asthmaticus should be the first-listed code. As a life-threatening condition, it is considered to be the diagnosis with the greatest severity and follows the sequencing rules that you learned in Chap. 3. In addition, status asthmaticus, being the more severe condition, will override an additional diagnosis of acute exacerbation of asthma.

Exacerbation

An increase in the severity of a disease or its symptoms.

Status asthmaticus

The condition of asthma that is life-threatening and does not respond to therapeutic treatments.

LET'S CODE IT! SCENARIO

Nita Kinnerson, a 57-year-old female, has a history of intermittent dyspnea and wheezing. She comes today to see Dr. Hall with complaints of tachypnea, chest tightness, and a cough with thick mucus. The results of Dr. Hall's PE, the chest x-ray, sputum culture, ECG, pulmonary function tests, and an arterial blood gas analysis indicate asthma with COPD, with exacerbation.

Let's Code It!

Nita's diagnosis is *asthma with COPD, with exacerbation.* Let's turn to the alphabetic index and look up *asthma:*

Asthma
With
Chronic obstructive pulmonary disease (COPD) 493.2

That matches Dr. Hall's notes exactly. Turn to the tabular list to confirm

√4th 493 Asthma

The EXCLUDES note only mentions wheezing so keep reading down the column to find the most accurate 4th digit.

√5th 493.2 Chronic obstructive asthma

You'll notice that the code requires a fifth digit. You may have to look up the column, right under the three-digit 493 code description to find the three choices for the fifth digit:

0 unspecified

KEYS TO CODING »»

Review the **ICD-9-CM Coding Guidelines, Section I. chapter 8. Disease of Respiratory System (460-519),** subsection **a. Chronic obstructive pulmonary disease (COPD) and asthma** for more input on identifying what to code, what not to code, and in what order to put multiple codes. Use this to support your reading here, and as a reminder booster later on.

1 with status asthmaticus

2 with (acute) exacerbation

The fifth-digit 2 adds the last portion of Dr. Hall's diagnosis of Nita, the exacerbation.

493.22 Chronic obstructive asthma with exacerbation

Good job!

«« CODING TIP

If both diagnoses are included in the notes–status asthmaticus *and* acute exacerbation of asthma–use only one asthma code, with the fifth-digit 1 for status asthmaticus. Do not use two asthma codes.

YOU CODE IT! CASE STUDY

Roger Samuels, a 57-year-old male, was brought into the emergency department (ED) by ambulance because he was having a severe asthma attack. His wife, Roxan, stated that he was diagnosed with asthma about 2 years prior. This attack began 5 days ago and has not responded to his inhaler, his regular asthma pills, or any other treatment. Dr. Hunter diagnosed Roger with acute exacerbation of late-onset asthma with status asthmaticus.

You Code It!

Go through the steps of coding, and determine the diagnosis code or codes that should be reported for this encounter between Dr. Hunter and Roger Samuels.

Step 1: Read the case completely.

Step 2: Abstract the notes: Which key words can you identify relating to why Dr. Hunter cared for Roger?

____

Step 3: Query the provider, if necessary.

Step 4: Code the diagnosis or diagnoses.

____

Step 5: Code the procedure(s): ED visit.

Step 6: Link the procedure codes to at least one diagnosis code to confirm medical necessity.

Step 7: Back code to double-check your choices.

Answer

Did you find the correct code?

493.11 Intrinsic asthma with status asthmaticus

You are really getting good at this!

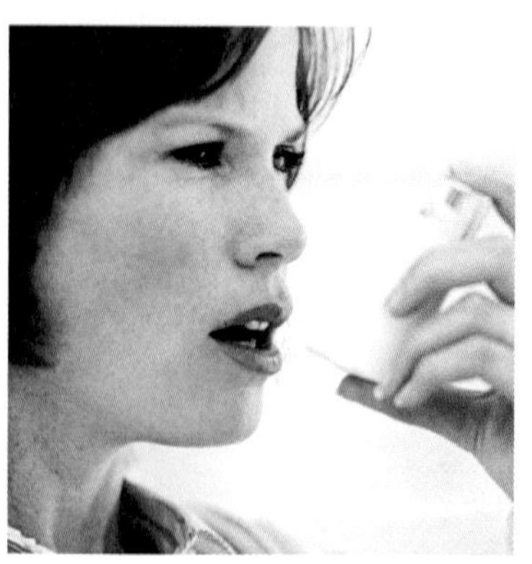

«« KEYS TO CODING

Why would you use the fifth-digit of 1 with status asthmaticus and not 2 with (acute) exacerbation, or report two codes–one with each? **Section I. chapter 8.a. 4 Acute exacerbation of asthma and status asthmaticus** states, "It is inappropriate to assign an asthma code with 5th digit 2 with acute exacerbation together with an asthma code with 5th digit 1 with status asthmaticus. Only the 5th digit 1 should be assigned."

CODING TIP »»

Do *not* use both 491.22 AND 466.0 on the same claim form for the same patient.

KEYS TO CODING »»

Review the **ICD-9-CM Coding Guidelines, Section I. chapter 8. Disease of Respiratory System (460-519),** subsection **b. Chronic obstructive pulmonary disease (COPD) and bronchitis** for more input on identifying what to code, what not to code, and in what order to put multiple codes. Use this to support your reading here, and as a reminder booster later on.

COPD with Bronchitis

When a patient is diagnosed with acute bronchitis, the ICD-9-CM will lead you to the code

466.0 Acute bronchitis

However, if this patient has also been diagnosed with COPD, you will, instead, use the code

491.22 Obstructive chronic bronchitis with acute bronchitis

If acute exacerbation is also documented in the patient with acute bronchitis and COPD, the 491.22 will report the entire situation, and you do not use code 491.21.

If the notes state the patient has acute exacerbation of COPD, with no mention of acute bronchitis, then you will use the code

491.21 Obstructive chronic bronchitis with (acute) exacerbation

It can get a little confusing, so take a look at Table 13-1 and see if it helps with your diagnostic coding for those conditions.

LET'S CODE IT! SCENARIO

Adrian Wicker, a 49-year-old male, diagnosed with COPD two years ago, comes in to Dr. Washington with complaints of a productive cough, with yellow white sputum, and dyspnea, particularly after he exerts himself to any great extent. Dr. Washington performs a complete PE and takes a chest x-ray, pulmonary function test, arterial blood gas analysis, and an ECG. He diagnoses Adrian with chronic tracheobronchitis with COPD.

Let's Code It!

Dr. Washington diagnosed Adrian with *chronic tracheobronchitis with COPD.* Turn to the alphabetic index, and look up *tracheobronchitis:*

Tracheobronchitis

Chronic 491.8

Turn to the tabular list to confirm the code:

√4th 491 Chronic bronchitis

The EXCLUDES note does not relate to Adrian's diagnosis, so keep reading to find the most accurate fourth-digit:

491.8 Other chronic bronchitis, chronic tracheobronchitis

Good work!

TABLE 13-1 **Bronchitis and COPD Combination Codes**

Code	Description
√4th 491	Chronic bronchitis
√5th 491.2	Obstructive chronic bronchitis
491.20	Bronchitis with COPD
491.21	Bronchitis with exacerbated COPD
491.22	Acute bronchitis with COPD

RESPIRATORY CONDITIONS REQUIRING E CODES

In Chap. 2 of this text, you learned about E codes and how to determine whether they are necessary. In addition, you practiced assigning E codes when you were coding poisonings (Chap. 6), burns (Chap. 7), and fractures (Chap. 8). There are respiratory conditions that may require E codes as well, to explain how, and sometimes where, an external condition was involved in causing this health problem. Some of these conditions are:

478.9 Cicatrix of trachea might need an E code to identify it as a late effect of an injury or poisoning.

495.0 Extrinsic allergic alveolitis, farmers' lung might need an E code for a workers' compensation claim.

495.7 "Ventilation" pneumonitis would need an E code to report "sick building syndrome" for workers' compensation.

√4th 506 Respiratory conditions due to chemical fumes and vapors would need an E code to identify the chemical.

√4th 508 Respiratory conditions due to other and unspecified external agents would need an E code to identify the external cause of the condition.

512.1 Iatrogenic pneumothorax would need an E code to identify that it was a postoperative condition.

518.5 Pulmonary insufficiency following trauma and surgery, adult respiratory distress syndrome would need an E code to identify the trauma, such as smoke inhalation from a building fire.

BRIDGE TO ICD-10-CM

ICD-10-CM provides a separate subsection titled, "Lung Diseases due to External Agents (J60-J70)."

LET'S CODE IT! SCENARIO

Corrine Alexander, a 28-year-old female, worked in a veterinary clinic. After a very sick stray animal was brought in, she was instructed by her boss to disinfect the floor of the clinic by mopping it with straight bleach. It was cold outside, so all the doors and windows were closed tightly, and Corrine began to have trouble breathing. She went immediately to Dr. Borman's office, where, after examination and tests, he diagnosed her with acute chemical bronchitis.

Let's Code It!

Dr. Borman diagnosed *acute chemical bronchitis.* In the alphabetic index:

Bronchitis

Chemical (acute) (subacute) 506.0

Will the tabular list confirm this suggested code?

√4th 506 Respiratory conditions due to chemical fumes and vapors

Did you notice that ICD-9-CM has reminded you to "Use additional E code to identify cause"? Keep reading down the column to

506.0 Bronchitis due to fumes and vapors, chemical bronchitis (acute)

As ICD-9-CM directed, you must report how and where Corrine was exposed to the chemical. Let's go the alphabetic index for E codes (volume 2, section 3) and look up how Corrine was injured by the bleach—she inhaled the chemical.

Inhalation

Liquid air, hydrogen, nitrogen E901.1

The above is not an exact match, but it appears to be the closest description. Let's turn to the tabular list and look under the heading Accidents Due to Natural and Environmental Factors (E900–E909).

√4th E901 Excessive cold

E901.1 Excessive cold, of man-made origin

It does not match Corrine's situation at all. Let's go back to the E code alphabetic listing:

Inhalation

Poisonous gas—*see* Table of Drugs and Chemicals

Turn to volume 2, section 2, the Table of Drugs and Chemicals, and look down the first column to find bleach:

Bleach NEC

Reading across this line, in the second column titled Poisoning you will see the suggested poisoning code. Remember that, if this was not an adverse reaction to properly prescribed and taken medication, this is reported as a poisoning. The code suggested on the line for Bleach is 983.9.

While you are here in the Table of Drugs and Chemicals, on this same line, you can also find the suggested code for how Corrine came to get poisoned. The next column to the right from the poisoning column is titled *Accident*. It was an accident that she had the reaction, so jot down code E864.3. Now, we need to turn to the tabular list to confirm the most accurate codes. Let's begin with the poisoning code:

√4th 983 Toxic effect of corrosive aromatics acids, and caustic alkalis

There are no notations or directives, so keep reading to find the most accurate 4th digit.

983.9 Toxic effect of corrosive aromatics, acids, and caustic alkalis, caustic unspecified

This does look like the best choice. However, before you report this for Corrine, look back to the beginning of the subsection:

Toxic Effects of Substances Chiefly Nonmedicinal as to Source (980–989)

EXCLUDES Burns from chemical agents (ingested) (947.0–947.9)
Localized toxic effects indexed elsewhere (001.0–799.9)
Respiratory conditions due to external agents (506.0–508.9)

This last exclusion notation instructs you *not* to include that poison code for Corrine's case. Instead we need to go check out code category 506.

√4th 506 Respiratory conditions due to chemical fumes and vapors

Use additional E code to identify cause

Sound familiar? You already have determined this code for Corrine. There is no reason to report it twice, so that's that. Good thing you didn't code directly from the alphabetic index including the Table of Drugs and Chemicals! Now, we need to turn to the E code tabular list to check the complete code description. Notice the subsection heading:

ACCIDENTAL POISONING BY OTHER SOLID AND LIQUID SUBSTANCES, GASES, AND VAPORS (E860–E869)

Remember, the Table of Drugs and Chemicals suggested

√4th E864 Accidental poisoning by corrosives and caustics, not elsewhere classified

Take a look at the EXCLUDES note: those as components of disinfectants (E861.4). Hmmm. Bleach was being used as a disinfectant when Corrine had her reaction. Let's take a look at E861.4, just to be certain.

√4th E861 Accidental poisoning by cleansing and polishing agents, disinfectants, paints, and varnishes

E861.4 Accidental poisoning by cleansing agents, disinfectants

This code is much more accurate. Another instance where the ICD-9-CM's redirection sends you to the most accurate code in the tabular list. It is really good that you checked the suggested codes from the Table of Drugs and Chemicals, isn't it?

In addition, Corrine was at work when it happened, so you will need an E code to report where she was at the time of her injury. The E code alphabetic index will direct you:

Place of occurrence if accident—see Accident (to), occurring (at) (in)

Turn to Accident, and find

Accident
    Occurring (at) (in)
        Hospital E849.7

There is no specific listing for veterinary clinic. However, *hospital* does come the closest. Let's turn to the code in the numeric list and check the description:

E849.7 Place of occurrence, residential institution

Well, that really does not hit the target. Remember, the code is being included to explain that Corrine was hurt at work, most often to support a workers' compensation claim. Therefore, it would be more accurate to report:

E849.3 Place of occurrence, industrial place and premises that includes shop (place of work)

The three codes on Corrine's report are 506.0, E861.4, and E849.3.

RESPIRATORY FAILURE

Respiratory failure identifies that a patient's lungs are not working efficiently. The result may be a reduced intake of oxygen or an excess of carbon dioxide that is not thoroughly being expelled from the lungs, or both. You have learned throughout this chapter about the problems that can occur in the body when it does not get enough oxygen, called hypoxemic respiratory failure, or when there is too much carbon dioxide, called hypercapnic respiratory failure.

Respiratory failure can be a manifestation of a respiratory disease such as COPD. In addition, certain injuries can affect a patient's ability to breathe. For example, a spinal cord injury may involve damage to the nerves that control breathing. A drug or alcohol overdose can also have an impact on the nervous system in a manner that affects the nervous system's ability to properly control respiration. Code choices include

581.81 Acute respiratory failure

581.83 Chronic respiratory failure

581.84 Acute and chronic respiratory failure

The physician may diagnose the patient with acute respiratory failure as a primary diagnosis when it meets the requirements to be first-listed as directed in the official guidelines. More typically, you will find that respiratory failure will be a secondary diagnosis, as mentioned previously.

KEYS TO CODING »»

Review the **ICD-9-CM Coding Guidelines, Section I. chapter 8. Disease of Respiratory System (460-519),** subsection **C. Acute respiratory failure** for more input on identifying what to code, what not to code, and in what order to put multiple codes. Use this to support your reading here, and as a reminder booster later on.

CHAPTER SUMMARY

Sadly, most people take breathing for granted . . . until they cannot do it without difficulty or pain. You have to know how to code respiratory conditions accurately whether working for a family physician, a pediatrician, or a pulmonologist. In addition, respiratory conditions might be present in a patient of an immunologist; allergist; or ear, nose, and throat (ENT) specialist.

Chapter 13 Review
Coding Respiratory Conditions

1. Respiratory disorders can be
   a Genetic.
   b. Environmental.
   c. Congenital.
   d. All of these.

2. When an infectious organism is involved in a respiratory condition, code
   a. Only the infectious organism.
   b. Both the organism and the respiratory condition.
   c. Only the respiratory condition.
   d. A personal history code.

3. When the cause of pneumonia is an underlying disease such as HIV or whooping cough, the codes should be sequenced:
   a. Pneumonia first, underlying disease second.
   b. Pneumonia only.
   c. Underlying disease only.
   d. Underlying disease first, pneumonia second.

4. COPD stands for
   a. Chronic obstructive pneumonia dyspnea.
   b. Chronic olfactory pharyngitis disease.
   c. Caustic other pneumonic disease.
   d. Chronic obstructive pulmonary disease.

5. One of the three types of COPD is
   a. Sinusitis.
   b. Pneumonia.
   c. Emphysema.
   d. Pharyngitis.

6. If the diagnostic statement includes both status asthmaticus and acute exacerbation of asthma,
   a. Code only the status asthmaticus.
   b. Code only the acute exacerbation of asthma.
   c. Code both status asthmaticus and acute exacerbation with two codes.
   d. These two diagnoses cannot be in the same patient at the same time.

7. A patient diagnosed with obstructive chronic bronchitis with acute bronchitis will get
   a. One code—acute bronchitis only.
   b. Two codes—obstructive chronic bronchitis and acute bronchitis.
   c. One code—bronchitis unspecified.
   d. One code—obstructive chronic bronchitis with acute bronchitis.

8. Respiratory conditions need E codes
   a. Never.
   b. Sometimes.
   c. Always.
   d. Only if there is an external cause for the condition.

9. An E code might be needed to support
   a. A workers' compensation claim.
   b. A liability claim.
   c. None of the above.
   d. Both (*a*) and (*b*).

10. Respiratory conditions affect
    a. Only the lungs.
    b. The lungs and bronchi.
    c. The entire respiratory system.
    d. The nose and mouth.

You Code It! Practice

Chapter 13. Coding Respiratory Conditions

1. Scott Merlman is admitted into the hospital with chest pain. After a thorough examination and the appropriate tests, he is diagnosed with chronic obstructive pulmonary disease.

   ____

2. Beth Ramos was brought into the ED suffering a severe asthma attack. Dr. Porter gave her an injection for rapid desensitization after determining that she was having an allergic reaction that affected her bronchial asthma.

   ____

3. Edward Agmata has been sneezing and has a stuffed nose. Dr. Kristine diagnosed him with allergic rhinitis and ordered testing to discover the allergen.

   ____

4. Ronine Fabrere is HIV positive, and was just admitted with organic pneumonia.

   ____

5. Gigi Warner was diagnosed with chronic bronchitis 6 months ago and is on medication. This morning, she came to see Dr. Lorrel because she was coughing and having difficulty breathing. Dr. Lorrel admitted her into the hospital with a diagnosis of obstructive chronic bronchitis with acute exacerbation.

   ____

6. Trudy Benington, a 3-year-old female, was brought to the ED by her mother. Trudy had a cough and fever, and her eyes were tearing. She was complaining that her eyes were itchy and burning. After a thorough examination and chest x-ray, Dr. Minister diagnosed her with an upper respiratory infection with bilateral acute conjunctivitis.

   ____

7. Gerald Fontaine came to see Dr. Brown with complaints of a fever and postnasal drip. After the exam, Dr. Brown diagnosed Gerald with chronic sinusitis.

   ____

8. Erin Bishoff, a 59-year-old female, was admitted to the hospital with a diagnosis of complete bilateral paralysis of the vocal cords.

   ____

9. Feona Fennell, a 41-year-old female, has had emphysema for over a year. Dr. Orton admits her today to the hospital with a diagnosis of aspiration pneumonia with pneumonia due to *Staphylococcus aureus*.

____

10. Garrett Church, a 33-year-old male, was diagnosed with pneumonia. He also has acute exacerbation of COPD.

____

11. Faith Dutton, a 21-year-old female, comes to see Dr. Fraiser with complaints of a headache and sinus congestion. Dr. Fraiser diagnoses her with acute and chronic maxillary sinusitis.

____

12. Sean Dublin has recurrent spontaneous pneumothorax.

____

13. Joy Carter came into the ambulatory care center to have a septoplasty to correct her deviated nasal septum (acquired).

____

14. Clay Logan, a 12-year-old male, is admitted into the Same Day Surgery Center to have a bilateral tonsillectomy to address his hypertrophic tonsillitis.

____

15. Meredith Chester had chest congestion and chest pain. Dr. Hayden diagnosed her with interlobar pleurisy.

____

You Code It! Simulation

Chapter 13. Coding Respiratory Conditions

On the following pages, you will see physicians' notes documenting encounters with patients at our textbook's health care facility, Taylor, Reader, & Associates. Carefully read through the notes and find the best ICD-9-CM code for each case.

TAYLOR, READER, & ASSOCIATES
A Complete Health Care Facility
975 CENTRAL AVENUE • SOMEWHERE, FL 32811 • 407-555-4321

PATIENT: COOPER, MARION
ACCOUNT/EHR #: COOPMA001
Date: 07/16/11

Attending Physician: Suzanne R. Taylor, MD

Pt presented to the ED normotensive with respirations of 10 and without any cyanosis. The pt is currently awake and alert. She is on the ACUD mode on the ventilator, breathing approximately ten times per minute. She does seem disoriented and does not appear to be as lucid as she had been when she first arrived, although there is no obvious focal neurologic deficit. The pt appears to be staring to the ceiling and was able to answer some questions, but was confused. She did speak over the ventilator but was following commands appropriately. She denied any pain and she was disoriented.

The patient's blood gases showed a compensated respiratory acidosis, and she was supporting stable vital signs and was afebrile. BP 153/71. Sinus tachycardia on the monitor at about 127 beats per minute. Lung fields are clear to auscultation and percussion.

DIAGNOSES: 1. Respiratory failure, chronic
2. Sinus tachycardia

PLAN/RECOMMENDATIONS:
1. 100% ventilator support for the time being
2. Continue nutrition with PulmoCare at 60 cc an hour
3. Follow up laboratory

Suzanne R. Taylor, MD

SRT/pw D: 07/16/11 09:50:16 T: 07/18/11 12:55:01

Find the best, most appropriate diagnosis code(s).

TAYLOR, READER, & ASSOCIATES
A Complete Health Care Facility
975 CENTRAL AVENUE • SOMEWHERE, FL 32811 • 407-555-4321

PATIENT: MCLEOD, WINSTON
ACCOUNT/EHR #: MCLEWI001
Date: 08/11/11

Attending Physician: Willard B. Reader, MD

S: Pt is a 23-month-old male who almost drowned in the swimming pool at his home 2 days ago. He is experiencing rapid, shallow breathing and dyspnea.

O: Hypoxemia is apparent. Chest sounds, crackles and rhonchi indicate fluid accumulation. Tachycardia and restlessness are also evident. ABG (arterial blood gas) analysis shows respiratory acidosis; serial chest x-rays show bilateral infiltrates.

A: Acute respiratory distress

P: Oxygen hood to supply warm, humidified, oxygen-enriched gases

---

Willard B. Reader, MD

WBR/pw D: 08/11/11 09:50:16 T: 08/13/11 12:55:01

Find the best, most appropriate diagnosis code(s).

___

___

___

TAYLOR, READER, & ASSOCIATES
A Complete Health Care Facility
975 CENTRAL AVENUE • SOMEWHERE, FL 32811 • 407-555-4321

PATIENT: CUMMINGS, LINDA
ACCOUNT/EHR #: CUMMLI001
Date: 07/16/11

Attending Physician: Suzanne R. Taylor, MD

S: This Pt is a 66-year-old female who presents today with complaints of dyspnea on exertion, and coughing.
I last saw this patient 1 year ago.

O: Ht 5′3″ Wt. 157 lb. R 15. BP 145/95 P90 thready. Chest: tachycardia, tachypnea, dependent crackles. HEENT: neck vein distention, Coughing produces frothy, bloody sputum. Skin is cold, clammy, diaphoretic, and cyanotic. ABG analysis shows hypoxia. Chest x-ray shows diffuse haziness of the lung fields.

A: Acute pulmonary edema

P: 1. Administer high concentrations of oxygen by a cannula
2. Rx Lasix

Suzanne R. Taylor, MD

SRT/pw D: 07/16/11 09:50:16 T: 07/18/11 12:55:01

Find the best, most appropriate diagnosis code(s).

TAYLOR, READER, & ASSOCIATES
A Complete Health Care Facility
975 CENTRAL AVENUE • SOMEWHERE, FL 32811 • 407-555-4321

PATIENT: CLYDE, NELSON
ACCOUNT/EHR #: CLYDNE001
Date: 09/15/11

Attending Physician: Willard B. Reader, MD

S: This new Pt is a 23-year-old male who presents with complaints of fever and recurrent chills. He states that he has a cough producing rusty, bloody, viscous sputum (pt states "like currant jelly"). He states his breathing is difficult and shallow, and he noticed that his lips and fingernails appear bluish. Pt recently moved here from Detroit. He was found to be HIV positive 2 years ago and is on pharmaceutical therapy.

O: HEENT: Cyanosis of lips confirms hypoxemia. Chest: respirations are shallow and grunting. Chest x-ray shows consolidation in the upper lobe causing bulging of fissures; WBC count is elevated; sputum culture and gram stain show gram-negative cocci Klebsiella

A: Pneumonia due to klebsiella, HIV positive

P: Oxygen hood to supply warm, humidified, oxygen-enriched gases

Willard B. Reader, MD

WBR/pw D: 09/15/11 09:50:16 T: 09/17/11 12:55:01

Find the best, most appropriate diagnosis code(s).

TAYLOR, READER, & ASSOCIATES
A Complete Health Care Facility
975 CENTRAL AVENUE • SOMEWHERE, FL 32811 • 407-555-4321

PATIENT: CONDRON, CLARENCE
ACCOUNT/EHR #: CONDCL001
Date: 11/25/11

Attending Physician: Willard B. Reader, MD

S: This new Pt is a 35-year-old male complaining of a cough with a foul-smelling sputum, dyspnea, excessive sweating, and chills.

PMH: Pt has poor oral hygiene. Missing teeth and inflamed gums have gone untreated for years due to his fear of the dentist. He states that a few months ago, he had a bout of pneumonia. He self-medicated but hasn't felt right since then.

O: Chest: Auscultation reveals crackles and decreased breath sounds. Chest x-ray shows localized infiltrate with one clear space containing air-fluid. Blood cultures, gram stain, and sputum culture identify leukocytosis.

A: Abscess of the lung, putrid

P: Begin antibiotic therapy immediately

Willard B. Reader, MD

WBR/pw D: 11/25/11 09:50:16 T: 11/27/11 12:55:01

Find the best, most appropriate diagnosis code(s).

Hospital (Inpatient) Diagnosis Coding

14

LEARNING OUTCOMES

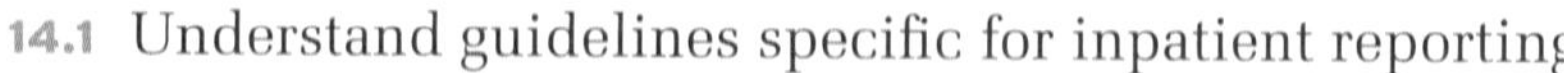

14.1 Understand guidelines specific for inpatient reporting

14.2 Determine the proper application of present on admission indicators

14.3 Identify complications and co-morbidities

14.4 Distinguish between inpatient and outpatient coding guidelines

14.5 Apply the correct POA indicator to each diagnosis code

KEY TERMS

Comorbidity

Complication

Concurrent coding

Diagnosis-related groups (DRG)

Hospital-acquired conditions (HAC)

Major complications and co-morbidities (MCC)

Present on admission (POA)

Uniform Hospital Discharge Data Set (UHDDS)

For the most part, coding hospital encounters and coding outpatient encounters use the same guidelines and the same coding process. However, emergency room and outpatient surgery departments, even though they may be under the same roof as the inpatient acute care facility, will typically be coded as outpatient encounters.

This chapter will review the few aspects of coding inpatient cases which differ somewhat from what you have learned throughout this book.

CONCURRENT AND DISCHARGE CODING

Concurrent Coding

Coding processes performed while a patient is still in the hospital receiving care.

Some acute care facilities have patients who may spend weeks or months in the hospital. In these cases, professional coding specialists may do what is called **concurrent coding.** This means that coders actually go up to the nurse's station on the floor of the hospital and code from the patient's chart while the patient is still in the hospital. Concurrent coding enables the hospital to gain reimbursement to date without having to wait until the patient is discharged, improving cash flow for the facility. Figure 14-1 shows you an example of progress notes that might be found in a patient's chart. A coder performing concurrent coding would read these, as well as other documentation, to determine what diagnoses to report.

Once a patient is discharged, you will go through the complete patient record. The most important documentation to look for will include

- Discharge summary or discharge progress notes signed by the attending physician

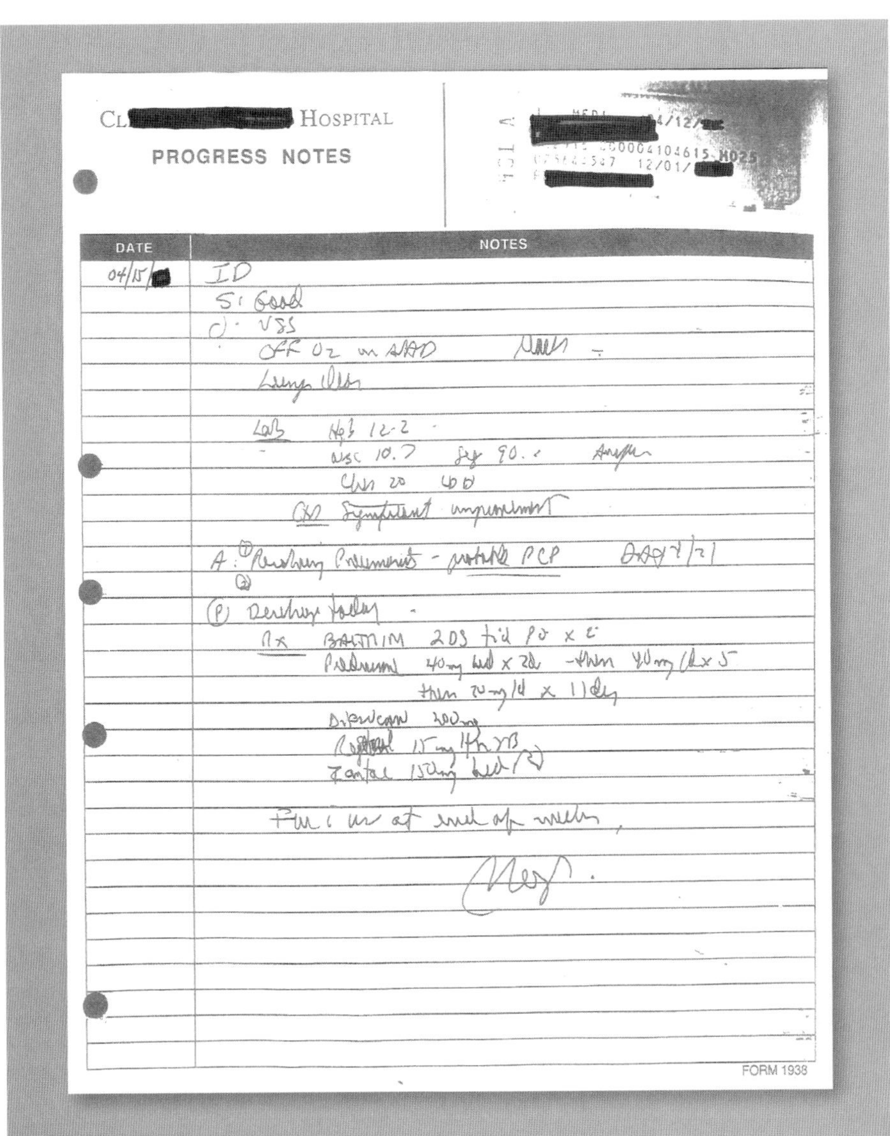

CL[redacted] HOSPITAL

PROGRESS NOTES

DATE	NOTES
04/15/	

FORM 1938

Figure 14-1 Progress Notes.

- Hospital course - a summary of the patient's hospital stay
- Discharge instructions - a copy of which is given to the patient
- Discharge disposition - that contains orders for the patient to be transferred home with special services, transferred to another facility, etc.
- The death/discharge summary - if the patient has expired prior to discharge

All of these documents should be reviewed to provide you with a complete picture of what procedures, services, and treatments were provided to the patient along with signs, symptoms, and diagnoses to support medical necessity.

LET'S CODE IT! SCENARIO

The attending physician, Milo Sternan, MD, included this in the discharge summary:

Admission Diagnosis: Abdominal pain, status post appendectomy

Final Diagnosis: Abdominal pain, unknown etiology, status post appendectomy

Brief History: Patient underwent an appendectomy for perforated appendicitis six weeks ago. . . . Three days prior to admission, she had a recurrent bout of diffuse, dull, abdominal pain in the right upper quadrant with associated nausea and anorexia. She was admitted to the hospital at the time for workup of this pain.

At this time, the patient has just had a regular meal without difficulty and feels like returning home. She will be discharged home at this time and can follow up with her primary MD. We will see her on an as-needed basis.

Let's Code It!

This discharge documentation provides you the information you need to code the diagnosis supporting this patient's stay in the hospital. (To code the procedures, you would have to review the complete record.)

You have the admitting diagnosis and the final diagnosis. Remember that the Official Guidelines state the principal diagnosis is "that condition established after study. . ." This tells you that the final diagnosis would be used. You have two conditions to report: *Abdominal pain, unknown etiology* and *status post appendectomy.*

As always, begin in the alphabetic index, and find

Pain

Abdominal 789.0

Turn to the tabular list to review the complete code description.

√4th 789 Other symptoms involving abdomen and pelvis

The EXCLUDES note does not appear to include any diagnosis documented in these notes, so continue reading down the column to find the most accurate fourth digit.

√5th 789.0 Abdominal pain

KEYS TO CODING »»

What about the part of the diagnosis where Dr. Sternan wrote. . . . Abdominal pain, *unknown etiology*? How is that reported? Notice that the code 789.01 for the abdominal pain is located in the "Symptoms, Signs, and Ill-Defined Conditions" chapter of ICD-9-CM volume 1. This is the part that reports the physician could not determine the cause (etiology) of the pain. Had the cause of the pain been identified, you would be reporting that with a different code.

Once you have read all the other fourth-digit choices, you will find that this is the most accurate, as per the physician's documentation. This code requires a fifth-digit, but there are none below, so you will have to read above to the box to review the fifth-digit choices.

Virtually all of the ten choices you have for the fifth digit are specific to the location of the pain in the abdomen. Dr. Sternan did state that when she was admitted she had *"abdominal pain in the right upper quadrant"* leading you to the fifth-digit 1. So, this diagnosis code will be reported as

789.01 Abdominal pain, right upper quadrant

Are you done? Do you need to report that the patient was status post appendectomy? Yes, you do. It is not known if the pain is related to the surgical procedure or the condition for which it was performed. So, let's turn back to the alphabetic index and look up

Status (post)

Appendectomy is not listed. What can you look up? Think about the patient status post . . . what exactly is an appendectomy? Surgery. No, surgery is not listed in this index either. Hmmmm. Try looking at post-surgical. Aha!

Status (post)
    Postsurgical NEC V45.89

(Postoperative NEC is also shown, leading to the same code.)
Let's turn to the V code section and check this code out.

√4th V45 Other postprocedural states

Neither of the EXCLUDES notes relate to this discharge summary, so continue reading down the column to find the correct fourth digit. No other fourth digit is accurate to report post appendectomy, so let's take a look at what the alphabetic index suggested:

√5th V45.8 Other postprocedural status
    V45.89 Other

When you review the other procedures included in this classification none seem to relate to an appendectomy. But the right code has to be here somewhere! Take a look back at

√5th V45.7 Acquired absence of organ
    V45.79 Other acquired absence of organ

An appendectomy is the surgical removal of the appendix. While the appendix may not be an organ like a heart or bladder, it is an organ. This code description is the most accurate of those available. So, the diagnosis codes you will report for this case are

789.01 Abdominal pain, right upper quadrant
V45.79 Other acquired absence of organ

Good job!

OFFICIAL CODING GUIDELINES

The Official Coding Guidelines located in your ICD-9-CM book will still provide you guidance. However, there are two instances where the guidelines direct inpatient coders differently than outpatient.

Uncertain Diagnosis

Remember that you learned for outpatient coding, that you are *not permitted* to ever code something identified by the physician in his or her documentation as "rule out," "probable," "possible," "suspected," or other similar terms of an unconfirmed nature. This guidance (as shown in Section IV, subsection I. Uncertain diagnosis) is different from that provided to inpatient coders.

The guidance for inpatient coders is that you *are permitted* to "code the condition as if it existed or was established." This is done so that medical necessity can be reported for tests, observation, or other services and resources used to care for the patient whether or not these efforts resulted in a confirmed diagnosis.

«« KEYS TO CODING

Review the **ICD-9-CM Coding Guidelines, Section II. Selection of Principal Diagnosis,** subsection **H. Uncertain diagnosis** for more input on identifying what to code, what not to code, and in what order to put multiple codes. Use this to support your reading here, and as a reminder booster later on.

Patient Receiving Diagnostic Services Only

In the outpatient world, the guidelines instruct you to wait until the test results have been determined and interpreted by the physician as documented in the final report before coding. At that time, confirmed diagnoses, or the signs and symptoms that were documented as the reason for ordering the test, are reported.

When coding for inpatient services, abnormal test results are not reported unless the physician has documented the clinical significance of those results. Interestingly, in this section of the guidelines, it is reiterated that if the coding professional notices abnormal test results and documentation is unclear from the physician, it is "appropriate to ask the provider whether the abnormal finding should be added."

«« KEYS TO CODING

Review the **ICD-9-CM Coding Guidelines, Section III. Reporting Additional Diagnoses,** subsection **B. Abnormal findings** for more input on identifying what to code, what not to code, and in what order to put multiple codes. Use this to support your reading here, and as a reminder booster later on.

YOU CODE IT! CASE STUDY

The attending physician, Oscar Medina, MD, included this in the discharge summary:

Admission Diagnosis: Acute cervical pain admitted through ED after MVA

Final Diagnosis: Acute cervical pain and radiculitis secondary to degenerative disc disease with post-traumatic activation of pain

Brief History: Patient is a 37-year old male who was involved in a motor vehicle accident, admitted after being brought to the ED by the ambulance that responded to the accident scene. Patient showed signs of neck and arm pain associated with cervical radiculopathy, radiating into the shoulders along with constant headaches. He has numbness and tingling into the hands and fingers.

Radiology: X-rays AP and lateral cervical spinal x-rays demonstrate evidence of significant degenerative disc disease at C5-6 and C6-7 levels. MRI of cervical spine demonstrates evidence of significant degenerate disc disease at the C5-6 and C6-7 levels with osteophyte formation and canal compromise with the spinal canal diameter reduced to approximately 9mm. Lumbar spine MRI demonstrates mild degenerative disc disease; otherwise normal.

Recommendation to patient is to undergo an anterior cervical diskectomy and fusion utilizing an autologous iliac bone grafting and placement of anterior titanium plate. After reviewing with patient regarding risks and benefits of surgery, the patient refused and requested to be discharged immediately.

You Code It!

In this case, the patient received only diagnostic services. Determine the most accurate diagnosis codes for this inpatient encounter. Did you find the accurate codes?

722.4 Degeneration of cervical intervertebral disc

723.4 Brachial neuritis or radiculitis NOS, (cervical radiculitis)

338.11 Acute pain due to trauma

E819.9 Motor vehicle traffic accident of unspecified nature, unspecified person

Good job!

PRESENT ON ADMISSION INDICATORS

Present on admission (POA) indicators are required for each diagnosis code reported on UB-04 and 837 Institutional claim forms. They are used to report additional detail about the patient's condition.

Centers for Medicare and Medicaid Services (CMS), in CR5499, requires a POA indicator for every diagnosis appearing on a claim from an acute care facility for all patients beginning with those discharged on or after January 1, 2008. After a grace period that ended on April 1, 2008, claims are now returned stamped "unpaid" to the facility if POA indicators are not included. Hospitals are permitted to enter the POA indicators and refile the claim; however, think about all the time and work wasted by having to do this.

Present on admission (POA)

A one-character indicator reporting the status of the diagnosis at the time the patient was admitted to the acute care facility.

KEYS TO CODING »»

Review the **ICD-9-CM Coding Guidelines, Appendix I. Present on Admission Reporting Guidelines** for more input on identifying what to code, what not to code, and in what order to put multiple codes. Use this to support your reading here, and as a reminder booster later on.

General Reporting Guidelines

According to CMS Publication 100-04, *"Present on admission is defined as present at the time the order for inpatient admission occurs—conditions that develop during an outpatient encounter, including emergency department, observation, or outpatient surgery, are considered as present on admission."*

What does this mean? This means professional coders must carefully review the admitting physician's submitted history and physical (H&P)—the documentation that supports the order to admit the patient into the hospital (see Figure 14-2 for an example)—to determine whether or not the condition was identified at that time. Then, you will assign the POA indicator to report this fact. Yes—this diagnosis was present when the patient was admitted; No—it was not present; etc.

One reason for the importance of gathering POA data is to identify **hospital-acquired conditions (HAC).** A hospital-acquired condition is exactly as it sounds. This is a circumstance under which a patient catches an illness or suffers an injury solely due to the fact that he or she was in

Hospital-acquired conditions (HAC)

A condition, illness, or injury contracted by the patient during his or her stay in an acute care facility; also known as a nosocomial condition.

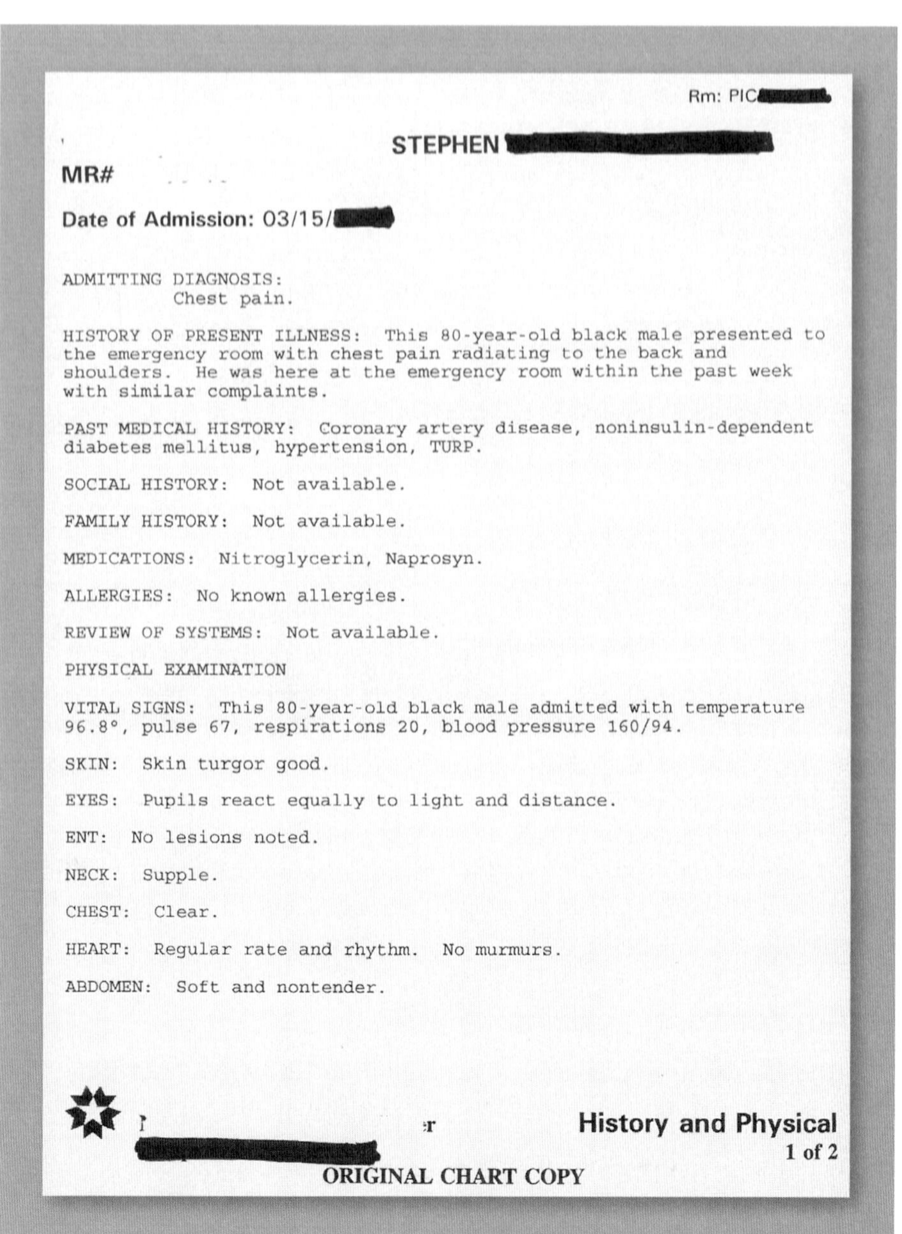
Rm: PIC

STEPHEN

MR#

Date of Admission: 03/15/

ADMITTING DIAGNOSIS:
Chest pain.

HISTORY OF PRESENT ILLNESS: This 80-year-old black male presented to the emergency room with chest pain radiating to the back and shoulders. He was here at the emergency room within the past week with similar complaints.

PAST MEDICAL HISTORY: Coronary artery disease, noninsulin-dependent diabetes mellitus, hypertension, TURP.

SOCIAL HISTORY: Not available.

FAMILY HISTORY: Not available.

MEDICATIONS: Nitroglycerin, Naprosyn.

ALLERGIES: No known allergies.

REVIEW OF SYSTEMS: Not available.

PHYSICAL EXAMINATION

VITAL SIGNS: This 80-year-old black male admitted with temperature 96.8°, pulse 67, respirations 20, blood pressure 160/94.

SKIN: Skin turgor good.

EYES: Pupils react equally to light and distance.

ENT: No lesions noted.

NECK: Supple.

CHEST: Clear.

HEART: Regular rate and rhythm. No murmurs.

ABDOMEN: Soft and nontender.

History and Physical
1 of 2

ORIGINAL CHART COPY

Figure 14-2 Admitting History & Physical (H&P).

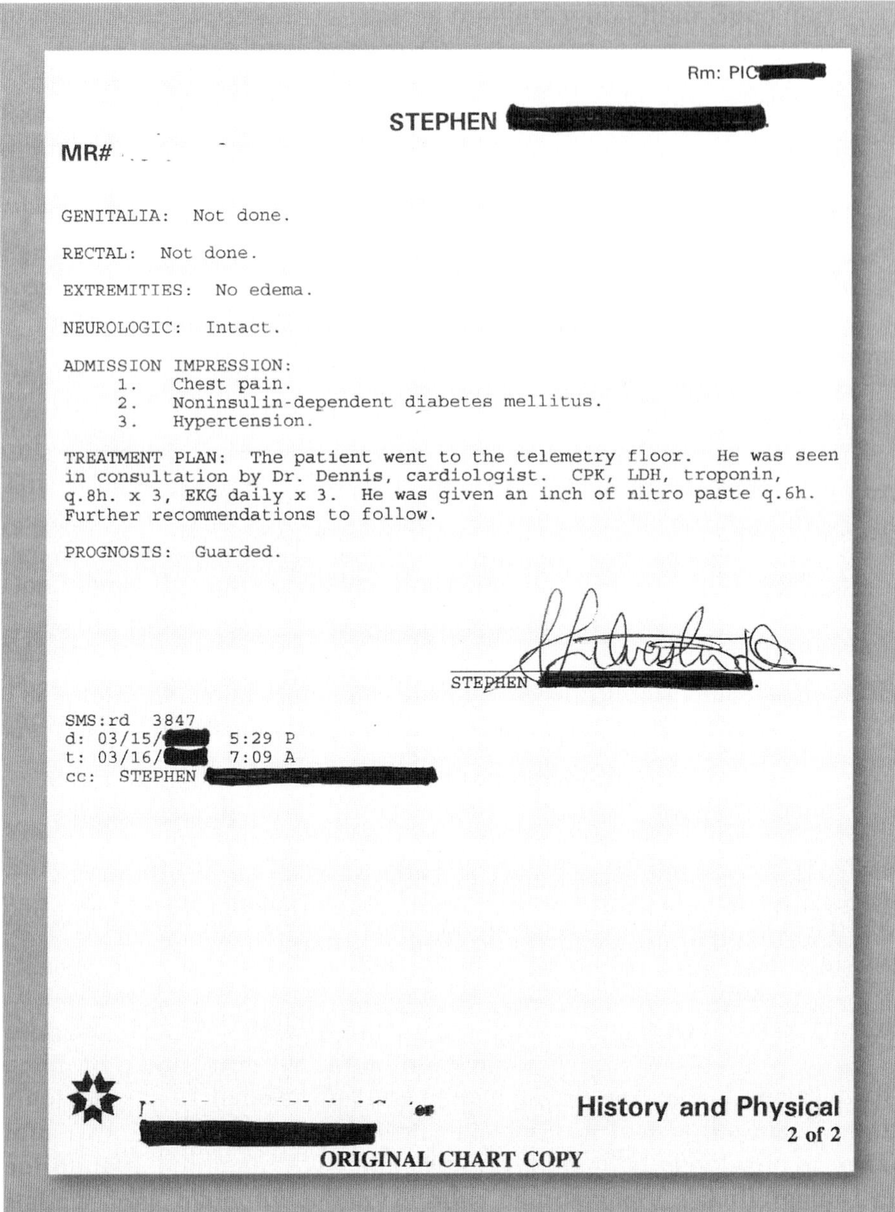

Rm: PIC

STEPHEN

MR#

GENITALIA: Not done.

RECTAL: Not done.

EXTREMITIES: No edema.

NEUROLOGIC: Intact.

ADMISSION IMPRESSION:
1. Chest pain.
2. Noninsulin-dependent diabetes mellitus.
3. Hypertension.

TREATMENT PLAN: The patient went to the telemetry floor. He was seen in consultation by Dr. Dennis, cardiologist. CPK, LDH, troponin, q.8h. x 3, EKG daily x 3. He was given an inch of nitro paste q.6h. Further recommendations to follow.

PROGNOSIS: Guarded.

STEPHEN

SMS:rd 3847
d: 03/15/ 5:29 P
t: 03/16/ 7:09 A
cc: STEPHEN

History and Physical
2 of 2
ORIGINAL CHART COPY

Figure 14-2 *(Continued)*

KEYS TO CODING »»

POA indicators are not required for E (external cause) codes unless the E code is being reported as an "other diagnosis."

the hospital at the time. Collecting HAC data is used for many different evaluations, including patient safety directives and limiting payment to a facility for errors they may have made that caused the problem.

POA Indicators

The POA indicators are used to clearly identify whether or not those signs, symptoms, and diagnoses reported on the claim form were documented by the admitting physician at the time the patient was admitted into the hospital.

The indicators are:

Y Yes This condition was documented by the admitting physician as present at the time of inpatient admission.

Example of POA Y Indicator

Serena is admitted to the hospital from the emergency department (ED) with severe angina (chest pains), dyspnea (shortness of breath), and parenthesia (tingling) in her left arm. After all the tests were run, Dr. Abaddi diagnoses her with an acute myocardial infarction (AMI) of the anterolateral wall, discusses diet, exercise, medications, and discharges her. Reported with code 410.01 Acute myocardial infarction of the anterolateral wall, initial episode of care would be POA indicator of Y because the signs and symptoms that caused her admission to the hospital are those of an AMI. Her heart attack was present on admission.

N No This condition was *not* present at the time of inpatient admission.

Example of POA N Indicator

Elijah is admitted with an esophageal ulcer that did not begin bleeding until after admission. Reported with code 530.21 Ulcer of esophagus with bleeding is POA indicator of N because the entire description of this code was not present at admission.

U Unknown Documentation from the admitting physician is insufficient to determine if condition is present on admission.

Example of POA U Indicator

Zach was admitted to the hospital to have his tonsils removed due to his chronic tonsillitis. The second day, the physician noted a diagnosis of urinary tract infection (UTI) and ordered antibiotics. Upon discharge, code 474.00 Chronic tonsillitis will get a POA indicator of Y; however the 599.0 Urinary tract infection, site not specified would receive a U because the documentation is not clear whether the UTI was not present and developed while he was in the hospital or present and not diagnosed when Zach was admitted.

W Clinically Undetermined Provider is unable to clinically determine whether condition was present on admission or not.

Example of POA W Indicator

Clarissa was admitted with diabetic gangrene. After a blood workup early on her third day in the hospital, the physician documented an additional diagnosis of septicemia. Upon discharge, the codes for the diabetes (250.73) and the gangrene (785.4) would both be reported with a POA of Y; however, the septicemia (038.9) would receive a POA indicator of W because the physician documented that there is no way to be certain clinically whether the septicemia was not present and developed while she was in the hospital or present and not diagnosed when Clarissa was admitted.

1 Exempt

You can find a list of the conditions, and their diagnosis codes, that are exempt from POA reporting in the Official Coding Guidelines in your ICD-9-CM book or on the CMS website. (Note: Some third-party payers prefer this box remain blank instead of using the numeral one.)

«« CODING TIP

If any part of the diagnosis code description was NOT present at the time of admission, report this with an N.

«« KEYS TO CODING

It is the responsibility of the physician or health care provider admitting the patient into the hospital to clearly document which conditions are POA. However, it is the professional coder's responsibility to query the physician if the documentation is incomplete with regard to this issue.

«« KEYS TO CODING

Review the **ICD-9-CM Coding Guidelines, Appendix I. Present on Admission Reporting Guidelines,** subsection **Categories and Codes Exempt from Diagnosis Present on Admission Requirement** for more input on identifying what to code, what not to code, and in what order to put multiple codes. Use this to support your reading here, and as a reminder booster later on.

Example of POA Exempt Diagnoses

Makenzie was admitted to the hospital in full labor and delivered a beautiful baby boy the next morning. Upon discharge, both codes 650 Normal delivery and V27.0 Outcome of delivery, single liveborn are reported with POA indicator 1. You will notice that both of these codes are on the Exempt list shown in the Official Coding Guidelines in ICD-9-CM.

LET'S CODE IT! SCENARIO

Roberta was admitted into the hospital because she was suffering acute exacerbation of her obstructive chronic bronchitis. After two days of treatment, while still in the hospital, she tried to get out of bed without help, fell, and broke her wrist.

Let's Code It!

The reason Roberta was admitted into the hospital was because she was having exacerbation of her bronchitis. Therefore, the documentation (the physician's H&P) identifies this as being present when she was admitted.

491.21 Obstructive chronic bronchitis with acute exacerbation POA: Y

When she was discharged, Roberta also had her wrist in a cast, due to the break suffered from her fall. This is very clearly a condition she did not have when she was admitted.

814.00 Fracture of carpal bone, closed, carpal bone unspecified POA: N

DIAGNOSIS-RELATED GROUPS

Diagnosis-related group (DRG)

An episodic-care payment system basing reimbursement to hospitals for inpatient services upon standards of care for specific diagnoses grouped by their similar usage of resources for procedures, services, and treatments.

In addition to dealing with diagnosis and procedure codes, hospitals must work with **diagnosis-related groups (DRG)** for Medicare reimbursement, under Medicare Part A—Hospital Insurance. To determine how much an acute care facility will be paid, the Inpatient Prospective Payment System (IPPS) was developed. Within IPPS, each and every patient case is sorted into a DRG.

Each DRG has a payment weight assigned to it determined by the typical resources used to care for the patient in that case. This calculation includes the labor costs, such as nurses and technicians, as well as non-labor costs, such as maintenance for equipment and supplies.

Typically, professional coding specialists do not have to worry about assigning the DRG for a patient's case. This is determined, most often, by a special software program known as a "DRG grouper."

Principal Diagnosis

So, why do you need to know all this? The *principal* diagnosis assigned is one of the factors used to determine which DRG is most accurate. Particularly when it comes to coding for reporting inpatient services to a Medicare beneficiary, the sequence in which you place the diagnosis codes can make a big difference in how accurately the hospital will be reimbursed.

Remember that the principal, or first-listed, diagnosis, as defined by the ICD-9-CM guidelines is "*that condition established after study to be chiefly responsible for occasioning the admission of the patient to the hospital for care.*" This is the diagnosis that explains the most serious reason for the patient to be in the hospital. This might be the reason for admission, it might be the most serious condition, or it might be the condition that required the greatest number of services, treatments, or procedures during the patient's stay in the hospital.

«« KEYS TO CODING

Review the **ICD-9-CM Coding Guidelines, Section II. Selection of Principal Diagnosis** for more input on identifying what to code, what not to code, and in what order to put multiple codes. Use this to support your reading here, and as a reminder booster later on.

Complications and Co-morbidities (CC)

As each diagnosis is evaluated for its standard of care, CMS understands that a patient in a hospital may have multiple conditions or concerns (signs, symptoms, diagnoses) that are interrelated and create a more complex need for care. These may be complications and/or comorbidities.

In some cases, regardless of the precautions that may be taken, **complications** of a procedure or treatment may arise during the patient's stay. This condition must also be coded and reported to support the medical necessity for the treatment provided to resolve the concern.

Complication

An unexpected illness or other condition that develops as a result of a procedure, service, or treatment provided during the patient's hospital stay.

Example

Curtis had surgery this morning and is now having a bronchospasm, a reaction to the general anesthesia. This bronchospasm is a complication of the administration of general anesthesia and must be coded and reported to identify the medical necessity for the treatments to help alleviate this condition.

You have learned throughout this textbook that a patient may have, or end up with, several different conditions treated during a stay in the hospital. The individual may also have pre-existing conditions that have nothing to do with the reason for admission but still need attention by hospital personnel.

Example

Bernard was admitted into the hospital with appendicitis. During his stay, the physician had to order and the nurses had to continue to give Bernard his Lipitor prescribed for his pre-existing hypercholesterolemia (high cholesterol). Even though this condition has nothing to do with the appendicitis or the appendectomy (surgery to remove the infected appendix), this **comorbidity** must be coded and reported to support the medical necessity for the hospital supplying the medication.

Comorbidity

A separate condition or illness present in the same patient at the same time as another unrelated condition or illness.

Major Complications and Comorbidities (MCC)

Conditions, illnesses, injuries come in all shapes and sizes, as well as severities, and so do complications and comorbidities. Typically, a **major complication or comorbidity (MCC)** is a condition that is systemic, making treatment for the principal diagnosis more complex and/or make the health concern life-threatening.

Major Complication and Comorbidity (MCC)

A complication or comorbidity that has an impact on the treatment of the patient and that makes care for that patient more complex.

KEYS TO CODING »»

Review the **ICD-9-CM Coding Guidelines, Section III. Reporting Additional Diagnoses** for more input on identifying what to code, what not to code, and in what order to put multiple codes. Use this to support your reading here, and as a reminder booster later on.

Uniform Hospital Discharge Data Set (UHDDS)

A compilation of data collected by acute care facilities and other designated health care facilities.

Example

Kenneth was admitted to the hospital with an open wound requiring complex repair. His admitting physician noted on his H&P that he also has cystic fibrosis with pulmonary exacerbation. These pancreatic and respiratory conditions will certainly make repair of the laceration more complicated and therefore need to be coded and reported.

Uniform Hospital Discharge Data Set (UHDDS)

The **Uniform Hospital Discharge Data Set (UHDDS)** is a collection of specific data gathered about hospital patients at discharge. No, this is not an invasion of privacy nor is it a collection of personal data. The information pulled from hospital claim forms are related to demographic and clinical details.

Demographic data includes:

- Gender
- Age
- Race and ethnicity
- Geographic location
- Provider information such as the hospital facility NPI (National Provider Identifier) as well as attending and operating physician(s)
- Expected sources of payment including primary and other sources of payment for this care
- Length of stay (LOS) determined by date of admission and date of discharge
- Total charges billed by the hospital for this admission (this will not include physician and other professional services billed)

Clinical data collected evaluates:

- Type of admission described as *scheduled* (planned in advance with preregistration at least 24 hours prior) or *unscheduled*
- Diagnoses including principal and additional diagnoses
- Procedures, services, and treatments provided during this admission period
- External causes of injury determined by the reporting of E codes

Definitions of these, and other, categories, as determined by the UHDDS are used by ICD-9-CM in the official coding guidelines. Over the years that the UHDDS has been in place, these definitions have been used to assist the reporting of patient data not only in acute care facilities (hospitals), but also for inpatient short-term care, long-term care, and psychiatric hospitals. Outpatient providers including home health agencies, nursing homes, and rehabilitation facilities also use these definitions for their data.

CHAPTER SUMMARY

The coding process remains the same for inpatient and outpatient services when determining and reporting accurate diagnosis codes. The same code set, ICD-9-CM, volumes 1 & 2, is used; the same guidelines are used (with the exception of those two specific guidelines). With the additional knowledge provided in this chapter, a professional coder can be successful in any type of facility.

Chapter 14 Review

Hospital (Inpatient) Diagnosis Coding

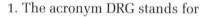

1. The acronym DRG stands for
   a. Diagnostic and Radiologic Guidelines.
   b. Discharge Restrictive Guidance.
   c. Diagnosis-Related Groups.
   d. Detailed Radiologic Groups.

2. All of the following are POA indicators except
   a. W.
   b. X.
   c. Y.
   d. 1.

3. The term "concurrent coding" means coding
   a. The case while the patient is still in the hospital.
   b. Diagnosis and procedure codes at the same time.
   c. Signs and symptoms along with confirmed diagnoses.
   d. All of the above.

4. Inpatient coders are not permitted to ever code something identified in the physician's notes as "suspected" or "probable."

   True

   False

5. The UHDDS is a new code set that will replace ICD-9-CM in 2013.

   True

   False

6. Felicia was admitted into the hospital with a compound fracture of the left femur head. Three days later, during her stay, she developed pneumonia. The POA indicator for the pneumonia is
   a. Y.
   b. N.
   c. W.
   d. 1.

7. The UHDDS collects all of these data elements except
   a. Gender.
   b. Principal diagnosis.
   c. Payment sources.
   d. Credit card numbers.

8. An example of a complication is
   a. Postoperative wound infection.
   b. Known allergy to penicillin.
   c. Family history of breast cancer.
   d. High-risk pregnancy.

9. DRGs are used for reimbursement from Medicare to
   a. Physician offices.
   b. Ambulatory Surgical Centers.
   c. Acute care facilities.
   d. Walk-in clinics.

10. POA indicators are appended to the data element related to the admitting procedure code.

    True

    False

YOU CODE IT! Simulation

Chapter 14. Hospital (Inpatient) Diagnosis Coding

Below and on the following pages, you will see physicians' notes documenting encounters with patients at our textbook's health care facility, Hillside Hospital. Carefully read through the notes and find the best ICD-9-CM diagnosis code or codes for each case.

HILLSIDE HOSPITAL
359 Mountain Pass Road
Langston, FL 33993

DISCHARGE SUMMARY

Patient: MASCONNI, ANGELO
DATE OF ADMISSION: 05/30/11
DATE OF SURGERY: 05/31/11
DATE OF DISCHARGE: 06/01/11

ADMITTING DIAGNOSIS: Right breast mass
DISCHARGE DIAGNOSIS: Malignant neoplasm of areola, right breast, estrogen receptor status negative; postsurgical respiratory congestion

This 39-year-old African-American male was admitted to the hospital with a palpable 2-cm nodule in the right breast in the superficial aspect of the right breast in the 5 o'clock axis near the periphery.

Excision of the right breast mass with an intermediate wound closure of 3 cm was accomplished. Patient tolerated the procedure well; however, some respiratory complications were realized as a result of the general anesthesia so the patient was kept in the facility for an extra day.

Patient is discharged home with his wife. Discharge orders instruct him to make a follow-up appointment with Dr. Facci, the oncologist, to discuss treatment.

Find the best, most appropriate diagnosis code(s).

____

____

____

HILLSIDE HOSPITAL
359 Mountain Pass Road
Langston, FL 33993

DISCHARGE SUMMARY

Patient:	COLLIER, ROBIN
DATE OF ADMISSION:	07/15/11
DATE OF SURGERY:	07/29/11
DATE OF DISCHARGE:	08/01/11

ADMITTING DIAGNOSIS:	Schizoaffective disorder
DISCHARGE DIAGNOSIS:	Schizoaffective disorder; hypothyroidism; hypercholestolemia; borderline hypertension

The patient is a 57-year-old white female with a long history of schizoaffective disorder with numerous hospitalizations, brought in by ambulance for increasing paranoia; increasing arguments with other people; and, in general, an exacerbation of her psychotic symptoms, which had been worsening over the previous two weeks.

She is now discharged to return to her home at the YMCA and also to return to her weekly psychiatric appointments with Dr. Yahia. The patient also is advised to follow up with her medical doctor for her hypertension.

The patient was advised during this admission to start on hydrochlorothiazide 12.5 mg daily, but she refused.

She has been compliant with her medication until the recently refused hydrochlorothiazide. She is irritable at times, but overall she is redirectable and is considered to be at or close to her best baseline. She is considered in no imminent danger to herself or to others at this time.

Find the best, most appropriate diagnosis code(s).

HILLSIDE HOSPITAL
359 Mountain Pass Road
Langston, FL 33993

DISCHARGE SUMMARY

Patient:	DRONICA, BRUCE
DATE OF ADMISSION:	03/05/11
DATE OF DISCHARGE:	03/17/11
ADMITTING DIAGNOSIS:	Major depressive disorder
DISCHARGE DIAGNOSIS:	Alcohol dependence; cocaine dependence; major depressive disorder, recurrent; HIV positive; hepatitis C; and history of asthma.

This 23-year-old single male was referred for this admission, his second lifetime rehabilitation. The patient has a history of alcohol and cocaine dependence since age 17.

During the course of admission, the patient was placed on hydrochlorothiazide 25 milligrams for hypertension to which he responded well. He participated in this rehabilitation program and worked rigorously throughout.

On discharge, the patient is alert and oriented ×3. Mood is euthymic. Affect is full range. The patient denies SI, HI, denies AH, VH. Thought process is organized. Thought content—no delusions elicited. There is no evidence of psychosis. There is no imminent risk of suicide or homicide.

Find the best, most appropriate diagnosis code(s).

____

____

____

HILLSIDE HOSPITAL
359 Mountain Pass Road
Langston, FL 33993

DISCHARGE SUMMARY

Patient:	PREGGER, LOUIS
DATE OF ADMISSION:	01/15/11
DATE OF DISCHARGE:	01/17/11

ADMITTING DIAGNOSIS:	Mass in bladder
DISCHARGE DIAGNOSIS:	High-grade transitional cell carcinoma of the left bladder wall; low-grade transitional cell carcinoma in situ, underlying mild chronic inflammation

This 63-year-old male was admitted with a suspicious mass identified in the lateral bladder. Biopsy was performed, and upon pathology report of malignancy, a transurethral resection of the bladder tumors was performed. Patient is kept overnight. Foley catheter removed second day, and discharged with orders to make appointment to be seen in the office in about two weeks to start weekly BCG bladder installation treatments for recurrent bladder tumors.

Find the best, most appropriate diagnosis code(s).

____

____

____

HILLSIDE HOSPITAL
359 Mountain Pass Road
Langston, FL 33993

DISCHARGE SUMMARY

Patient:	WOLSZCZAK, LEE
DATE OF ADMISSION:	10/07/11
DATE OF DISCHARGE:	10/09/11
ADMITTING DIAGNOSIS:	Hematuria
DISCHARGE DIAGNOSIS:	Benign prostatic hypertrophy; hematuria

This 45-year-old male had a transurethral resection of prostate 10 years ago, complicated by a postoperative bleed as well as evaluation with an attempted ureteroscopy for persistent hematuria. This hematuria is secondary to prostatic varices.

Flexible cystoscopy demonstrated a normal urethra and obstructed bladder outlet secondary to a very large nodular regrowth of the prostate at the medium lobe.

A transurethral resection of prostate was performed with success.

Find the best, most appropriate diagnosis code(s).

____

____

____

HILLSIDE HOSPITAL
359 Mountain Pass Road
Langston, FL 33993

DISCHARGE CLINICAL RESUME

Patient: BOLIVAR, STEPHEN
DATE OF ADMISSION: 05/09/11
DATE OF DISCHARGE: 05/14/11

ADMITTING DIAGNOSES:
1. Dyspnea
2. Congestive heart failure (CHR) exacerbation
3. Hypertension
4. Heart murmur
5. Inferior vena cava filter placed July 2010 secondary to lower extremity deep venous thrombosis (DVT)
6. Hypothyroidism with TSH 9.1
7. Peripheral vascular disease—peripheral arterial disease

DISCHARGE DIAGNOSES:
1. Dyspnea, resolved
2. Diastolic CHR, ejection fraction 70%
3. Hypertension, controlled
4. Severe aortic stenosis
5. Catheter placed secondary to deep venous thrombosis, on Coumadin, INR in 2 on discharge
6. Hypothyroidism
7. Peripheral vascular disease
8. Renal ultrasound with medical disease

HISTORY: An 88-year old male who was admitted with dyspnea. He was found with diastolic CHF exacerbation. The patient was seen by Dr. Patel, vascular surgeon, who believed that he had some mild arterial insufficiency and continued anticoagulation. He wants to see him in his office as an outpatient. During admission, on and off he was having numbness in bilateral feet and hands and cyanosis that resolved by themselves with no problems. Probably Raynaud phenomenon. During the admission also was seen by cardiologist, who diuresed the patient with no complications. He believes that the patient needs to be started on 1mg po Bumex. Weigh every day. If the weight gain is more than 3 pounds Bumex is to be increased by 1 mg po. The patient also was seen by Dr. Bommineni, who believed that the patient can go home and continue follow-up as an outpatient. Pulmonology saw the patient as well and believed the same thing. The patient has been stable. Vital signs stable, afebrile, 98% 02 stat on room air. He was complaining of some biting itching. The daughter had taken him to the dermatologist and wants to continue follow-up with the dermatologist as an outpatient.

RECOMMENDATIONS: Discharge patient home. Follow up with Dr. Yablakoff in the nursing home.

Continued

DISCHARGE MEDICATIONS

1. The patient is going with alendronate 70 mg every week, bumetanide 1 mg twice a day if the weight gain is more than 3 pounds.
2. Diovan 80 mg once a day
3. Levothyroxine was increased to 200 mcg every day, and check TSH in 4 weeks with Dr. Yablakoff
4. Metolazone 2.5 mg once a day
5. Potassium 20 prn every day
6. Warfarin 5 mg every day. Check INR every day and let Dr. Yablakoff know if the INR is more than 2.5
7. Medrol Dosepak as directed

The case was discussed with the patient and his daughter, the plan out of the hospital. They understood, had no questions, agreed with the plan.

Roger Casey, MD – 9999
556842/mt98328 05/14/11 12:13:56 05/14/11 17:51:58
cc. Carole Yablakoff, MD

Find the best, most appropriate diagnosis code(s).

____

____

____

HILLSIDE HOSPITAL
359 Mountain Pass Road
Langston, FL 33993

DISCHARGE CLINICAL RESUME

Patient:	NATUZZI, BARRY
DATE OF ADMISSION:	06/03/11
DATE OF DISCHARGE:	06/06/11

ADMITTING DIAGNOSIS:
Ischemia transient ischemic attack, rule out myocardial infarction, arrythmia

DISCHARGE DIAGNOSES:
Transient ischemic attack, history of paroxysmal supraventricular tachycardia and status post cardioversion
Hyperlipidemia
Coronary artery disease, status post coronary artery bypass graft
Urinary tract infection

CONSULTATIONS: Dr. Falkner for neurology and Dr. Mathias for cardiology

PROCEDURES: Echocardiogram, TEE, Thallium stress test

COMPLICATIONS: None

INFECTIOUS: None

HISTORY: Seventy-one-year old white male with significant history of coronary artery disease, status post coronary artery bypass graft three years ago and cardioversion in February 2011, who presented with difficulty speaking. He stated that he had difficulty obtaining the right words when he spoke. This lasted about 15 minutes; however, when the patient came to the emergency room he was completely okay. He did not have any deficits. The patient was admitted and consultants were called in to provide evaluation of possible TIA with rule out cardiac source. Carotid Doppler was done. Echocardiogram was done. This showed dilated left ventricle, severe global left ventricular dysfunction, estimated ejection fraction 20% and left atrial enlargement, mitral annular calcification with severe mitral regurgitation, aortic sclerosis with moderate aortic insufficiency and severe tricuspid regurgitation with estimated pulmonary study pressure of 70mm. Thallium stress test was uneventful. Persantine infusion protocol and no clinical EKG changes of ischemia and radionuclide showed fixed defect anteroseptal, anteroapical, and adjacent inferior wall with hypokinesis; no ischemia seen. The ejection fraction was calculated 40%. CT of the brain showed white matter ischemic changes and atrophy, no acute intracranial abnormalities. MRI showed extensive periventricular white matter ischemia changes. MRA was normal. EKG was within normal limits, showing sinus bradycardia with average of 50 to 56.

The patient went to TEE to rule out cardiac source. The TEE was not conclusive and there was no hypokinesis, as described in the previous echocardiogram and it was considered the patient needs to have lifetime Coumadin because of previous events.

Continued

The hospital course was uneventful. He never presented with any other new deficit or any new symptoms.

Today, the patient is asymptomatic; vital signs are stable. Monitor shows sinus rhythm, and he is discharged in stable condition to be followed by Dr. Roman in 1 week; by Dr. Falkner in 2 weeks and by Dr. Mathias in 2 weeks. He will have home health nurse to inject him Lovenox until PT and INR reach therapeutic levels of 2/3. He will be on Coumadin for 5 mg po qd, and home health nurse will draw PT and INR daily until Dr. Roman thoroughly assesses the patient. He will receive the last dose of Bactrim today for urine; however, urine culture has been negative.

Roger Casey, MD – 9999
556842/mt98328 06/06/11 1:23:36 06/06/11 10:11:59
cc. Kevin Roman, MD

Find the best, most appropriate diagnosis code(s).

____

____

____

HILLSIDE HOSPITAL
359 Mountain Pass Road
Langston, FL 33993

DISCHARGE DOCUMENT SUMMARY

Patient: BRINKLEY, CAROLE
DATE OF ADMISSION: 02/09/11
DATE OF DISCHARGE: 02/10/11

ADMISSION DIAGNOSIS:
Abdominal pain, status postappendectomy

DISCHARGE DIAGNOSIS:
Abdominal pain, unknown etiology, status postappendectomy

BRIEF HISTORY: The patient is an 18-year-old female who, 6 weeks ago, underwent an appendectomy for perforated appendicitis. About 3 weeks following that, she had episodes of nausea and vomiting and diffuse abdominal pain. This was worked up at McGraw Medical Center, including CT scan, Meckel scan, and laboratory, which were unremarkable. It resolved spontaneously over a 3-day period. Three days prior to admission, she had a recurrent bout of diffuse, dull, abdominal pain with associated nausea and anorexia. She was admitted to the hospital at the time for workup of this pain.

CLINICAL COURSE: On examination, the patient was found to have a diffuse, mild tenderness without any rebound or peritoneal signs. Plain radiographs of the abdomen were obtained, which were within normal limits. A CT scan of the abdomen and pelvis was also obtained, which was unremarkable. She was without leukocytosis. Dr. Andrews of GI saw the patient in consultation, and an upper GI with small bowel follow-through was obtained. This was performed today and was found to be normal.

At this time, the patient has just had a regular meal without difficulty and feels like returning home. She will be discharged home at this time and can follow up with her primary MD. We will see her on an as-needed basis.

Gail Robbins, MD – 7777
6582411/mt98328 02/10/11 12:13:56 02/10/11 17:51:58

Find the best, most appropriate diagnosis code(s).

____

____

____

HILLSIDE HOSPITAL
359 Mountain Pass Road
Langston, FL 33993

DISCHARGE DOCUMENT SUMMARY

Patient: LOWENSON, MARC
DATE OF ADMISSION: 08/01/11
DATE OF DISCHARGE: 08/22/11

FINAL DIAGNOSES:

1. Alcohol dependence, cocaine dependence
2. Major depressive disorder, recurrent
3. HIV
4. History of positive PPD
5. Hepatitis C
6. History of asthma

DISCHARGE MEDICATIONS:

1. Zoloft 100 milligrams, po, qam
2. Seroquel 50 mg po qhs
3. Truvade 1 tab qam
4. Regataz 300 mg po qam
5. Norvir 100 mg po qam with breakfast
6. Dapsone 100 mg po qam
7. Hydrochlorothiazide 25 mg po qam

DISPOSITION: The patient will return to his residence at the Midtown Hotel. He will attend the hospital continuing day treatment program.

PROGNOSIS: Guarded

HISTORY: He is noted to have significant immunosuppression related to his HIV. Currently there is no stigmata of opportunistic infection.

During the course of admission, the patient was placed on hydrochlorothiazide 25 mg for hypertension, which he responded well to.

CONDITION ON DISCHARGE: The patient is a 54-year-old single black male referred for his first BRU admission, his second lifetime rehabilitation. The patient has a history of alcohol and cocaine dependence since age 17. Prior to this admission he had attained no significant period of sobriety other than time spent incarcerated.

The patient participated in a 21-day MICA rehabilitation program. He worked rigorously throughout the entire program. He had perfect attendance and participated well as a peer support provider. The patient attended eight groups daily. He worked well in individual therapy with his nurse practitioner and social worker.

Continued

On discharge, the patient is alert and oriented ×3. Mood is euthymic. Affect is full range. The patient denies SI, HI, denies AH, VH. Thought process is organized. Thought content—no delusions elicited. There is no evidence of psychosis. There is no imminent risk of suicide or homicide.

Keith Masters, MD – 5555
517895221/mt98328 08/22/11 12:13:56 08/22/11 17:51:58

Find the best, most appropriate diagnosis code(s).

____

____

____

HILLSIDE HOSPITAL
359 Mountain Pass Road
Langston, FL 33993

DISCHARGE CLINICAL RESUME

Patient:	WYLER, WENDY
DATE OF ADMISSION:	11/05/11
DATE OF DISCHARGE:	11/18/11

This is a 36-37 week female delivered to a 22-year-old, gravida 2, para 1, who was a known breech presentation. She presented with complaint of vaginal bleeding, rupture of membranes, and abdominal pain and cramping. On exam found to be complete with large fecal impaction. Fetal heart rate 120 by monitor. To c-section room for disimpaction and cesarean section for beech. Delivered precipitously immediately after impaction was removed, breech presentation. OB moved baby to warmer. She was pale with no respiratory effort or heart rate. Ambu bagged with mask for 30 seconds. Intubation attempted. Code called. UAC was placed. ENT in place and bagged. No heart rate, no breath sounds, pale, cyanotic. Reintubated with chest rise, heart rate about 60. Chest compression stopped when heart rate above 120, color improved. Apgar 0 at 1 minute, 1 at 5 minutes, and 4 at 10 minutes. No spontaneous respiratory effort. Received sodium bicarbonate, epinephrine and calcium. No grimace, no spontaneous movements. Pupils midpoint, nonreactive to light. NG placed for distended abdomen. Cord pH 7.33. Mother noted to have 50% abruptio placenta. Transferred to Neo. UAC was removed and replaced. UVC also placed.

Physical exam: weight 2,620 grams, pink, fontanelle soft, significant clonus of extremities, tone decreased. Pupils 2 cm and round, nonreactive to light. No movement, no grimace, no suck, good chest rise. Equal breath sounds, no murmur. Pulses 2+. Perfusion good. Abdomen soft and full. No masses. Normal female genitalia externally. Anus patent. Extremities no edema. Skin—Mongolian spot sacrum and both arms, single café-au-lait spot left flank 1.5 cm × 0.5 cm. Palate intact.

IMPRESSION:
1. 36–37 week AGA female
2. Status postcardiopulmonary arrest
3. Rule out sepsis
4. At risk for hypoxic ischemic encephalopathy

PHYSICAL EXAM: 43 days of age, weight 2,520 grams, head circumference 35, pink. Anterior fontanelle soft. Heart—II/VI murmur radiating to the axilla. Chest clear. Abdomen soft, positive bowel sounds, gastrostomy tube intact, wound is okay. Neuro—irritable. The infant has an anal fissure at 12 o'clock which has caused some blood streaks in the stool.

Continued

FINAL DIAGNOSES:

1. 36–37 week appropriate for gestational age female
2. Status postcardiopulmonary arrest
3. Transient respiratory distress
4. Rule out sepsis
5. Hypoxic ischemic encephalopathy
6. Seizures
7. Gastroesophageal reflux and feeding difficulty
8. Postoperative wound infection

Gary Benjamin, MD – 3333
2564821/mt98328 11/18/11 12:13:56 11/18/11 17:51:58

Find the best, most appropriate diagnosis code(s).

____

____

____

15 You Code It! Practice and Simulation

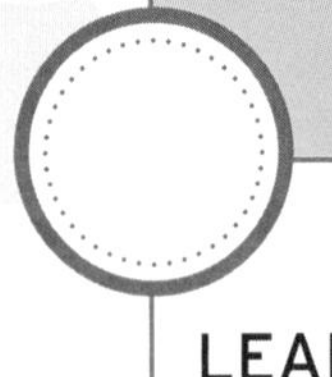

Complete Diagnostic Coding Review

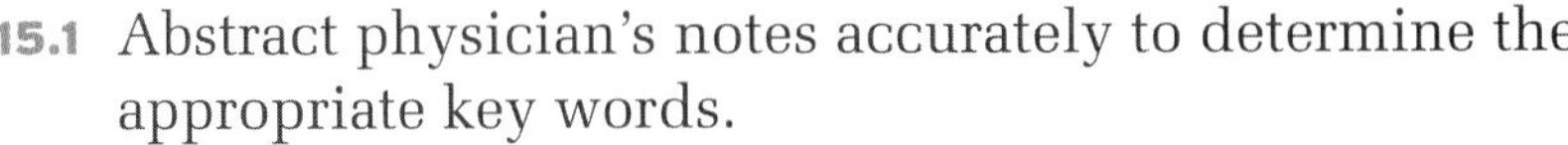

LEARNING OUTCOMES

15.1 Abstract physician's notes accurately to determine the appropriate key words.

15.2 Assess the reasons the patient came to see the health care professional.

15.3 Correctly apply the guidelines to find the most accurate diagnosis code or codes.

15.4 Identify the circumstances under which an E code is required.

15.5 Apply the rules and policies in determining if additional codes are needed.

15.6 Determine the correct sequencing when multiple codes are required.

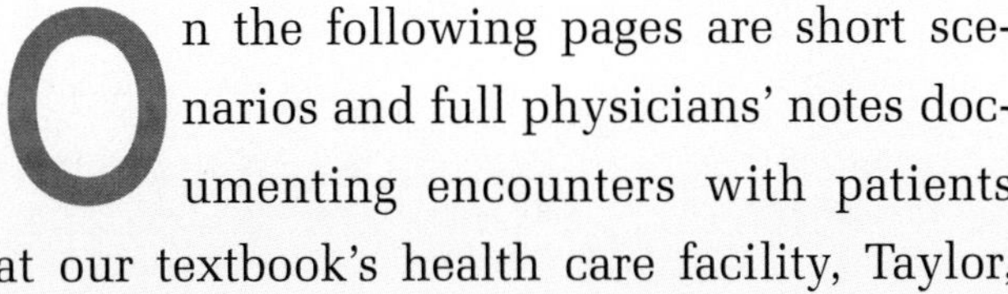

On the following pages are short scenarios and full physicians' notes documenting encounters with patients at our textbook's health care facility, Taylor, Reader, & Associates. Carefully read through the notes, and find the best ICD-9-CM diagnosis code or codes for each case.

YOU CODE IT! Scenarios

1. Karyn Cassey, a 3-year-old female, sees Dr. Fahey, a pediatrician, for the first time because of itchy spots all over her body. After a detailed history and a detailed examination, Dr. Fahey diagnoses her with chickenpox.

____

2. Isaac Thomas, a 73-year-old male, is admitted to the observation unit today after collapsing at church during services. He continues to have an irregular heartbeat.

____

3. Johanna Arthur, a 7-year-old female, is admitted to the hospital with severe poison ivy contracted while on a field trip with the Girl Scouts.

____

4. Dr. Maxwell calls in Dr. Frizzola for a consultation on 8-year-old David Harrison to determine if a tonsillectomy should be performed. David is currently in the hospital for treatment of his previously diagnosed acute lymphoid leukemia. Dr. Frizzola gathers a comprehensive history, performs a comprehensive examination in the hospital room, and spends time reviewing all prior test results. He then confirms the diagnosis of tonsillitis and schedules the procedure.

____

5. Dr. Anthony spent approximately one hour on a conference call talking with an oncologist in Texas and a reconstructive specialist in California. The three professionals were discussing treatment plans and options for Zena Johnson, a 37-year-old female, who was recently diagnosed with parosteal osteogenic sarcoma.

____

6. Jamie Farmer came into the hospital for initial observation for lower right quadrant pain, accompanied by nausea, vomiting, and a low-grade fever. Dr. Wadhwa was brought in for a surgical consultation, and he recommended that Jamie stay in the hospital overnight to rule out the possibility of a ruptured appendix.

____

7. Randy Taylor, a 2-year-old male, is admitted into the hospital with bacterial pneumonia after 5 days of antibiotic therapy. At admittance, his vitals show a temperature of 38.3°C (101°F) with a mild rash on his torso.

____

8. Loretta Gerbil, a 47-year-old female, was sent to Dr. Harrington, an OB-GYN, for an office consultation. She had been suffering with moderate pelvic pain, a heavy sensation in her lower pelvis, and marked discomfort during sexual intercourse. In a detailed history, Dr. Harrington noted the location, severity, and duration of her pelvic pain and related symptoms. In the review of systems, Loretta had positive findings related to her gastrointestinal, genitourinary, and endocrine body systems. Dr. Harrington noted that her past medical history was noncontributory to the present problem. The detailed physical examination centered on her gastrointestinal and genitourinary systems with a complete pelvic exam. Dr. Harrington ordered lab tests and a pelvic ultrasound in order to consider uterine fibroids, endometritis, or other internal gynecological pathology.

____

9. Martin Mazzenthorp went to see Dr. Appleton for a confirmatory consultation regarding his own physician's recommendation for surgical repair of a hiatal hernia. After a brief problem-focused history of present illness and a problem-focused exam of the affected body area and organ system, Dr. Appleton made a straightforward medical decision to support the original recommendation for surgery.

____

10. Carolina Tanner came into the emergency department (ED) with a wrist sprain where a ball had hit her. She had been playing at the baseball field and got hurt during a baseball game. She was in obvious pain, and the wrist was swollen and too painful upon attempts to flex. Dr. Ramada performed an expanded problem-focused history and exam before ordering radiographs. Reports confirmed a fracture of the distal radius.

____

11. Bernard Kristenson, an 82-year-old male, was diagnosed with advanced Alzheimer's disease about one year ago. Today he is being seen by the nursing facility's physician, Dr. Mintz, over concern of the development of urinary and fecal incontinence, as well as an increase in Bernard's hypertension. In addition to the detailed interval history, the physician spoke with family members and the nursing staff and reviewed the patient's record to create an extended history necessary for an extended review of systems (ROS). Dr. Mintz performed a comprehensive physical exam to assess all body systems. Afterward, he wrote all new orders due to the patient's dramatic change in his physical and mental condition. A new treatment plan was created.

____

12. Verniece Dantini, a 61-year-old female, comes to see Dr. Smallerman for her regular annual physical. She has insulin-dependent diabetes mellitus with retinal edema and nephrosis. In addition, she suffers from hypertensive heart disease with episodes of congestive heart failure. Dr. Smallerman completes an age-appropriate physical examination. After the exam, Dr. Smallerman spends some time talking with Verniece about her day-to-day activities, her diet and overall eating habits, whether or not she is engaging in regular exercise, and her overall mental attitudes as well as physical well-being. The patient states it can be difficult to get around by herself due to the problems with her eyes, and she is finding it more and more difficult to give herself the insulin injections. Dr. Smallerman provides her with some information about an insulin pump and she states she will go over it and discuss it with her son.

____

13. Karina Wilmington, a 33-year-old female, came to the office to see Dr. Grace for the first time because of a cough, fever, excessive sputum production, and shortness of breath. She had been reasonably well until now. Dr. Grace did a detailed exam of the respiratory system, as well as a review of the patient's cardiovascular and gastrointestinal systems. A detailed history of the present illness was performed. Dr. Grace ordered a chest x-ray to rule out pneumonia and told Karina to come back in a week to discuss the test results.

____

14. George Carter, a 17-month-old male, was admitted to the hospital by his pediatrician, Dr. Mitchell, after Dr. Mitchell confirmed via chest x-ray that the child had pneumonia. The initial hospital care included a detailed history and detailed physical exam with an extended problem-focused ROS completed with Petula Carter, the child's mother.

____

15. Tricia Thornwell, a 27-year-old female, is admitted to the hospital for observation after falling from the roof of her carport (approximately 8 feet high). Tricia has complaints of pain in multiple areas, and numerous x-rays were ordered.

____

16. Ellen Onoton, a 45-year-old female, recently diagnosed with asthma, comes to see Dr. Pashma for a routine office visit with a complaint of severe headaches.

____

17. Frank Childers, a 72-year-old male in good health, came to see his regular family physician, Dr. Rappoport, for his yearly physical exam. No problems were found during the examination.

____

18. Raymond Catertell, a 20-year-old male, was admitted into the hospital two days ago for bronchitis. Raymond requested that his family physician, Dr. Kaminsky, perform a circumcision, so Dr. Kaminsky called Dr. Longwell, a urologist, in for a consultation. Dr. Longwell performed a problem-focused history and problem-focused physical exam and made the straightforward decision to recommend that Raymond have the surgical procedure done as an outpatient at a later date. Code for Dr. Longwell's consultation.

____

19. Maribelle Johannsen, a 75-year-old female, lives in Sun City Extended Nursing Facility where she is seen by Dr. Modesta as a part of Maribelle's annual assessment. Dr. Modesta completes a detailed interval history with a comprehensive, head-to-toe physical exam. He reviews and affirms the medical plan of care developed by the multidisciplinary care team at Sun City. Maribelle's condition is stable, her hypertension and diabetes (type 2) are in good control, and she has no new problems. There are minimal data for Dr. Modesta to review and few diagnoses to consider.

____

20. With a diagnosis of intrinsic asthma with status asthmaticus, Wilson McGraw was admitted into the hospital the day before yesterday from the ED. For the last 30 hours, he has been receiving extensive respiratory therapy and is now seen by his family physician, Dr. Avenavour. Dr. Avenavour performs a detailed interval history and a detailed physical exam and reviews an extensive amount of documentation, lab tests, and other test results that have been added to Wilson's record. Wilson's respiratory condition is still unstable, and Dr. Avenavour is concerned that pneumonia may develop and complicate Wilson's asthma.

____

21. Premier Life & Health Insurance Company required Tom Cavellini, a 31-year-old male, to have Dr. Louisman, his regular physician, complete a certificate confirming that Tom's current disability prevents him from working at his regular job and that Tom is eligible for disability insurance.

____

22. Oscar Unger, a 27-year-old male, goes to his family physician, Dr. Carter, for a tetanus shot after stepping on a rusty nail at the beach. While there, Oscar asked Dr. Carter to look at a cut on his left hand. Dr. Carter examines the wound and tells him to keep the wound clean and bandaged.

____

23. Dr. Pittman goes to see his patient, Matilda Grinowski, a 78-year-old female, who is homebound since having a stroke one year ago. Matilda has essential benign hypertension, peripheral vascular disease, and is post-CVA hemiplegic on her dominant side. Dr. Pittman does an expanded problem-focused interval history and a problem-focused examination. Due to his familiarity with Matilda and her concerns, his medical decision-making is straightforward. He renews her prescriptions.

____

24. Ronald Walden, a 53-year-old male, was admitted to the hospital with precordial chest pain. A detailed history was documented in his chart. Later that same day, after the results of a comprehensive group of tests were all within normal limits, he was discharged.

____

25. A 15-year-old female, Lakeesha Jones, sprained her left ankle and was brought to the emergency department by her mother. Lakeesha had been rollerblading and tripped, falling sideways. Lakeesha was in pain and unable to flex her ankle, which had already begun to swell. Dr. Carole talked with the girl about her ankle, gathered a brief history of the incident that caused the sprain, as well as any history relating to her legs and feet. He then performed a limited examination of her left leg, ankle, and foot. The imaging confirmed a sprained calcaneofibular ligament and a sprained anterior tibiofibular ligament.

____

YOU CODE IT! Case Studies

TAYLOR, READER, & ASSOCIATES
A Complete Health Care Facility
975 CENTRAL AVENUE • SOMEWHERE, FL 32811 • 407-555-4321

PATIENT: GONZALEZ, RENITA
ACCOUNT/EHR #: GONZRE001
Date: 09/16/11

Attending Physician: Suzanne R. Taylor, MD

S: This new Pt is a 72-year-old female brought in by her daughter. She has been anxious, hyperventilating, labored breath, short of breath—worse since taking medication for anxiety. She is allergic to PCN, Biaxin, and ASA.

Patient has a history of asthma, tinnitus, kidney stones, and hypertension. She is retired. Patient is extremely anxious. She states her husband died 2 years ago, and she has been having trouble. She started seeing a psychiatrist one week ago, and he prescribed Zoloft 50 mg bid. She is also taking Liseropril 1 tab qd, potassium 20 mg qd. She denies pain but has trouble breathing at times when she is anxious.

O: Wt. 160 lb. Ht 5′6″ T 97.5 P 95 R 26 BP 155/83. Lungs clear. Pt calmed down with reassurance and emotional support. EKG abnormal, cardiac enzyme in normal range. Automated differential, PT, PTT, EKG show normal sinus rhythm. Left ventricular hypertrophy with repolarization abnormality, Chest x-rays (PA and Lat) show no acute intrathoracic abnormality. CBC: Glucose is elevated; sodium, potassium, and chloride are low. All other labs are unremarkable.

A: Anxiety

P: 1. Rx Xanax 1 mg PO tid
2. Follow-up with psychiatrist

Suzanne R. Taylor, MD

SRT/pw D: 09/16/11 09:50:16 T: 09/18/11 12:55:01

Find the best, most appropriate diagnosis code(s).

____

____

____

TAYLOR, READER, & ASSOCIATES
A Complete Health Care Facility
975 CENTRAL AVENUE • SOMEWHERE, FL 32811 • 407-555-4321

PATIENT: STARKER, SHARON
ACCOUNT/EHR #: STARSH001
Date: 08/11/11

Attending Physician: Willard B. Reader, MD

S. Patient is a 41-year-old female, who comes in with a complaint of severe neck pain and difficulty turning her head. She states she was in a car accident two days ago, her car struck from behind when she was driving home from work.

O: PE reveals tightness upon palpitation of ligaments in neck and shoulders, most pronounced C3 to C5. X-rays are taken of head and neck including the cervical vertebrae. Radiologic review denies any fracture.

A. Anterior longitudinal cervical sprain

P: 1. Applied cervical collar to be worn during all waking hours.
2. Rx Vicodin (hydrocodone) 500 mg po prn
3. 1,000 mg aspirin qid
4. Pt to return in 2 weeks for follow-up

Willard B. Reader, MD

DRC/pw D: 08/11/11 09:50:16 T: 08/13/11 12:55:01

Find the best, most appropriate diagnosis code(s).

TAYLOR, READER, & ASSOCIATES
A Complete Health Care Facility
975 CENTRAL AVENUE • SOMEWHERE, FL 32811 • 407-555-4321

PATIENT:	WESTERBY, ELMO
ACCOUNT/EHR #:	WESTEL001
Date:	09/16/11
Attending Physician:	Suzanne R. Taylor, MD
Preoperative DX:	Orbital mass, OD
Postoperative DX:	Herniated orbital fat pad, OD
Procedure:	Excision of mass and repair, right superior orbit
Surgeon:	Raul Sanchez, MD
Anesthesia:	Local

PROCEDURE: After proparacaine was instilled in the eye, it was prepped and draped in the usual sterile manner, and 2% lidocaine with 1:200,000 epinephrine was injected into the superior aspect of the right orbit. A corneal protective shield was placed in the eye. The eye was placed in down-gaze.

The upper lid was everted and the fornix examined. The herniating mass was viewed and measured at 0.75 cm in diameter. Westcott scissors were used to incise the fornix conjunctiva. The herniating mass was then clamped, excised, and cauterized. It appeared to contain mostly fat tissue, which was sent to pathology.

The superior fornix was repaired using running suture of 6-0 plain gut. Bacitracin ointment was applied to the eye followed by an eye pad. The patient tolerated the procedure well and left the operating room in good condition.

Suzanne R. Taylor, MD

SRT/pw D: 09/16/11 09:50:16 T: 09/18/11 12:55:01

Find the best, most appropriate diagnosis code(s).

TAYLOR, READER, & ASSOCIATES
A Complete Health Care Facility
975 CENTRAL AVENUE • SOMEWHERE, FL 32811 • 407-555-4321

PATIENT: CAPOZZI, VINCENT
ACCOUNT/EHR #: CAPOVI001
Date: 08/11/11

Attending Physician: Willard B. Reader, MD

Patient is a 62-year-old male previously seen by Dr. David Bush 18 months ago. The patient has a history of coronary artery disease and hyperlipidemia. He underwent coronary bypass surgery in 1973, by Dr. Howard that involved a left internal mammary artery to left anterior descending. In 1989, he underwent a redo operation consisting of a right internal mammary artery to left anterior descending, saphenous vein graft to circumflex, and saphenous vein graft to right coronary artery.

He did well until yesterday afternoon when he developed an episode of moderate retrosternal chest pressure radiating to the right shoulder, which was prolonged and lasted until 3:00 A.M., at which time he presented to the ED. He apparently was given one nitroglycerin sublingual, with resolution of symptoms. The patient is currently asymptomatic on examination, and his review of systems is noncontributory.

PE: He is alert, oriented times three, in no acute distress. HEENT: unremarkable. Lungs: clear. Cardiovascular: Regular rate and rhythm. No murmurs and no gallops. Abdomen: Benign. Extremities: No edema. EKG: Normal sinus rhythm with myocardial changes. Lipid Panel: all unremarkable except for a cholesterol of 255. CBC: within normal limits. PT and PTT within normal limits. Cardiac enzymes times one: negative. Chest x-ray: unremarkable.

Admitting DX: Prolonged chest pain with negative electrocardiogram and negative enzymes times one. Admit for observation to telemetry. In view of the atypical nature of prolonged chest pain, we will proceed with a screening Cardiolite stress test later today. Nitroglycerin paste was applied on admission; however, it will be held until the stress test is completed. One aspirin a day was started. Further recommendation and interventions will depend on the results from the stress test.

Discharge DX: Coronary atherosclerosis of native coronary artery

Willard B. Reader, MD

DRC/pw D: 08/11/11 09:50:16 T: 08/13/11 12:55:01

Find the best, most appropriate diagnosis code(s).

TAYLOR, READER, & ASSOCIATES
A Complete Health Care Facility
975 CENTRAL AVENUE • SOMEWHERE, FL 32811 • 407-555-4321

PATIENT: GAYLORD, NITA
ACCOUNT/EHR #: GAYLNI001
Date: 09/16/11

Attending Physician: Suzanne R. Taylor, MD

The patient is a 61-year-old female with a very long history of schizoaffective disorder with numerous hospitalizations who was brought in by ambulance from the YMCA where she resides for increasing paranoia, increasing arguments with other people, and in general an exacerbation of her psychotic symptoms, which had been worsening over the previous two weeks.

Initially, the patient was very agitated and uncooperative. She refused medications. She wanted to leave the hospital. A 2PC* was done, and the patient had a court hearing that resulted in retention. Eventually, the patient agreed to a trial of Risperdal. She showed fairly rapid improvement once she was started on Risperdal 2 mg twice daily. At the time of discharge compared with admission, the patient is much improved. She is usually pleasant and cooperative with occasional difficult moments, some continuing mild paranoia. She has no hallucinations. She has no thoughts of harming herself or anyone else. She is compliant with her medication until the recently refused hydrochlorothiazide. She is irritable at times, but overall she is redirectable and is considered to be at or close to her best baseline. She is considered no imminent danger to herself or to others at this time.

Final DX: Schizoaffective disorder; hypothyroidism; hypercholesterolemia; borderline hypertension.

Prescriptions for 30-day supplies were given: Ativan 2 mg po tid; Celexa 40 mg po daily; Risperdal 2 mg po bid; Synthroid 0.088 mg po qam; Zocor 40 mg po qhs

---

Suzanne R. Taylor, MD

SRT/pw D: 09/16/11 09:50:16 T: 09/18/11 12:55:01

*2PC is the acronym used for "two physician certified". This is the legal requirement of an involuntary commitment of a patient who holds that, prior to the admission of this patient to a mental health facility or ward, two physicians have certified that the individual has a significant mental illness and may be at risk of harm to himself/herself or others.

Find the best, most appropriate diagnosis code(s).

____

____

____

TAYLOR, READER, & ASSOCIATES
A Complete Health Care Facility
975 CENTRAL AVENUE • SOMEWHERE, FL 32811 • 407-555-4321

PATIENT: KELLO, JOAN
ACCOUNT/EHR #: KELLJO001
Date: 09/16/11

Attending Physician: Suzanne R. Taylor, MD

The patient is a 25-year-old female with a history of recurrent sinus infections and was well until 5 days ago. She presents with fever, severe frontal headache, facial pain, and runny nose. Patient states she has been having difficulty concentrating.

T 101.5° HEENT: Tenderness over frontal and left maxillary sinuses. Nasal congestion visible.

CT scan reveals opacification of both frontal and left maxillary, sphenoid sinuses and a possible large nonenhanced lesion in the brain.

Parasagittal MRI and axial MRI show a large (7-cm) well-circumscribed epidural collection compressing the left frontal lobe.

DX: Epidural abscess with frontal lobe lesions caused by significant compression on frontal lobe. Recommendation for surgery to evacuate the abscess.

Rx antibiotics and pseudoephedrine.

Suzanne R. Taylor, MD

SRT/pw D: 09/16/11 09:50:16 T: 09/18/11 12:55:01

Find the best, most appropriate diagnosis code(s).

____

____

____

TAYLOR, READER, & ASSOCIATES
A Complete Health Care Facility
975 CENTRAL AVENUE • SOMEWHERE, FL 32811 • 407-555-4321

PATIENT: RUBEN, BETTY
MRN: RUBEBE01
DATE: 09/23/11

Attending Physician: James Healer, MD

Preoperative Diagnosis: C5 compression fracture

Postoperative Diagnosis: same

Procedure: C5 corpectomy and fusion fixation with fibular strut graft and Atlantis plate

Anesthesia: General endotracheal

This is a 25-year-old female status post assault. The pt sustained a C5 compression fracture. MRI scan showed compression with evidence of posterior ligamentous injury. The patient was subsequently set up for the surgical procedure. The procedure was described in detail including the risks. The risks included but were not limited to bleeding, infection, stroke, paralysis, death, cerebrospinal fluid (CSF) leak, loss of bladder and bowel control, hoarse voice, paralyzed vocal cord, death and damage to adjacent nerves and tissues. The pt understood the risks. The pt also understood that back bone instrumentation would be used and that the back bone could collapse and the instrumentation could fail, break, or the screws could pull out. The pt provided consent.

The pt was taken to the OR. Endotracheal tube was placed. A Foley was placed. The pt was given preoperative antibiotics. The pt was placed in slight extension. The right neck was prepped and draped in the usual manner. A linear incision was made over the C5 vertebral body. The platysma was divided. Dissection was continued medial to the sternocleidomastoid to the prevertebral fascia. This was cauterized and divided.

The longus colli was cauterized and elevated. The fracture was visualized. A spinal needle was used to verify the location using fluoroscopy. The C5 vertebral body was drilled out. The bone was saved. The disk above and below were removed. The posterior longitudinal ligament was removed. The bone was quite collapsed and fragmented. Distraction pins were then packed with bone removed from the C5 vertebral body prior to implantation. A plate was then placed with screws in the C4 and C6 vertebral bodies. The locking screws were tightened. The wound was irrigated. Bleeding was helped with the bipolar. The retractors were removed. The incision was approximated with simple interrupted Vicryl. The subcutaneous tissue was approximated and skin edges approximated subcuticularly. Steri-Strips were applied. A dressing was applied. The pt was placed back in an Aspen collar. The pt was extubated and transferred to recovery.

James Healer, MD

JH/mgr D: 09/23/11 12:33:08 PM T: 09/25/11 3:22:54 PM

Find the best, most appropriate diagnosis code(s).

____

____

____

TAYLOR, READER, & ASSOCIATES
A Complete Health Care Facility
975 CENTRAL AVENUE • SOMEWHERE, FL 32811 • 407-555-4321

PATIENT: KLOTSKY, STACY
MRN: KLOTST01
Admission Date: 5 October 2011
Discharge Date: 5 October 2011
Date: 5 October 2011

Preoperative DX: Rule out bladder tumor
Postoperative DX: same
Procedure: Cystoscopy, biopsy, and fulguration of bladder

Surgeon: Leonard Dupont, MD

Assistant: None
Anesthesia: Spinal

Indications: The pt is a 73-year-old female with a history of grade II superficial transitional cell carcinoma of the bladder. Cystoscopy showed a suspicious erythematous area on the right trigone. She presented today for cystoscopy, biopsy, and fulguration. Findings—the urethra was normal, the bladder was 1+ trabeculated, the mid and right trigone areas were slightly erythematous and hypervascular. No papillary tumors were noted; no mucosal abnormalities were noted.

Procedure: The pt was placed on the table in supine position. Satisfactory spinal anesthesia was obtained. She was placed in dorsolithotomy position. She was prepped sterilely with Hibiclens and draped in the usual manner. A #22 French cystoscopy sheath was passed per urethra in atraumatic fashion. The bladder was resected with the 70-degree lens with findings as noted above. Cup biopsy forceps were placed, and three biopsies were taken of the suspicious areas of the trigone. These areas were fulgurated with the Bugby electrode; no active bleeding was seen. The scope was removed; the pt was returned to recovery having tolerated the procedure well. Estimated blood loss was minimal.

Pathology report: Chronic cystitis (cystica) with squamous cell metaplasia.
10/05/11 11:47:39

Find the best, most appropriate diagnosis code(s).

TAYLOR, READER, & ASSOCIATES
A Complete Health Care Facility
975 CENTRAL AVENUE • SOMEWHERE, FL 32811 • 407-555-4321

PATIENT:	RUDERMAN, LILLIE ANN
MRN:	RUDELI01
Admission Date:	15 October 2011
Discharge Date:	15 October 2011
Date:	15 October 2011
Preoperative DX:	Augmentation of lips
Postoperative DX:	same
Procedure:	Collagen injections
Surgeon:	Wayne Fleeter MD
Assistant:	None
Anesthesia:	Local

Indications: The patient is a 41-year-old female with a low self-image. She presents today for enhancement of her lips.

Procedure: The patient was placed on the table in supine position. Local anesthesia was administered. As soon as patient stated a complete loss of feeling in the area, the injections were given subcutaneously—a total of 2.3 cc.

10/15/11 11:47:39

Find the best, most appropriate diagnosis code(s).

___

___

___

TAYLOR, READER, & ASSOCIATES
A Complete Health Care Facility
975 CENTRAL AVENUE • SOMEWHERE, FL 32811 • 407-555-4321

PATIENT:	JABELONE, JAMAL
MRN:	JABEJA01
Admission Date:	9 October 2011
Discharge Date:	9 October 2011
Date:	9 October 2011
Preoperative DX:	Lacerations of arm, hand, and leg
Postoperative DX:	same
Procedure:	Layered repair of leg laceration; simple repair of arm and hand lacerations
Surgeon:	Geoff Conner, MD
Assistant:	None
Anesthesia:	General

Indications: The patient is a 4-year-old male brought to the emergency room by his father. He was helping his father install a new window when the window fell and shattered. The boy suffered lacerations on his left hand, left arm, and left leg.

Procedure: The patient was placed on the table in supine position. Satisfactory anesthesia was obtained. The area was prepped, and attention to the deeper laceration of the left thigh, right above the patella, was first. A layered repair was performed and the 5.1 cm laceration was closed successfully with sutures. The lacerations on the upper extremity, 2 cm laceration on the left hand at the base of the fifth metacarpal, and the 3 cm laceration on the left arm, just below the joint capsule in the posterior position, were successfully closed with 4-0 Vicryl as well. The patient tolerated the procedures well, and was transported to the recovery room.

10/09/11 11:47:39

Find the best, most appropriate diagnosis code(s).

TAYLOR, READER, & ASSOCIATES
A Complete Health Care Facility
975 CENTRAL AVENUE • SOMEWHERE, FL 32811 • 407-555-4321

PATIENT: BACHELDER, JEFFREY
MRN: BACHJE01
Admission Date: 13 October 2011
Discharge Date: 13 October 2011
Date: 13 October 2011

Preoperative DX: Malignant neoplasm, scrotum, CA in situ
Postoperative DX: same
Procedure: Resection of scrotum, needle biopsy of testis, laparoscopy with a ligation of spermatic veins

Surgeon: Daniel Macintosh, MD

Assistant: None
Anesthesia: General

Indications: The pt is a 59-year-old male with a recent diagnosis of malignancy of the scrotum.

Procedure: The pt was placed on the table in supine position. Dr. Cattan administered general anesthesia. The pt was placed in proper position. A needle biopsy was taken of the testis, and then a surgical resection of the scrotum was performed. Before closing, a surgical laparoscopy with a ligation of the spermatic veins was performed as well.

10/13/11 11:47:39

Find the best, most appropriate diagnosis code(s).

____

____

____

TAYLOR, READER, & ASSOCIATES
A Complete Health Care Facility
975 CENTRAL AVENUE • SOMEWHERE, FL 32811 • 407-555-4321

PATIENT: DENNISON, DANIEL
MRN: DENNDA01
Date: 23 November 2011

Procedure Performed: Vasectomy

Physician: Sunil Kaladuwa, MD

Indications: Elective sterilization

Procedure: The pt was given Versed for anxiety, and local anesthesia was administered. Removal of a segment of the deferent duct was accomplished bilaterally. Pt tolerated the procedure well.

Impression: Successful outcome

Plan: Postoperative semen examination is scheduled for 1 week.

Sunil Kaladuwa, MD

MA/mg D: 11/23/11 09:50:16 T: 11/25/11 12:55:01

Find the best, most appropriate diagnosis code(s).

___

___

___

TAYLOR, READER, & ASSOCIATES
A Complete Health Care Facility
975 CENTRAL AVENUE • SOMEWHERE, FL 32811 • 407-555-4321

PATIENT: KLACKSON, KEVIN
MRN: KLACKE01
Date: 15 September 2011

Diagnosis: Primary cardiomyopathy with chest pain
Procedure: Arterial catheterization

Physician: Frank Vincent, MD

Anesthesia: Local

Procedure: The pt was placed on the table in supine position. Local anesthesia was administered. Once we were assured that the pt had achieved no nervous stimuli, the incision was made and the catheter was introduced percutaneously. The incision was sutured with a simple repair. The pt tolerated the procedure well and was transferred to the recovery room.

Frank Vincent, MD

FV/mg D: 09/15/11 09:50:16 T: 09/15/11 12:55:01

Find the best, most appropriate diagnosis code(s).

___

___

___

TAYLOR, READER, & ASSOCIATES
A Complete Health Care Facility
975 CENTRAL AVENUE • SOMEWHERE, FL 32811 • 407-555-4321

PATIENT:	UNDERWOOD, PRICILLA
MRN:	UNDEPR01
Date:	25 September 2011
Diagnosis:	Medulloblastoma at the temporal lobe
Procedure:	Central venous access device (CVAD) insertion
Physician:	Frank Vincent, MD
Anesthesia:	Conscious sedation

Procedure: Pt is a 4-year-old female, with a recent diagnosis of malignancy. Due to an upcoming course of chemotherapy, the CVAD is being inserted to ease administration of the drugs. The pt was placed on the table in supine position. The pt was given Versed to achieve conscious sedation. The incision was made to insert a central venous catheter, centrally. During the placement of the catheter, a short tract (non-tunneled) is made as the catheter is advanced from the skin entry site to the point of venous cannulation. The catheter tip is set to reside in the subclavian vein. The pt was gently aroused from the sedation and was awake when transported to the recovery room.

Frank Vincent, MD

FV/mg D: 09/25/11 09:50:16 T: 09/25/11 12:55:01

Find the best, most appropriate diagnosis code(s).

TAYLOR, READER, & ASSOCIATES
A Complete Health Care Facility
975 CENTRAL AVENUE • SOMEWHERE, FL 32811 • 407-555-4321

PATIENT: FERRARO, MADONNA
MRN: FERRMA01
Date: 25 September 2011

HPI: Pt is a 91-year-old nursing home patient, examined bedside. She has lost weight and is not eating, and protein-calorie malnutrition is evident.

PMH: Her past medical history includes chronic pain syndrome; status post fracture of the hip on the right; constipation; status post cataract surgery

CURRENT MEDICATION: Lorazepam, Lasix, Ecotrin 1 tab daily; Cipro 500 mg PO bid

REVIEW OF SYSTEMS: The pt denies any chest pain or abdominal pain; denies dysuria or hematuria. There are no melana, and there is no nausea or vomiting. There is no history of diarrhea. There is history of constipation.

PE: BP 138/60 P 68 R 20 T98.3

Pt appears in no acute distress. Facial changes over the upper lip are notes. Mild asymmetry is present. Pupils react to light and accommodation. Conjunctivae are pink. Neck is supple, and lungs are clear. Cardiovascular review shows S1, S2, with a I/VI ejection murmur.

ABDOMEN: Bowel sounds present. Right upper quadrant scar noted. Right hip scar noted. Abdomen soft, nontender

INDICATIONS: Surveillance endoscopy for percutaneous endoscopic gastrostomy placement

IMPRESSION:

1. Weight loss, a documented 20-pound loss per the nursing home.
2. Protein-calorie malnutrition
3. Organic brain syndrome
4. Status post hip fracture
5. History of constipation, on bed rest.

GASTROENTEROLOGY ASSESSMENT: Normal surveillance esophagogastroduodenoscopy followed by a percutaneous endoscopic gastrostomy tube with a 20-French Bard gastrostomy tube.

PLAN: Hygience, upkeep of the gastrostomy tube, and feeding orders as well as analgesia are given. She will be followed with a KUB in the morning and will begin feedings in the morning.

Lionell Harrison, MD

LH/mg D: 09/25/11 09:50:16 T: 09/25/11 12:55:01

Find the best, most appropriate diagnosis code(s).

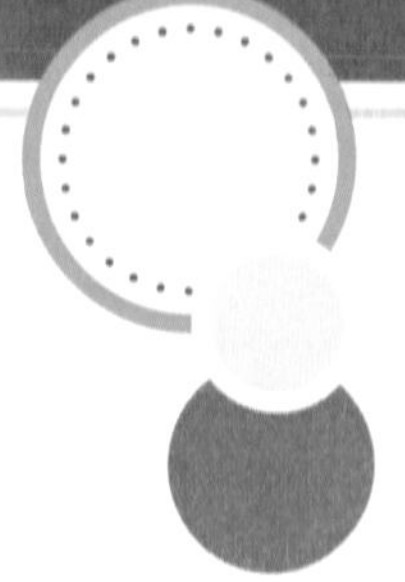

Glossary

A

Abortion The expulsion of an embryo or fetus, prior to 20 weeks gestation, from the uterus.

Acute Severe; serious.

Adverse effect An unexpected, bad result; also known as an adverse reaction. The harm a patient experiences by a medication that has been prescribed by a health care professional and taken as instructed; an unexpected reaction to a drug taken for therapeutic purposes.

Aftercare Follow-up monitoring of the patient's condition after the primary treatment has been completed.

Anatomical site A specific location or part of the human body.

Anomaly Abnormal, or unexpected, condition.

Antepartum Before the onset of labor.

Apgar Assessment of a neonate's condition based on five areas: muscle tone, heart rate, reflex response, skin color, and breathing.

Asymptomatic No symptoms or manifestations.

B

Bacteremia The presence of bacteria in the blood; an abnormal blood culture.

Benign Nonmalignant characteristic of a neoplasm; not infectious or spreading.

Benign hypertension Hypertension kept under control with diet and medication.

Burn Injury by heat, fire, or a chemical.

C

Carcinoma A malignant neoplasm or cancerous tumor.

Cartilage Tough, connective, nonvascular tissue.

Cerebrovascular accident (CVA) Rupture of a blood vessel in the brain; also known as *stroke*.

Chemicals Substances used in, or made by, the process of chemistry. Examples include benzene, turpentine, and bleach.

Chronic Long duration; continuing over a long period of time.

Chronic obstructive pulmonary disease (COPD) An ongoing obstruction of the airway.

Clinically significant Signs, symptoms, and/or conditions present at birth that may impact the child's future health status.

Closed fracture A fracture in which the broken bone has not protruded through the skin.

Coding for coverage Choosing a code on the basis of what the insurance company will cover (pay for) rather than accurately reflecting the truth.

Co-morbidity A separate condition or illness present in the same patient at the same time as another unrelated condition or illness.

Complication An unexpected illness or other condition that develops as a result of a procedure, service, or treatment provided during the patient's hospital stay.

Concurrent coding Coding processes performed while a patient is still in the hosptial receiving care.

Condition A health-related situation.

Confirmed Found to be true or definite.

Congenital A condition existing at the time of birth.

Contracture An abnormal tightening or shortening, often resulting in a deformity.

Controlled hypertension Hypertension that is successfully being treated.

D

Diabetes mellitus A chronic systemic disease that causes the body to improperly metabolize carbohydrates, proteins, and fats.

Diagnosis A physician's determination of a patient's condition, illness, or injury.

Diagnosis-related group (DRG) An episodic-care payment system basing reimbursement to hospitals for inpatient services upon standards of care for specific diagnoses grouped by their similar usage of resources for procedures, services, and treatments.

Dislocation The displacement of a limb, bone, or organ from its customary position.

Double billing Sending a claim for the second time to the same insurance company, for the same procedure or service, provided to the same patient on the same date of service.

Drugs Substances, natural or combined, created to treat or prevent illness or disease. Examples include aspirin, Lipitor, and Prozac.

Dyslipidemia Abnormal lipoprotein metabolism.

E

E codes Codes that report *how* and/or *where* an injury or poisoning happened.

Elevated blood pressure An occurrence of high blood pressure; an isolated or infrequent reading of a systolic blood pressure above 140 mm/Hg and/or a diastolic blood pressure above 90 mm/Hg.

Eponym A condition named after a person.

Exacerbation An increase in the severity of a disease or its symptoms.

Expiration The physical process of expulsing carbon dioxide.

Extent The percentage of the body that has been affected by the burn.

External cause An event, outside the body, that causes injury, poisoning, or an adverse reaction.

F

First degree Redness of the epidermis (skin).

Fracture Broken cartilage or bone.

Functional activity Glandular secretion in abnormal quantity.

G

Gestation The length of time for the complete development of a baby from conception to birth; on average 40 weeks.

Gestational diabetes mellitus Usually a temporary diabetes occurring during pregnancy; however, patients with GDM do have an increased risk of developing diabetes later on.

Gestational hypertension Hypertension that develops during pregnancy and typically goes away once the pregnancy has ended.

Gravida An alphanumeric (G1, G2, G3, etc.) that indicates how many times a woman has been pregnant in her life.

Gynecologist A physician specializing in the care of the female reproductive organs.

H

Histology The study of the microscopic composition of tissues.

Hospital-acquired conditions (HAC) A condition, illness, or injury contracted by the patient during his or her stay in an acute care facility; also known as a nosocomial condition.

Human immunodeficiency virus (HIV) A condition affecting the immune system.

Hyperglycemia Abnormally high levels of glucose.

Hypertension High blood pressure, usually a chronic condition; often identified by a systolic blood pressure above 140 mm/Hg and/or a diastolic blood pressure above 90 mm/Hg.

Hypoglycemia Abnormally low glucose levels.

I

ICD-9-CM The acronym for International Classification of Diseases, Ninth Revision, Clinical Modification.

ICD-10-CM The acronym for International Classification of Diseases, Tenth Revision, Clinical Modification.

Infarction Tissue or muscle that has deteriorated or died (necrotic).

Infectious A condition that can be transmitted from one person to another.

Influenza An acute infection of the respiratory tract caused by the influenza virus.

Inpatient facility An establishment that provides acute care services to individuals who stay overnight on the premises.

Inspiration The physical process of acquiring oxygen.

Intent The reason behind the cause of the incident.

Interaction The mixture of two or more substances that change the effect of any of the individual substances.

L

Late effect Cause-and-effect relationship between an original condition, illness, or injury and an additional problem caused by the existence of that original condition. Time is not a requirement for a diagnosis as a late effect because the additional concern may be present at any time.

Low birth weight (LBW) A baby born weighing less than 5 lb 8 oz, or 2,500 grams.

M

Major Complication and Comorbidity (MCC) A complication or comorbidity that has an impact on the treatment of the patient and that makes care for that patient more complex.

Malignant Invasive and destructive characteristic of a neoplasm; possibly causing damage or death.

Malignant hypertension Hypertension accompanied by optic nerve swelling and other serious manifestations.

Malunion A fractured bone that did not heal correctly; healing of bone that was not in proper position or alignment.

Manifestation A condition caused or developed from the existence of another condition.

Mass Abnormal collection of tissue.

Medical necessity The determination that the health care professional was acting according to standard practices in providing a particular procedure for an individual with a particular diagnosis. Also referred to as *medically necessary.*

Metastasize To proliferate, reproduce, or spread.

Morbidity The status of being diseased.

Morphology The study of the configuration or structure of living organisms.

Mortality Cause of death.

Myocardial Infarction (MI) Malfunction of the heart due to necrosis or deterioration of a portion of the heart muscle; also known as a heart attack.

N

Necrosis The death of the tissue.

Neonate An infant from birth to 1 month of age.

Neoplasm Abnormal tissue growth; tumor.

Nonessential modifiers Descriptors that are not absolutely necessary to have been included in the physician's notes and are provided simply to further clarify a code description; optional terms.

Nonunion A fractured bone that did not heal back together; no mending or joining together of the broken segments.

Not elsewhere classifiable (NEC) Specifics that are not described in any other code in the book; also known as *not elsewhere classified.*

Not otherwise specified (NOS) The absence of additional details documented in the notes.

O

Obstetrics A health care specialty focusing on the care of women during pregnancy and the puerperium.

Open fracture A fracture in which the broken bone has protruded through the skin; fracture with a wound.

Other specified Additional information that the physician specified and isn't included in any other code description.

Outpatient services Health care services provided to individuals without an overnight stay in the facility.

Overlapping boundaries Multiple sites of carcinoma without identifiable borders.

P

Para An alphanumeric that identifies the number of times a woman has given birth, designated on the chart as P1, P2, etc.; had a fetus reach viability.

Pathogen An element, such as bacteria or virus, that may cause disease.

Pathologic Related to, or caused by, disease.

Perinatal The time period from before birth to the 28th day after birth.

Physician's Desk Reference (PDR) A series of reference books identifying all aspects of prescription and over-the-counter medications, as well as herbal remedies.

Pneumonia An inflammation of the lungs.

Pneumothorax A condition by which air or gas is present within the chest cavity but outside the lungs.

Poisoned A condition produced by a substance that harms or causes death.

Polydipsia Excessive thirst.

Polyuria Excessive urination.

Postpartum The first 6 weeks after childbirth.

Prematurity Birth occurring prior to the completion of 37 weeks gestation.

Prenatal Prior to birth; also antenatal.

Present on admission (POA) A one-character indicator reporting the status of the diagnosis at the time the patient was admitted to the acute care facility.

Principal diagnosis The condition that is the primary, or main, reason for the encounter.

Puerperium The time period from the end of labor until the uterus returns to normal size, typically 3 to 6 weeks.

R

Respiration The physical process of acquiring oxygen and releasing carbon dioxide.

Respiratory disorder A malfunction of the organ system relating to respiration.

Rule of nines A general division of the whole body portioned out to represent 9 percent used for estimating the extent of a burn.

S

Second degree Blisters on the skin; involvement of the epidermis and the dermis layers.

Secondary hypertension The condition of hypertension caused by another condition or illness.

Sepsis Condition typified by two or more systemic responses to infection; a specified pathogen.

Septicemia Generalized infection spread through the body via the bloodstream; blood infection.

Septic shock Severe sepsis with hypotension, unresponsive to fluid resuscitation.

Severe sepsis Sepsis with signs of acute organ dysfunction.

Severity The level of seriousness.

Sign Objective evidence of a disease or condition.

Site The location on or in the human body; the anatomical part.

Sprain A partially torn or overstretched ligament.

Status asthmaticus The condition of asthma that is life-threatening and does not respond to therapeutic treatments.

Subluxation A partial dislocation.

Supporting documentation The paperwork in the patient's file that corroborates the codes presented on the claim form for a particular encounter.

Symptom A subjective sensation or departure from the norm as related by the patient.

Systemic inflammatory response syndrome (SIRS) A definite physical reaction, such as fever, chills, etc., to an unspecified pathogen.

T

Therapeutic Intended to restore good health or reduce the effect of disease or negative condition.

Third degree Destruction of all layers of the skin, with possible involvement of the subcutaneous fat, muscle, and bone.

Thrombosis The formation of a blood clot in a blood vessel (plural = thrombi).

Toxic effect Poisonous substance causing a health-related reaction.

Tuberculosis An infectious condition that causes small rounded swellings on mucous membranes throughout the body.

Type 1 diabetes mellitus A sudden onset of insulin deficiency. May occur at any age but most often in childhood and adolescence. Also known as insulin-dependent diabetes mellitus (IDDM), juvenile diabetes, or type I.

Type 2 diabetes mellitus A form of diabetes mellitus with a gradual onset. May develop at any age but most often in adults over the age of 40. Also known as non-insulin-dependent diabetes mellitus (NIDDM) or type II.

U

Unbundling Coding the individual parts of a specific diagnosis or procedure rather than one combination or bundle that includes all of those components.

Uncontrolled Diabetes for which current therapies and/or treatments are not maintaining a proper blood sugar level in the patient.

Uncontrolled hypertension Hypertension that is either untreated or not responding to therapy.

Underlying condition One disease that affects or encourages another condition.

Uniform Hospital Discharge Data Set (UHDDS) A compilation of data collected by acute care facilities and other designated health care facilities.

Unspecified The absence of additional specifics in the physician's documentation.

Upcoding Using a code on a claim form that indicates a higher level of service, or a more severe aspect of disease or injury, than that which was actual and true.

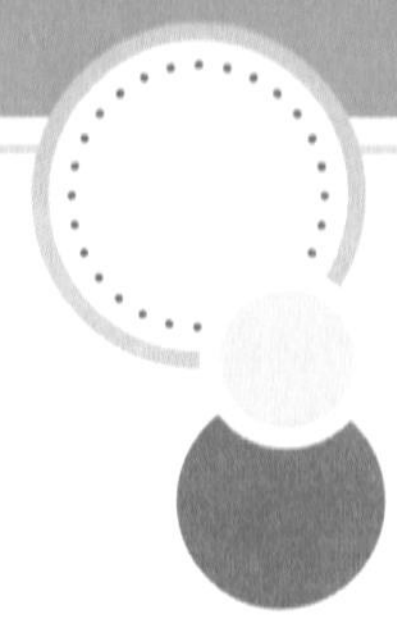

Photo Credits

Page 34: © The McGraw-Hill Companies, Inc./Jill Braaten, photographer; **p. 35:** © Getty RF; **5.1a-c:** © SPL/Photo Researchers, Inc.; **p. 183:** © The McGraw-Hill Companies, Inc./Rick Brady, photographer; **p. 217:** © BrandX/ Punchstock RF; **p. 224:** © Comstock RF; **p. 245:** © Getty RF; **pp. 250, 252, 254:** © Corbis RF; **p. 268:** © The McGraw-Hill Companies, Inc./Chris Kerrigan, photographer; **p. 299:** © Total Care Programming; **p. 301:** © Vol. 40 PhotoDisc/Getty Images RF; **p. 306:** © Vol. 40 PhotoDisc/Getty Images RF; **p. 336:** © Corbis RF; **p. 337:** © Stockdisk/Punchstock RF.

Index

Note: Page numbers followed by *f* designate figures; *b*, boxes; and *t*, tables. A page number in **boldface** indicates the definition of the term on that page.

D

Q

R

S